Hospital Statistics™

2004 Edition

AHA Institutional Members $155
Nonmembers $235
AHA Catalog NUMBER 082004
Telephone ORDERS 1-800-AHA-2626

ISSN 0090-6662
ISBN 0-87258-793-2

Contents

Acknowledgements & Advisements

Acknowledgments

The 2004 edition of Hospital Statistics is published by Health Forum an affiliate of the American Hospital Association, Richard J. Davidson, President.

Advisements

The data published here should be used with the following advisements: The data are based on replies to an annual survey that seeks a variety of information, not all of which is published in this book. The information gathered by the survey includes specific services, but not all of each hospital's services. Therefore, the data do not reflect an exhaustive list of all services offered by all hospitals. For information on the availability of additional data, please contact Health Forum, (800) 821-2039.

Health Forum does not assume responsibility for the accuracy of information voluntarily reported by the individual institutions surveyed. The purpose of this publication is to provide basic data reflecting the delivery of health care in the United States and associated areas, and is not to serve an official and all-inclusive list of services offered by individual hospitals.

Introduction

For more than five decades, *Hospital Statistics*™ has reported aggregate hospital data derived from the AHA Annual Survey and is the definitive source when doing trend analysis with data by bed size category, U.S. Census Divisions, States, and Metropolitan Statistical Areas (MSAs). As the health care delivery system changes, so have the data tracked by the survey and presented in this report. Recent additions include:

- **Community health indicators** that offer readers a connection to the community for their analysis and planning: the data are broken down into beds, admissions, inpatient days, ER outpatient visits, and other indicators per 1000 population, as well as expense per capita.

- **Utilization, personnel and finance** by all MSAs in the United States.

- **Five-year trend data** on physician models, insurance products, and managed care contracts enable you to identify changes in relationships between hospitals and other health care systems and providers.

- **Tables 3 through 6 have been organized** to show breakdowns between inpatient and outpatient care to better reflect market shifts toward outpatient-centered care. Additional clarity is gained by the breakdown between total facility data (which includes nursing home type units under the control of the hospital) and hospital units (which exclude the nursing home data).

TABLE 6	**Sample State**				
	U.S. Registered Community Hospitals				
	(Nonfederal, short-term general and other special hospitals)				
	Overview 1998-2002				
	2002	2001	2000	1999	1998
Physician Models					
Independent Practice Association	14	17	17	17	14
Group Practice without Walls	4	5	5	8	4
Open Physician-Hospital Organization	20	21	24	23	18
Closed Physician-Hospital Organization	21	17	18	17	11
Management Service Organization	14	18	20	14	9
Integrated Salary Model	35	29	30	26	24
Equity Model	4	3	4	6	3
Foundation	9	8	23	21	19
Insurance Products					
Health Maintenance Organization	20	22	23	24	19
Preferred Provider Organization	39	47	52	53	37
Indemnity Fee for Service	7	12	14	12	6
Managed Care Contracts					
Health Maintenance Organization	64	67	62	49	42
Preferred Provider Organization	97	93	92	87	72

Example of five-year trend data

- **Facilities and Services information** on more than 90 categories of hospital facilities and services in Table 7. At a glance, you can determine the number and percentage of hospitals offering a specific service such as Oncology, Angioplasty, Palliative Care Program, Complementary Medicine, Women's Health Services and Tobacco Cessation.

- **Plus, System and Network involvement along with Group Purchasing Organizations** that demonstrate ways in which organizations are linked.

The survey instrument and the glossary

A good place to begin your analysis is the AHA Annual Survey instrument. Found on page 197, it includes the instructions, questions, and terms that were used to gather the data for fiscal year 2002. This can be extremely valuable for a clearer understanding of the data we collect and the tables presented in *Hospital Statistics*.

Please also review the glossary in the back of the book. The glossary contains complete definitions for specific terms used in the tables and text of *Hospital Statistics*. These definitions will clarify how terminology is being used.

As mentioned above, it is important to note that the primary focus of the most detailed data contained in *Hospital Statistics* is community hospitals. As defined, community hospitals are all non-federal, short-term general and special hospitals whose facilities and services are available to the public. If the majority of a hospital's patients are admitted to units where the average length of stay is 30 days or less, a hospital may still be classified as short-term even if it includes a nursing- home-type unit. (For a more complete definition of community hospitals, please see the glossary definition, located on page 189.)

Getting the most out of *Hospital Statistics*

This section of the book provides an introduction for getting the most out of your *Hospital Statistics* 2004 edition. Here, you'll find a guide to the book, with insights into each table.

Equity model: An arrangement that allows established practitioners to become shareholders in a professional corporation in exchange for tangible and intangible assets of their existing practices.

Expenses: Includes all expenses for the reporting period including payroll, non-payroll, bad debt, and all nonoperating expenses. *Payroll expenses* include all salaries and wages. *Non-payroll expenses* are all professional fees and those salary expenditures excluded from payroll. *Labor related expenses* are defined as payroll expenses plus employee benefits. *Non-labor related expenses* are all other non-payroll expenses. *Bad debt* has been reclassified from a "reduction in revenue" to an expense in accordance with the revised AICPA Audit Guide. However, for purposes of historical consistency, the expense total that appears throughout *Hospital Statistics does not include "bad debt" as an expense item.* Note: Financial data may not add due to rounding.

Extracorporeal shock wave lithotripter (ESWL): A medical device used for treating stones in the kidney or ureter. The device disintegrates kidney stones noninvasively through the transmission of acoustic shock waves directed at the stones.

Fitness center: Provides exercise, testing, or evaluation programs and fitness activities to the community and hospital employees.

Example of Glossary definitions.

CLASSIFICATION	YEAR	HOSPITALS	BEDS (in thousands)	ADMISSIONS (in thousands)
Total United States	1946	6,125	1,436	15,675
	1950	6,788	1,456	18,483
	1955	6,956	1,604	21,073
	1960	6,876	1,658	25,027
	1965	7,123	1,704	28,812
	1970	7,123	1,616	31,759
	1971	7,097	1,556	32,664
	1972	7,061	1,550	33,265
	1973	7,123	1,535	34,352
	1974	7,174	1,513	35,506
	1975	7,156	1,466	36,157
	1976	7,082	1,434	36,776
	1977	7,099	1,407	37,060
	1978	7,015	1,381	37,243
	1979	6,988	1,372	37,802
	1980	6,965	1,365	38,892
	1981	6,933	1,362	39,169
	1982	6,915	1,360	39,095
	1983	6,888	1,350	38,887
	1984	6,872	1,339	37,938
	1985	6,872	1,318	36,304
	1986	6,841	1,290	35,219
	1987	6,821	1,267	34,439
	1988	6,780	1,248	34,107
	1989	6,720	1,226	33,742
	1990	6,649	1,213	33,774
	1991	6,634	1,202	33,567
	1992	6,539	1,178	33,536
	1993	6,467	1,163	33,201
	1994	6,374	1,126	33,125
	1995	6,291	1,081	33,282
	1996	6,201	1,062	33,307
	1997	6,097	1,035	33,624
	1998	6,021	1,013	33,766
	1999	5,890	994	34,181
Total nonfederal short-term general and other special	1946	4,444	473	13,655
	1950	5,031	505	16,663
	1955	5,237	568	19,100
	1960	5,407	639	22,970
	1965	5,736	741	26,463
	1970	5,859	848	29,252
	1971	5,865	867	30,142
	1972	5,843	884	30,777
	1973	5,891	903	31,761
	1974	5,977	931	32,943
	1975	5,979	947	33,519
	1976	5,956	961	34,068
	1977	5,973	974	34,353
	1978	5,935	980	34,575
	1979	5,923	988	35,160
	1980	5,904	992	36,198
	1981	5,879	1,007	36,494
	1982	5,863	1,015	36,429
	1983	5,843	1,021	36,201
	1984	5,814	1,020	35,202
	1985	5,784	1,003	33,501
	1986	5,728	982	32,4..
	1987	5,659	961	3...
	1988	5,579	940	

Example of Table 1

Table 1 — Historical Trends in Utilization, Personnel and Finances for Selected Years from 1946 through 2002

Table 1 at a Glance

This table is used to evaluate historical data and allows you to examine long-term trends in health care with data dating back more than fifty years. Table 1 reports on all AHA registered hospitals in the United States. One important note: To be considered an AHA-registered hospital, a hospital does not need to be an AHA member. Rather, the hospital must meet particular certification or satisfy a number of requirements. These Registration Requirements immediately follow this section and begin on page xiv.

This table segments the data into various organizational structure categories. Here's a brief look at these different classifications:

- Total United States Hospitals.
- Total Non-Federal Short-term and other special hospitals.
- Community hospitals
- Non-government not-for-profit community hospitals
- Investor-owned (for-profit) community hospitals
- State and local government community hospitals

Table 1 also provides input on nationwide utilization, personnel and finance trends. You'll find answers to questions such as: *Over the past 25 years, what trends do I see comparing the average length of stay at government and non-government not-for-profit community hospitals and investor-owned for-profit community hospitals?* or *What has been the trend in outpatient visits?*

Table 2 — 2002 U.S. Registered Hospitals: Utilization, Personnel and Finances

Table 2 at a Glance

This table takes a closer look at U.S. Registered Hospitals for 2002. It offers a snapshot of utilization, personnel and finance statistics, and breaks down this information for specialty hospitals. In addition, this is the only table that outlines data on federal hospitals. You'll be able to use this table to better understand the number of beds set-up and staffed, how many personnel and trainees are on the payroll, and what the financial implications of these may be.

TABLE 3

TOTAL UNITED STATES

U.S. Registered Community Hospitals
(Nonfederal, short-term general and other special hospitals)

Utilization, Personnel, Revenue and Expenses, Community Health Indicators 1998-2002

	2002	2001	2000	1999	1998
TOTAL FACILITY (Includes Hospital and Nursing Home Units)					
Utilization - Inpatient					
Beds	839,988	853,287	862,352	872,736	902,061
Admissions	31,811,673	31,576,960	31,098,959	30,945,357	30,718,136
Inpatient Days	191,430,450	192,504,015	193,747,004	199,876,367	207,180,278
Average Length of Stay	6.0	6.1	6.2	6.5	6.7
Inpatient Surgeries	9,735,705	9,509,081	9,545,612	9,700,613	9,833,938
Births	3,726,233	3,742,191	3,723,871	3,764,698	3,809,367
HOSPITAL UNIT (Excludes Separate Nursing Home Units)					
Utilization - Inpatient					
Beds	758,186	769,505	782,504	794,502	824,969
Admissions	31,265,867	31,047,930	30,652,820	30,577,564	30,403,766
Inpatient Days	165,644,176	165,605,620	168,189,130	174,898,504	182,702,882
Average Length of Stay	5.3	5.3	5.5	5.7	6.0
Personnel					
Total Full Time	3,235,153	3,183,730	3,154,603	3,166,729	3,147,922
Total Part Time	1,213,426	1,214,232	1,153,790	1,146,082	1,122,957
Revenue and Expenses - Totals					
(Includes Inpatient and Outpatient)					
Total Net Revenue	$333,054,828,642	$322,459,942,930	$310,513,291,998	$298,519,717,355	$285,858,018,951
Total Expenses	314,709,758,455	301,905,101,393	290,128,641,153	282,372,557,487	272,840,121,437

Example of Table 3. Helps contrast acute and long-term care

Table 3 — Total United States

Table 3 at a Glance

This table provides a look at all U .S. Registered Community Hospitals, in terms of general overview with utilization by inpatient and outpatient, personnel, revenue, expenses and community health indicators. It provides a snapshot of the past five years, allowing you to track emerging trends.

This national information can be compared to local or regional trends, for benchmarking

- Both inpatient and outpatient information is included, for better evaluation of data.

- Reporting by total facility *Includes hospital and Nursing Home Units* and hospital unit only *Excludes Separate Nursing Home Units* helps contrast acute and long-term care.

- Community health indicators can help uncover trends and help determine future facility needs

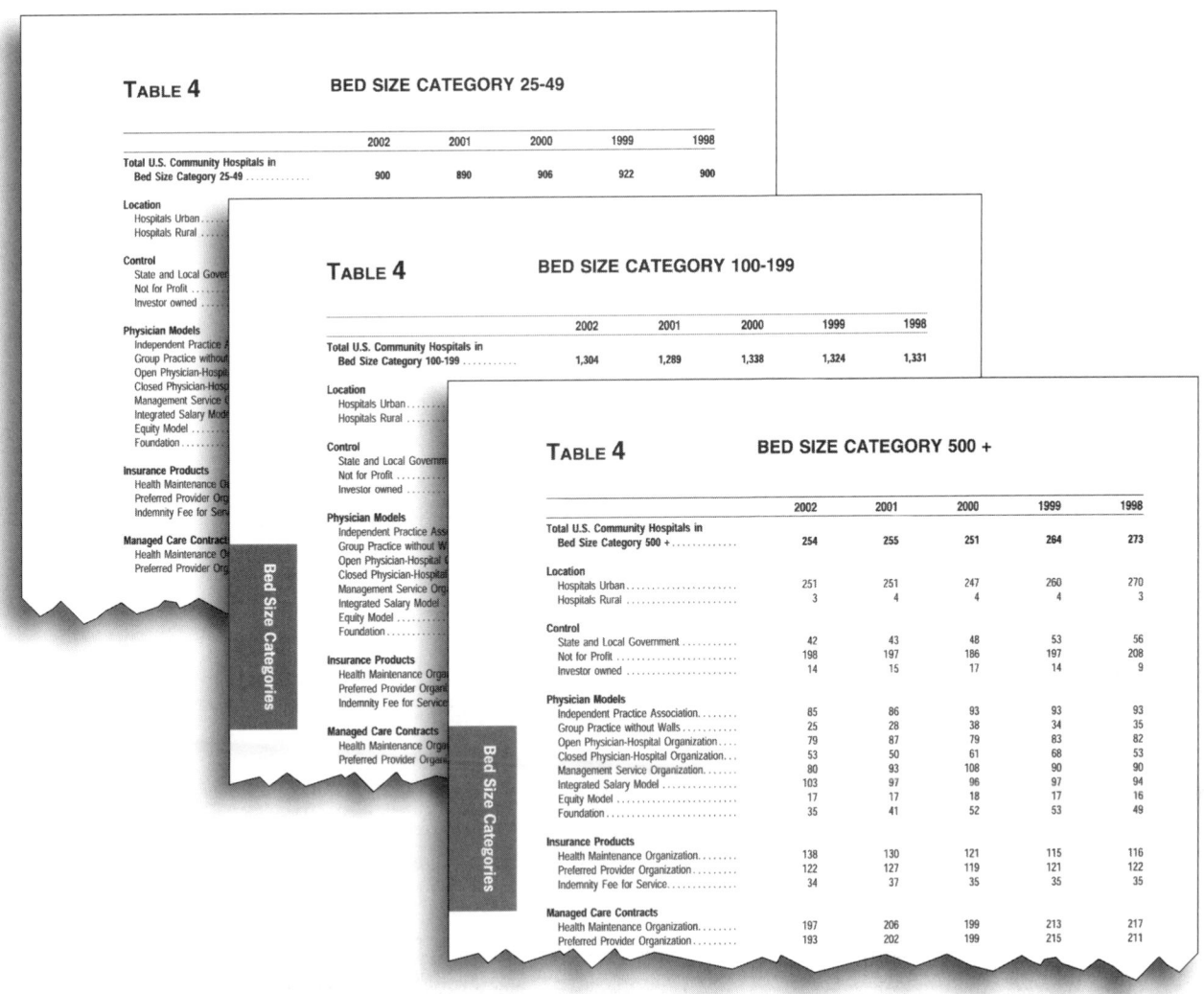

Example of Table 4. Compares facilities with peers.

Table 4 — Bed Size Categories

Table 4 at a Glance
This table provides a look at all U.S. Registered Community Hospitals, broken down by bed size. The table includes general overview, utilization, personnel, and revenue and expense information. These categories of bed sizes were developed by the AHA, and have become an industry standard. By categorizing each facility into a peer group, this table provides a snapshot of the past five years allowing you to compare facilities with their peers.

TABLE 5

TABLE 5

U.S. CENSUS DIVISION 2: MIDDLE ATLANTIC

U.S. Registered Community Hospitals
(Nonfederal, short-term general and other special hospitals)

Utilization, Personnel, Revenue and Expenses, Community Health Indicators 1998-2002

	2002	2001	2000	1999	1998
COMMUNITY HEALTH INDICATORS PER 1000 POPULATION					
Total Population (in thousands)...	38,292	38,216	38,184	38,147	38,108
Inpatient					
Beds.........................	3.6	3.8	3.9	4.0	4.1
Admissions....................	135.8	136.7	136.2	138.3	137.4
Inpatient Days.................	963.5	988.8	1,019.0	1,093.8	1,145.0
Inpatient Surgeries.............	42.2	41.4	41.2	42.7	43.6
Births........................	13.0	13.2	13.6	13.7	14.3
Outpatient					
Emergency Outpatient Visits......	367.7	362.0	363.4	379.5	360.1
Other Outpatient Visits..........	1,970.9	1,802.3	1,767.7	1,680.3	1,573.9
Total Outpatient Visits...........	2,338.6	2,164.3	2,131.1	2,059.8	1,934.0
Outpatient Surgeries.............	67.8	62.4	59.9	55.4	53.5
Expense per Capita (per person)....	$1,494.9	$1,462.7	$1,428.6	$1,429.8	$1,369.2

Example of Table 5. Uncovers trends to determine future facility needs.

Table 5 — U.S. Census Divisions

Table 5 at a Glance
This table provides a look at all U.S. Registered Community Hospitals, broken down by Census Division. The table includes general overview, utilization, personnel, and expenses, and community health indicator information. It provides a snapshot of the past five years, allowing you to track trends on a regional level. In addition, this allows you to compare this data to other population based health indicators, offering a more comprehensive look than the survey data alone. Community health indicators can help uncover trends and help determine future facility needs.

Table 6 — States

Table 6 at a Glance
This table provides a look at all U.S. Registered Community Hospitals, broken down by State. The table includes general overview, utilization, personnel, revenue and expenses, and community health indicator information. It provides a snapshot of the past five years, allowing you to track trends on a state level.

Note:
You can use the information in tables 3,4,5 and 6 to make accurate comparisons across Total U.S., Bed Size Category, Census Division and State.

Table 7 — 2002 Facilities and Services in the U.S. Census Divisions and States

Table 7 at a Glance

This table examines facilities and services by both Census Division and State. A comprehensive alphabetical guide helps make each facility or service easy to find. This table will allow you to better understand what service lines are emerging and how many facilities offer a particular service in a discrete state or region.

This collection of facilities and services information data is unique to *Hospital Statistics* and the list is continually growing. Recent additions include:

- Pain Management Programs
- Complementary Medicine (i.e. Alternative Medicine)
- Chiropractic Services
- Acute Long Term Care
- Auxiliary
- Ambulance Services
- Enabling Services
- Palliative Care Program
- Enrollment Assistance Services
- Hemodialysis
- Sleep Center
- Tobacco Treatment/Cessation Program

Table7 (Continued)

CLASSIFICATION	HOSPITALS REPORTING	CASE MANAGEMENT Number	CASE MANAGEMENT Percent	CHILDREN WELLNESS PROGRAM Number	CHILDREN WELLNESS PROGRAM Percent	CHIROPRACTIC SERVICES Number	CHIROPRACTIC SERVICES Percent	COMMUNITY OUTREACH Number	COMMUNITY OUTREACH Percent
UNITED STATES	4,797	2,980	62.1	780	16.3	61	1.3	2,725	56.8
COMMUNITY HOSPITALS	4,113	2,820	68.7	742	18.0	53	1.3	2,491	60.5
CENSUS DIVISION 1, NEW ENGLAND	230	157	68.3	63	27.4	6	2.6	169	73.5
Connecticut	42	32	76.2	15	35.7	3	7.1	32	76.2
Maine	39	20	51.3	9	23.1	0	0.0	30	76.9
Massachusetts	85	64	75.3	21	24.7	2	2.4	62	72.9
New Hampshire	31	20	64.5	10	32.3	0	0.0	23	74.2
Rhode Island	16	12	75.0	4	25.0	1	6.3	11	68.8
Vermont	17	9	52.9	4	23.5	0	0.0	11	64.7
CENSUS DIVISION 2, MIDDLE ATLANTIC	461	344	74.6	149	31.0	7	1.5	345	74.8
New Jersey	71	65	93.0	29	40.8	2	2.8	60	84.5
New York	194	146	75.3	61	31.4	2	1.0	140	72.2
Pennsylvania	196	132	67.3	53	27.0	3	1.5	145	74.0
CENSUS DIVISION 3, SOUTH ATLANTIC	724	484	66.9	123	17.0	8	1.1	450	62.2
Delaware	9	5	55.6	4	44.4	0	0.0	5	55.6
District of Columbia	17	13	76.5	3	17.6	2	11.8	10	58.8
Florida	138	117	84.8	23	16.7	3	2.2	89	64.5
Georgia	144	87	60.4	19	13.2	0	0.0	75	52.1
Maryland	64	47	73.4	10	15.6	1	1.6	46	71.9
North Carolina	119	84	70.6	20	16.8	1	0.8	71	59.7
South Carolina	71	25	35.2	25	35.2	0	0.0	64	90.1
Virginia	98	72	73.5	9	9.2	0	0.0	55	56.1
West Virginia	64	34	53.1	10	15.6	1	1.5	35	54.7
CENSUS DIVISION 4, EAST NORTH CENTRAL	741	478	64.5	140	18.9	15	2.0	464	62.6
Illinois	193	126	65.3	45	23.3	5	2.6	132	68.4
Indiana	110	68	61.8	20	18.2	1	0.9	76	69.1
Michigan	148	92	62.2	32	21.6	0	0.0	101	68.2
Ohio	156	108	69.2	34	21.8	9	5.8	109	69.9
Wisconsin	134	82	61.2	9	6.7	0	0.0	46	34.3
CENSUS DIVISION 5, EAST SOUTH CENTRAL	403	229	56.8	26	6.5	3	0.7	198	49.1
Alabama	94	60	63.8	5	5.3	1	1.1	52	55.3
Kentucky	104	64	61.5	12	11.5	0	0.0	49	47.1
Mississippi	106	45	42.5	0	0.0	0	0.0	56	52.8
Tennessee	99	60	60.6	9	9.1	2	2.0	41	41.4
CENSUS DIVISION 6, WEST NORTH CENTRAL	703	308	43.8	85	12.1	11	1.6	370	52.6
Iowa	125	68	54.0	35	19.8	2	1.6	68	54.0
Kansas	139	48	34.5	12	8.6	3	2.2	46	33.1
Minnesota	115	33	28.7	9	7.8	1	0.9	74	64.3
Missouri	151	106	70.2	23	15.2	4	2.6	97	64.2
Nebraska	81	28	34.6	5	6.2	0	0.0	45	55.6
North Dakota	35	7	20.0	5	14.3	1	2.9	16	45.7
South Dakota	56	18	32.1	6	10.7	0	0.0	24	42.9
CENSUS DIVISION 7, WEST SOUTH CENTRAL	777	492	63.1	76	9.8	4	0.5	316	40.7
Arkansas	65	44	67.7	5	7.7	0	0.0	27	41.5
Louisiana	111	70	63.1	18	16.2	1	0.9	44	39.6
Oklahoma	115	60	52.2	9	7.8	1	0.9	49	42.6
Texas	486	318	65.4	44	9.1	2	0.4	196	40.3
CENSUS DIVISION 8, MOUNTAIN	333	194	58.3	47	14.1	2	0.6	162	48.6
Arizona	54	44	81.5	8	14.8	0	0.0	25	46.3
Colorado	59	40	67.8	10	16.9	1	1.7	41	69.5
Idaho	36	17	48.6	5	14.3	0	0.0	19	54.?
Montana	54	12	22.2	7	13.0	0	0.0	14	25.?
Nevada	20	15	75.0	3	15.0	0	0.0	10	50.?
New Mexico	40	22	55.0	7	17.5	0	0.0	18	45.0
Utah	44	26	59.1	6	13.6	1	2.3	20	45.5
Wyoming	27	18	66.7	1	3.7	0	0.0	15	55.?
CENSUS DIVISION 9, PACIFIC	425	294	69.2	80	18.8	5	1.2	251	59.?
Alaska	15	9	60.0	1	6.7	0	0.0	6	40.0
California	260	209	74.6	55	19.6	3	1.1	173	61.8
Hawaii	16	10	62.5	3	18.8	0	0.0	8	50.?
Oregon	52	28	63.8	11	21.2	0	0.0	31	59.?
Washington	82	38	61.3	10	16.1	2	3.2	33	

Example of Table 7.

These new categories reflect the trends as hospitals expand their service lines to reflect the needs of their patients. For example, services such as acupuncture or massage therapy are now accounted for in the Complementary Medicine service item.

This table can answer questions such as: *What percentage of hospitals in the United States offer complementary medicine or chiropractic services?* or *How are these new services distributed by state?*

Table 8 — Utilization, Personnel and Finances in Community Hospitals by MSAs for 2002.

Table 8 at a Glance

This table provides a look at all U.S. Registered Community Hospitals, broken down by Metropolitan Statistical Area (MSA). The table includes general overview, utilization, personnel, and finance information. It provides a snapshot of the past year.

Additional Resources

Again, in the back of the book you will find the comprehensive glossary and the 2002 annual survey questionnaire. The survey itself can be a valuable resource to understanding what was asked in order to gather the data in the book. This survey is also used to produce the *AHA Guide®* and AHA Annual Survey Database™.

Registration Requirements for Hospitals

AHA-Registered Hospitals

Any institution that can be classified as a hospital according to the requirements may be registered if it so desires. Membership in the American Hospital Association is not a prerequisite.

The American Hospital Association may, at the sole discretion of the Executive Committee of the Board of Trustees, grant, deny, or withdraw the registration of an institution.

An institution may be registered by the American Hospital Association as a hospital if it is accredited as a hospital by the Joint Commission on Accreditation of Healthcare Organizations or is certified as a provider of acute services under Title 18 of the Social Security Act and has provided the Association with documents verifying the accreditation or certification.

In lieu of the preceding accreditation or certification, an institution licensed as a hospital by the appropriate state agency may be registered by AHA as a hospital by meeting the following alternative requirements:

Function: The primary function of the institution is to provide patient services, diagnostic and therapeutic, for particular or general medical conditions.

1. The institution shall maintain at least six inpatient beds, which shall be continuously available for the care of patients who are nonrelated and who stay on the average in excess of 24 hours per admission.

2. The institution shall be constructed, equipped, and maintained to ensure the health and safety of patients and to provide uncrowded, sanitary facilities for the treatment of patients.

3. There shall be an identifiable governing authority legally and morally responsible for the conduct of the hospital.

4. There shall be a chief executive to whom the governing authority delegates the continuous responsibility for the operation of the hospital in accordance with establish policy.

5. There shall be an organized medical staff of fully licensed physicians* that may include other licensed individuals permitted by law and by the hospital to provide patient care services independently in the hospital. The medical staff shall be accountable to the governing authority for maintaining proper standards of medical care, and it shall be governed by bylaws adopted by said staff and approved by the governing authority.

6. Each patient shall be admitted on the authority of a member of the medical staff who has been granted the privilege to admit patients to inpatient services in accordance with state law and criteria for standards of medical care established by the individual medical staff. Each patient's general medical condition is the responsibility of a qualified physician member of the medical staff. When nonphysician members of the medical staff are granted privileges to admit patients, provision is made for prompt medical evaluation of these patients by a qualified physician. Any graduate of a foreign medical school who is permitted to assume responsibilities for patient care shall possess a valid license to practice medicine, or shall be certified by the Educational Commission for Foreign Medical Graduates, or shall have qualified for and have successfully completed an academic year of supervised clinical training under the direction of a medical school approved by the Liaison Committee on GAT Medical Education.

7. Registered nurse supervision and other nursing services are continuous.

8. A current and complete‡ medical record shall be maintained by the institution for each patient and shall be available for reference.

9. Pharmacy service shall be maintained in the institution and shall be supervised by a registered pharmacist.

10. The institution shall provide patients with food service that meets their nutritional and therapeutic requirements; special diets shall also be available.

Types of Hospitals

In addition to meeting these 10 general registration requirements, hospitals are registered as one of four types of hospitals: general, special, rehabilitation and chronic disease, or psychiatric. The following type of hospital and special requirements for registration are employed:

General

The primary function of the institution is to provide patient services, diagnostic and therapeutic, for a variety of medical conditions. A general hospital also shall provide:

- diagnostic x-ray services with facilities and staff for a variety of procedures
- clinical laboratory service with facilities and staff for a variety of procedures and with anatomical pathology services regularly and conveniently available
- operating room service with facilities and staff.

Special

The primary function of the institution is to provide diagnostic and treatment services for patients who have specified medical conditions, both surgical and nonsurgical. A special hospital also shall provide:

- such diagnostic and treatment services as may be determined by the Executive Committee of the Board of Trustees of the American Hospital Association to be appropriate for the specified medical conditions for which medical services are provided shall be maintained in the institution with suitable facilities and staff. If such conditions do not normally require diagnostic x-ray service, laboratory service, or operating room service, and if any such services are therefore not maintained in the institution, there shall be written arrangements to make them available to patients requiring them.
- clinical laboratory services capable of providing tissue diagnosis when offering pregnancy termination services.

Rehabilitation and Chronic Disease

The primary function of the institution is to provide diagnostic and treatment services to handicapped or disabled individuals requiring restorative and adjustive services. A rehabilitation and chronic disease hospital also shall provide:

- arrangements for diagnostic x-ray services, as required, on a regular and conveniently available basis
- arrangements for clinical laboratory service, as required on a regular and conveniently available basis
- arrangements for operating room service, as required, on a regular and conveniently available basis
- a physical therapy service with suitable facilities and staff in the institution
- an occupational therapy service with suitable facilities and staff in the institution
- arrangements for psychological and social work services on a regular and conveniently available basis

---

* Physician–Term used to describe an individual with an M.D. or D.O. degree who is fully licensed to practice medicine in all its phases.

‡ The completed records in general shall contain at least the following: the patient's identifying data and consent forms, medical history, record of physical examination, physicians' progress notes, operative notes, nurses' notes, routine x-ray and laboratory reports, doctors' orders, and final diagnosis.

- arrangements for educational and vocational services on a regular and conveniently available basis
- written arrangements with a general hospital for the transfer of patients who require medical, obstetrical, or surgical services not available in the institution.

Psychiatric

The primary function of the institution is to provide diagnostic and treatment services for patients who have psychiatric-related illnesses. A psychiatric hospital also shall provide:

- arrangements for clinical laboratory service, as required, on a regular and conveniently available basis
- arrangements for diagnostic x-ray services, as required on a regular and conveniently available basis
- psychiatric, psychological, and social work service with facilities and staff in the institution
- arrangements for electroencephalograph services, as required, on a regular and conveniently available basis.
- written arrangements with a general hospital for the transfer of patients who require medical, obstetrical, or surgical services not available in the institution.

The American Hospital Association may, at the sole discretion of the Executive Committee of the Board of Trustees, grant, deny, or withdraw the registration of an institution.

AOHA-Listed Hospitals

The list of osteopathic hospitals includes both members and nonmembers of the American Osteopathic Healthcare Association.

Data Comparability

The economic climate, demographic characteristics, personnel issues, and health care financing and payment policies differ by region, state, and city across the country. *Differences in these factors must be taken into account when using the data.* In addition, the profiles of hospitals across comparison groups vary. For example, states will differ in terms of the number and percentage of hospitals by size, ownership, services provided, types of patients treated, and so forth. *Differences in these variables must also be taken into consideration when doing a comparative analysis.*

Notes on the Survey

The 2004 edition of *Hospital Statistics*™ draws its data from the 2002 AHA Annual Survey of Hospitals. It is the statistical complement to the 2003-2004 edition of the *AHA Guide®*, which contains selected data about individual hospitals.

The AHA Survey was mailed to all hospitals, both AHA-registered and nonregistered, in the U.S. and its associated areas: American Samoa, Guam, the Marshall Islands, Puerto Rico, and the Virgin Island. U.S. government hospitals located outside the U.S. were not included. Overall, the average response rate over the past five years has been approximately 83 percent.

Reporting Period

In completing the survey, hospitals were requested to report data for a full year, in accord with their fiscal year, ending in 2002. The statistical table present data reported or estimated for a 12-month period, except for data on personnel, which represent situations as they existed at the end of the reporting period.

Respondents

Data for Tables 1 and 2 include 5,794 AHA-registered hospitals in the U.S. Data on community hospitals (nonfederal, short-term general and other special hospitals) only are presented in Tables 3-6, and Table 8.

It is important to note that the AHA-registered hospitals included in *Hospital Statistics* are not necessarily identical to those included in *AHA Guide*. The institutions listed in the 2003-2004 edition of *AHA Guide* include all of those institutions registered as of April 2002. Tables 1-6 in *Hospital Statistics* present data for AHA-registered hospitals that were in operation during the 12-month reporting period ending 2002.

Estimates

Estimates were made of data for nonreporting hospitals and for reporting hospitals that submitted incomplete AHA Annual Survey questionnaires. Estimates were not made for beds, bassinets and facilities and services. Data for beds and bassinets of nonreporting hospitals were based on the most recent information from those hospitals. (Note that in all statistical tables, whenever bed-size categories are listed, all eight categories appear, whether or not there are hospitals in every category.)

Missing revenue, expenses, admissions, births, inpatient days, surgical operations, outpatient visits, and full-time-equivalent personnel values are estimates from regression models. For all other variables the estimates were based on ratios such as per bed averages derived from data reported by hospitals similar in size, control, major service provided, length of stay, and geographical characteristics to the hospitals that did not report this information.

Tables 1–2

Table

1

Historical Trends in Utilization, Personnel, and Finances for Selected Years from 1946 through 2002

Data are for all AHA-registered hospitals in the United States. Data are estimated for nonreporting hospitals with the exception of newborn and outpatient data before 1972. Personnel data exclude residents, interns, and students from 1952 on; personnel data include full-time personnel and full-time equivalents for part-time personnel from 1954 on. As a result of the AHA Annual Survey validation process, the New York state expense data from 1976 were revised after the 1977 edition was published. The revised figures are included below. In order to provide trend data on a consistent basis, the 1970 and 1971 psychiatric and long-term data have been slightly modified. The 1982 FTE figures have been updated to provide the most accurate data possible.

CLASSIFICATION / YEAR	HOSPITALS	BEDS (in thousands)	ADMISSIONS (in thousands)	AVERAGE DAILY CENSUS (in thousands)	ADJUSTED AVERAGE DAILY CENSUS (in thousands)	AVERAGE STAY (days)	OUTPATIENT VISITS (in thousands)	NEWBORNS Bassinets	NEWBORNS Births	FTE PERSONNEL Number (in thousands)	FTE PERSONNEL Per 100 Adjusted Census	TOTAL EXPENSES Amount (In Millions of dollars)	TOTAL EXPENSES Adjusted per Inpatient Stay (dollars)	TOTAL EXPENSES Adjusted per Inpatient Day (dollars)
Total United States														
1946	6,125	1,436	15,675	1,142	—	—	—	85,585	2,135,327	830	—	$1,963	—	—
1950	6,788	1,456	18,483	1,253	—	—	—	90,101	2,742,780	1,058	—	$3,651	—	—
1955	6,956	1,604	21,073	1,363	—	—	—	98,823	3,476,753	1,301	—	$5,594	—	—
1960	6,876	1,658	25,027	1,402	—	—	—	102,764	3,835,735	1,598	—	$8,421	—	—
1965	7,123	1,704	28,812	1,403	—	—	125,793	101,287	3,565,344	1,952	—	$12,948	—	—
1970	7,123	1,616	31,759	1,298	—	—	181,370	97,128	3,537,000	2,537	—	$25,556	—	—
1971	7,097	1,556	32,664	1,237	—	—	199,725	94,344	3,464,513	2,589	—	$28,812	—	—
1972	7,061	1,550	33,265	1,209	—	—	219,182	92,960	3,231,875	2,671	—	$32,667	—	—
1973	7,123	1,535	34,352	1,189	—	—	233,555	90,071	3,087,210	2,769	—	$36,290	—	—
1974	7,174	1,513	35,506	1,167	—	—	250,481	88,269	3,043,386	2,919	—	$41,406	—	—
1975	7,156	1,466	36,157	1,125	—	—	254,844	86,875	3,091,629	3,023	—	$48,706	—	—
1976	7,082	1,434	36,776	1,090	—	—	270,951	85,284	3,067,063	3,108	—	$56,005	—	—
1977	7,099	1,407	37,060	1,066	—	—	263,775	83,193	3,223,699	3,213	—	$63,630	—	—
1978	7,015	1,381	37,243	1,042	—	—	263,606	80,650	3,250,373	3,280	—	$70,927	—	—
1979	6,988	1,372	37,802	1,043	—	—	262,009	79,720	3,376,467	3,382	—	$79,796	—	—
1980	6,965	1,365	38,892	1,060	—	—	262,951	79,842	3,500,043	3,492	—	$91,886	—	—
1981	6,933	1,362	39,169	1,061	—	—	265,332	78,823	3,558,274	3,661	—	$107,146	—	—
1982	6,915	1,360	39,095	1,053	—	—	313,667	77,998	3,615,751	3,746	—	$123,219	—	—
1983	6,888	1,350	38,887	1,028	—	—	273,168	77,837	3,596,146	3,707	—	$136,315	—	—
1984	6,872	1,339	37,938	970	—	—	276,566	77,845	3,563,106	3,630	—	$144,114	—	—
1985	6,872	1,318	36,304	910	—	—	282,140	77,202	3,630,961	3,625	—	$153,327	—	—
1986	6,841	1,290	35,219	883	—	—	294,634	76,002	3,680,178	3,647	—	$165,194	—	—
1987	6,821	1,267	34,439	873	—	—	310,707	74,770	3,698,294	3,742	—	$178,662	—	—
1988	6,780	1,248	34,107	863	—	—	336,208	72,568	3,794,369	3,839	—	$196,704	—	—
1989	6,720	1,226	33,742	853	—	—	352,248	71,491	3,920,384	3,937	—	$214,886	—	—
1990	6,649	1,213	33,774	844	—	—	368,184	70,539	4,046,704	4,063	—	$234,870	—	—
1991	6,634	1,202	33,567	827	—	—	387,675	69,464	4,047,504	4,165	—	$258,508	—	—
1992	6,539	1,178	33,536	807	—	—	417,874	69,052	4,007,179	4,236	—	$282,531	—	—
1993	6,467	1,163	33,201	783	—	—	435,619	67,911	3,949,788	4,289	—	$301,538	—	—
1994	6,374	1,128	33,125	745	—	—	453,584	67,311	3,886,667	4,270	—	$310,834	—	—
1995	6,291	1,081	33,282	710	—	—	483,195	66,256	3,833,132	4,273	—	$320,252	—	—
1996	6,201	1,062	33,307	685	—	—	505,455	65,138	3,790,678	4,276	—	$330,531	—	—
1997	6,097	1,035	33,624	673	—	—	520,600	64,649	3,811,522	4,333	—	$342,334	—	—
1998	6,021	1,013	33,766	662	—	—	545,481	63,485	3,795,212	4,407	—	$355,450	—	—
1999	5,890	994	34,181	657	—	—	573,461	62,714	3,829,881	4,369	—	$372,933	—	—
2000	5,810	984	34,891	650	—	—	592,673	61,915	3,940,017	4,454	—	$395,391	—	—
2001	5,801	987	35,644	658	—	—	612,276	61,527	3,929,733	4,535	—	$426,849	—	—
2002	5,794	976	36,326	662	—	—	640,515	62,151	3,934,421	4,610	—	$462,222	—	—

Table 1 (Continued)

CLASSIFICATION: Total nonfederal short-term general and other special

YEAR	HOSPITALS	BEDS (in thousands)	ADMISSIONS (in thousands)	AVERAGE DAILY CENSUS (in thousands)	ADJUSTED AVERAGE DAILY CENSUS (in thousands)	AVERAGE LENGTH OF STAY (days)	OUTPATIENT VISITS (in thousands)	NEWBORNS Bassinets	NEWBORNS Births	FTE PERSONNEL Number (in thousands)	FTE PERSONNEL Per 100 Adjusted Census	EXPENSES Amount (In Millions of dollars)	EXPENSES Adjusted per Inpatient Stay (dollars)	EXPENSES Adjusted per Inpatient Day (dollars)
1946	4,444	473	13,655	341	—	9.1	—	80,987	2,087,503	505	—	$1,169	—	—
1950	5,031	505	16,663	372	—	8.1	—	86,019	2,660,982	662	—	$2,120	—	—
1955	5,237	568	19,100	407	—	7.8	—	93,868	3,304,451	826	—	$3,434	—	—
1960	5,407	639	22,970	477	—	7.6	—	98,127	3,678,051	1,080	—	$5,617	—	—
1965	5,736	741	26,463	563	620	7.8	92,631	96,782	3,413,370	1,386	224	$9,147	$316.37	$40.56
1970	5,859	848	29,252	662	727	8.2	133,545	93,079	3,403,064	1,929	265	$19,560	$604.59	$73.73
1971	5,865	867	30,142	665	736	8.0	148,423	90,444	3,337,605	1,999	272	$22,400	$667.44	$83.43
1972	5,843	884	30,777	664	739	7.9	166,983	89,315	3,119,446	2,056	278	$25,549	$747.42	$94.61
1973	5,891	903	31,761	681	768	7.8	178,939	86,851	2,987,089	2,149	280	$28,496	$793.88	$101.78
1974	5,977	931	32,943	701	793	7.8	194,838	85,208	2,947,342	2,289	289	$32,751	$883.04	$113.21
1975	5,979	947	33,519	708	806	7.7	196,311	83,834	2,998,590	2,399	298	$39,110	$1,024.72	$133.08
1976	5,956	961	34,068	715	816	7.7	207,725	82,307	2,962,305	2,483	304	$45,402	$1,172.25	$152.24
1977	5,973	974	34,353	717	820	7.6	204,238	80,228	3,117,756	2,581	315	$51,832	$1,316.70	$173.25
1978	5,935	980	34,575	720	841	7.6	204,461	78,090	3,156,570	2,662	323	$58,348	$1,470.13	$193.81
1979	5,923	988	35,160	729	841	7.6	203,873	77,277	3,287,157	2,762	328	$66,184	$1,631.16	$215.75
1980	5,904	992	36,198	748	861	7.6	206,752	77,539	3,408,699	2,879	334	$76,970	$1,844.19	$244.44
1981	5,879	1,007	36,494	764	876	7.6	206,729	76,567	3,465,683	3,039	347	$90,739	$2,167.70	$283.94
1982	5,863	1,015	36,429	763	882	7.6	250,888	75,739	3,514,761	3,110	353	$105,094	$2,493.09	$326.68
1983	5,843	1,021	36,201	750	869	7.6	213,995	75,471	3,490,629	3,102	357	$116,632	$2,775.55	$368.01
1984	5,814	1,020	35,202	703	824	7.3	216,474	75,587	3,456,467	3,023	367	$123,550	$2,984.00	$409.85
1985	5,784	1,003	33,501	650	780	7.1	222,773	74,899	3,521,296	3,003	385	$130,700	$3,238.94	$459.57
1986	5,728	982	32,410	631	774	7.1	234,270	73,688	3,584,530	3,032	392	$140,907	$3,529.60	$499.19
1987	5,659	961	31,633	624	780	7.2	247,704	72,516	3,602,416	3,120	400	$152,909	$3,848.79	$536.96
1988	5,579	949	31,480	622	795	7.2	271,436	70,361	3,706,748	3,209	404	$168,941	$4,194.39	$581.08
1989	5,497	936	31,141	619	805	7.3	287,909	69,436	3,831,051	3,307	411	$185,204	$4,572.23	$630.59
1990	5,420	929	31,203	620	820	7.3	302,691	68,443	3,958,646	3,423	417	$203,927	$4,929.93	$681.52
1991	5,370	926	31,084	612	828	7.2	323,202	67,440	3,965,489	3,539	427	$225,230	$5,345.63	$745.37
1992	5,321	923	31,053	606	832	7.1	349,397	67,095	3,925,024	3,624	436	$248,318	$5,788.52	$815.99
1993	5,289	921	30,770	593	834	7.0	368,358	66,060	3,870,392	3,681	441	$266,382	$6,120.94	$874.98
1994	5,256	904	30,739	569	814	6.8	384,880	65,728	3,809,367	3,697	454	$276,148	$6,230.33	$929.65
1995	5,220	874	30,966	549	811	6.5	415,710	64,742	3,764,756	3,718	458	$286,073	$6,220.54	$966.79
1996	5,160	864	31,116	531	800	6.2	440,845	63,646	3,723,907	3,728	466	$293,920	$6,225.95	$1,005.45
1997	5,082	855	31,595	529	813	6.1	450,907	63,247	3,742,240	3,794	467	$306,088	$6,266.24	$1,031.68
1998	5,039	842	31,830	527	821	6.0	474,366	62,162	3,726,234	3,835	467	$319,035	$6,387.53	$1,064.93
1999	4,977	831	32,377	527	835	5.9	495,850	61,534	3,760,295	3,840	460	$335,405	$6,512.44	$1,101.47
2000	4,934	825	33,102	527	850	5.8	522,970	60,845	3,880,166	3,916	461	$356,757	$6,650.68	$1,147.99
2001	4,927	828	33,834	534	866	5.8	539,316	60,454	3,873,395	3,990	461	$383,911	$6,979.29	$1,216.04
2002	4,949	823	34,501	541	887	5.7	557,336	59,974	3,870,191	4,072	459	$416,791	$7,353.17	$1,288.63

Table 1 (Continued)

CLASSIFICATION	YEAR	HOSPITALS	BEDS (in thousands)	ADMISSIONS (in thousands)	AVERAGE DAILY CENSUS (in thousands)	ADJUSTED AVERAGE DAILY CENSUS (in thousands)	AVERAGE LENGTH OF STAY (days)	OUTPATIENT VISITS (in thousands)	NEWBORNS Bassinets	NEWBORNS Births	FTE PERSONNEL Number (in thousands)	FTE PERSONNEL Per 100 Adjusted Census	Amount (in Millions of dollars)	EXPENSES Adjusted per Inpatient Stay (dollars)	EXPENSES Adjusted per Inpatient Day (dollars)
Total community hospitals	1975	5,875	942	33,435	706	798	7.7	190,672	83,829	2,998,552	2,392	300	$38,962	$1,030.34	$133.81
	1976	5,857	956	33,979	713	810	7.7	201,247	82,296	2,962,216	2,475	306	$45,240	$1,176.25	$152.76
	1979	5,842	984	35,099	727	833	7.6	198,778	77,266	3,287,012	2,756	331	$66,004	$1,641.67	$217.34
	1980	5,830	988	36,143	747	857	7.6	202,310	77,522	3,408,482	2,873	335	$76,851	$1,851.04	$245.12
	1981	5,813	1,003	36,438	763	873	7.6	202,768	76,561	3,465,401	3,033	347	$90,572	$2,171.20	$284.33
	1982	5,801	1,012	36,379	762	878	7.6	248,124	75,733	3,514,457	3,103	353	$104,876	$2,500.52	$327.37
	1983	5,783	1,018	36,152	749	864	7.6	210,044	75,465	3,490,254	3,096	358	$116,438	$2,789.18	$369.49
	1984	5,759	1,017	35,155	702	820	7.3	211,961	75,581	3,456,308	3,017	368	$123,336	$2,995.38	$411.10
	1985	5,732	1,001	33,449	649	777	7.1	218,716	74,893	3,521,135	2,997	386	$130,499	$3,244.74	$460.19
	1986	5,678	978	32,379	629	770	7.1	231,912	73,682	3,584,408	3,025	393	$140,654	$3,532.51	$500.81
	1987	5,611	958	31,601	622	776	7.2	245,524	72,510	3,602,296	3,114	401	$152,585	$3,850.16	$538.96
	1988	5,533	947	31,453	620	787	7.2	269,129	70,325	3,706,402	3,205	407	$168,722	$4,206.73	$586.33
	1989	5,455	933	31,116	618	796	7.2	285,712	69,405	3,830,615	3,303	415	$184,898	$4,587.87	$636.96
	1990	5,384	927	31,181	619	813	7.2	301,329	68,412	3,958,263	3,420	421	$203,693	$4,946.68	$686.83
	1991	5,342	924	31,064	611	820	7.2	322,048	67,434	3,965,396	3,535	431	$225,023	$5,359.56	$752.10
	1992	5,292	921	31,034	604	827	7.1	348,522	67,089	3,924,944	3,620	437	$248,095	$5,794.43	$819.83
	1993	5,261	919	30,748	592	828	7.0	366,885	66,054	3,870,376	3,677	444	$266,089	$6,132.06	$880.52
	1994	5,229	902	30,718	568	812	6.7	382,924	65,722	3,809,367	3,692	455	$275,779	$6,229.83	$930.71
	1995	5,194	873	30,945	548	809	6.5	414,345	64,736	3,764,698	3,714	459	$285,588	$6,215.51	$967.69
	1996	5,134	862	31,099	531	799	6.2	439,863	63,640	3,723,871	3,725	466	$293,755	$6,224.94	$1,006.14
	1997	5,057	853	31,577	528	811	6.1	450,140	63,241	3,742,191	3,790	467	$305,763	$6,261.93	$1,032.70
	1998	5,015	840	31,812	525	819	6.0	474,193	62,156	3,726,233	3,831	468	$318,834	$6,385.99	$1,066.96
	1999	4,956	830	32,359	526	833	5.9	495,346	61,528	3,760,295	3,838	461	$335,246	$6,511.72	$1,102.61
	2000	4,915	824	33,089	526	849	5.8	521,404	60,839	3,880,166	3,911	461	$356,564	$6,648.82	$1,149.40
	2001	4,908	826	33,814	533	865	5.7	538,480	60,448	3,873,395	3,987	461	$383,735	$6,979.53	$1,217.27
	2002	4,927	821	34,478	540	886	5.7	556,404	59,974	3,870,191	4,069	459	$416,591	$7,354.60	$1,289.87
Nongovernment not-for-profit community hospitals	1975	3,339	658	23,722	510	574	7.8	131,435	57,496	2,131,057	1,712	298	$27,938	$1,040.21	$133.36
	1976	3,345	670	24,082	517	586	7.9	140,914	56,442	2,100,917	1,791	306	$32,764	$1,208.23	$152.94
	1979	3,330	690	24,874	528	603	7.7	139,565	52,859	2,308,548	1,999	332	$47,937	$1,684.40	$218.06
	1980	3,322	692	25,566	542	621	7.7	142,156	52,659	2,389,478	2,086	336	$55,780	$1,901.64	$245.74
	1981	3,340	706	25,945	555	636	7.8	143,380	52,302	2,455,033	2,213	399	$66,267	$2,225.17	$285.64
	1982	3,338	712	25,898	553	637	7.8	176,245	51,566	2,483,345	2,265	355	$76,806	$2,572.93	$330.41
	1983	3,347	718	25,827	544	629	7.7	150,839	51,649	2,465,604	2,270	362	$85,637	$2,868.80	$373.78
	1984	3,351	716	25,236	512	598	7.4	153,281	51,491	2,446,540	2,222	372	$90,814	$3,072.51	$415.04
	1985	3,349	707	24,179	476	569	7.2	158,953	51,424	2,507,288	2,216	389	$96,150	$3,307.41	$462.69
	1986	3,323	689	23,483	460	563	7.2	167,633	50,885	2,547,170	2,241	398	$103,524	$3,589.64	$503.64
	1987	3,274	673	22,937	455	566	7.2	177,413	50,133	2,557,294	2,298	406	$112,325	$3,914.23	$543.67
	1988	3,242	668	22,939	456	577	7.3	195,363	48,828	2,653,794	2,373	412	$124,703	$4,272.95	$591.13
	1989	3,220	661	22,792	455	584	7.3	209,191	48,305	2,751,426	2,454	420	$136,889	$4,649.22	$642.45
	1990	3,191	657	22,878	455	596	7.3	221,073	47,441	2,833,204	2,533	424	$150,673	$5,001.24	$692.36
	1991	3,175	656	22,964	451	603	7.2	238,204	47,229	2,845,995	2,624	435	$166,806	$5,393.30	$758.21
	1992	3,173	656	23,056	445	606	7.1	257,887	47,185	2,846,386	2,692	443	$183,793	$5,808.80	$828.44
	1993	3,154	651	22,749	432	602	6.9	270,138	46,214	2,802,164	2,711	451	$197,187	$6,177.69	$897.70
	1994	3,139	637	22,704	413	589	6.6	282,653	46,381	2,792,116	2,719	462	$204,219	$6,256.72	$950.31
	1995	3,092	610	22,557	393	578	6.4	303,851	45,198	2,725,641	2,702	468	$209,614	$6,279.17	$994.39
	1996	3,045	598	22,542	379	567	6.1	320,746	44,650	2,683,750	2,711	478	$215,950	$6,344.05	$1,042.04
	1997	3,000	591	22,905	376	575	6.0	330,215	44,484	2,698,086	2,765	481	$225,287	$6,392.74	$1,074.26
	1998	3,026	588	23,282	377	587	5.9	352,114	44,087	2,715,958	2,834	483	$237,978	$6,525.68	$1,110.50
	1999	3,012	587	23,871	381	605	5.8	370,784	44,172	2,746,453	2,862	473	$251,534	$6,607.51	$1,139.89
	2000	3,003	583	24,452	382	618	5.7	393,168	43,655	2,833,615	2,919	472	$267,051	$6,717.48	$1,182.32
	2001	2,998	585	24,983	385	628	5.6	404,901	43,640	2,829,691	2,971	473	$292,250	$7,051.76	$1,255.25
	2002	3,025	582	25,425	391	646	5.6	416,910	43,241	2,820,159	3,039	471	$312,726	$7,457.84	$1,328.81

Table 1 (Continued)

CLASSIFICATION	YEAR	HOSPITALS	BEDS (in thousands)	ADMISSIONS (in thousands)	AVERAGE DAILY CENSUS (in thousands)	ADJUSTED AVERAGE DAILY CENSUS (in thousands)	AVERAGE LENGTH OF STAY (days)	OUTPATIENT VISITS (in thousands)	NEWBORNS Bassinets	NEWBORNS Births	FTE PERSONNEL Number (in thousands)	FTE PERSONNEL Per 100 Adjusted Census	EXPENSES Amount (in Millions of dollars)	EXPENSES Adjusted per Inpatient Stay (dollars)	EXPENSES Adjusted per Inpatient Day (dollars)
Investor-owned (for-profit) community hospitals	1975	775	73	2,646	48	53	6.6	7,713	4,062	141,392	139	263	$2,561	$876.48	$132.80
	1976	752	76	2,734	50	54	6.6	8,048	4,044	144,751	147	272	$3,085	$1,031.91	$156.35
	1979	727	83	2,963	53	59	6.6	9,289	4,110	174,843	174	300	$4,820	$1,476.42	$225.87
	1980	730	87	3,165	57	62	6.5	9,696	4,439	199,722	189	304	$5,847	$1,675.85	$257.12
	1981	729	88	3,239	58	63	6.5	9,961	4,523	207,405	203	322	$6,856	$1,952.56	$299.02
	1982	748	91	3,316	60	66	6.6	13,193	4,736	219,675	212	320	$8,177	$2,224.75	$340.03
	1983	757	94	3,299	59	66	6.5	10,389	5,039	228,883	213	323	$9,208	$2,517.53	$385.42
	1984	786	100	3,314	57	64	6.3	11,090	5,807	242,088	214	335	$10,251	$2,748.51	$438.30
	1985	805	104	3,242	54	63	6.1	12,378	6,117	266,839	221	350	$11,486	$3,033.06	$500.48
	1986	834	107	3,231	54	65	6.1	14,896	6,305	291,112	229	354	$12,987	$3,341.79	$552.40
	1987	828	106	3,157	54	66	6.2	16,566	6,391	306,492	242	367	$14,067	$3,617.19	$585.01
	1988	790	104	3,090	53	66	6.2	17,926	6,254	308,828	249	379	$15,545	$4,022.77	$649.33
	1989	769	102	3,071	53	67	6.3	19,341	6,354	325,711	261	390	$17,240	$4,406.20	$707.90
	1990	749	101	3,066	54	69	6.4	20,110	6,261	340,555	273	396	$18,822	$4,727.27	$751.55
	1991	738	100	3,016	52	69	6.3	21,174	6,358	359,115	281	409	$20,516	$5,133.53	$820.19
	1992	723	99	2,969	51	69	6.3	22,900	6,519	357,776	285	412	$22,496	$5,548.24	$888.73
	1993	717	99	2,946	51	69	6.2	24,936	6,395	363,358	289	417	$23,077	$5,643.21	$914.39
	1994	719	101	3,035	50	70	6.1	26,443	6,329	354,477	302	434	$23,445	$5,528.91	$923.90
	1995	752	106	3,428	55	77	5.8	31,940	7,164	408,339	343	443	$26,653	$5,425.20	$946.99
	1996	759	109	3,684	56	82	5.6	37,347	7,441	444,697	359	437	$28,385	$5,207.44	$945.49
	1997	797	115	3,953	60	89	5.5	40,919	8,026	465,919	385	433	$31,179	$5,218.69	$961.96
	1998	771	113	3,971	60	90	5.5	42,072	7,895	466,025	383	425	$31,732	$5,262.44	$968.00
	1999	747	107	3,905	58	86	5.5	39,896	7,486	467,585	362	422	$31,179	$5,350.07	$999.03
	2000	749	110	4,141	61	90	5.4	43,378	7,792	503,497	378	418	$34,969	$5,642.18	$1,057.32
	2001	754	109	4,197	63	92	5.4	44,706	7,413	494,669	379	413	$37,348	$5,971.81	$1,121.31
	2002	766	108	4,365	64	93	5.3	45,215	7,467	496,988	380	407	$40,082	$6,161.44	$1,180.83
State and local government community hospitals	1975	1,761	210	7,067	148	171	7.6	51,525	22,271	726,103	540	316	$8,463	$1,030.86	$135.64
	1976	1,760	210	7,163	146	170	7.5	52,286	21,810	716,548	537	315	$9,391	$1,132.50	$151.00
	1979	1,785	211	7,262	146	171	7.4	49,924	20,297	803,621	583	341	$13,247	$1,561.04	$211.89
	1980	1,778	209	7,413	149	174	7.3	50,459	20,424	819,282	598	343	$15,204	$1,750.13	$238.63
	1981	1,744	210	7,255	150	174	7.6	49,427	19,736	802,963	618	354	$17,449	$2,071.57	$274.25
	1982	1,715	210	7,165	149	175	7.6	58,685	19,431	811,437	627	320	$19,893	$2,364.09	$311.56
	1983	1,679	207	7,025	145	170	7.6	48,816	18,777	795,767	613	360	$21,593	$2,621.28	$347.56
	1984	1,622	201	6,606	133	158	7.3	47,590	18,283	767,680	581	368	$22,271	$2,823.13	$385.17
	1985	1,578	189	6,028	119	145	7.2	47,386	17,352	747,008	561	387	$22,863	$3,106.14	$432.84
	1986	1,521	182	5,665	114	142	7.4	49,383	16,492	746,126	555	391	$24,143	$3,404.69	$466.17
	1987	1,509	180	5,507	113	144	7.5	51,544	15,986	738,510	573	399	$26,192	$3,717.77	$499.33
	1988	1,501	175	5,424	112	145	7.6	55,840	15,243	743,780	583	403	$28,474	$4,033.67	$538.63
	1989	1,466	170	5,253	110	145	7.7	57,179	14,746	753,478	589	406	$30,769	$4,430.12	$582.15
	1990	1,444	169	5,236	111	148	7.7	60,146	14,710	784,504	614	415	$34,198	$4,837.76	$634.45
	1991	1,429	168	5,084	108	148	7.8	62,670	13,847	760,286	630	424	$37,701	$5,339.75	$695.89
	1992	1,396	166	5,008	108	152	7.9	67,734	13,385	720,782	643	424	$41,806	$5,870.76	$753.92
	1993	1,390	169	5,054	109	157	7.8	71,811	13,445	704,854	676	430	$45,825	$6,205.52	$799.73
	1994	1,371	164	4,979	104	154	7.6	73,828	13,012	662,774	672	438	$48,115	$6,513.39	$858.62
	1995	1,350	157	4,961	100	154	7.4	78,554	12,374	630,718	670	435	$49,322	$6,445.18	$877.85
	1996	1,330	155	4,873	96	150	7.2	81,770	11,549	595,424	654	437	$49,420	$6,418.65	$903.41
	1997	1,260	148	4,720	92	148	7.1	79,007	10,731	578,186	640	433	$49,298	$6,475.07	$913.62
	1998	1,218	139	4,559	87	142	7.0	80,008	10,174	544,250	614	433	$49,123	$6,612.23	$949.36
	1999	1,197	136	4,583	86	143	6.9	84,667	9,870	546,257	614	430	$52,534	$6,923.35	$1,006.91
	2000	1,163	131	4,496	83	140	6.7	84,858	9,392	543,054	614	438	$54,544	$7,106.05	$1,063.75
	2001	1,156	132	4,634	85	145	6.7	88,873	9,395	549,035	637	438	$59,137	$7,400.01	$1,113.79
	2002	1,136	130	4,688	84	147	6.6	94,280	9,266	553,044	651	442	$63,783	$7,772.93	$1,188.12

Table **2**

2002 U.S. Registered Hospitals: Utilization, Personnel, and Finances

Excludes U.S.-Associated Areas, Puerto Rico, and nonregistered hospitals.

CLASSIFICATION	HOSPITALS	BEDS	ADMISSIONS	INPATIENT DAYS	ADJUSTED PATIENT DAYS	AVERAGE DAILY CENSUS	ADJUSTED AVERAGE DAILY CENSUS	AVERAGE STAY (days)	SURGICAL OPERATIONS	OUTPATIENT VISITS Emergency	OUTPATIENT VISITS Total	NEWBORNS Bassinets	NEWBORNS Births
UNITED STATES	5,794	975,962	36,325,693	241,224,085	—	661,804	—	—	28,338,946	114,207,460	640,515,076	62,151	3,934,421
6-24 Beds	375	6,572	183,753	814,882	—	2,235	—	—	197,444	1,434,709	9,783,216	1,692	13,558
25-49	1,043	37,183	1,151,648	6,167,127	—	16,936	—	—	1,041,635	6,349,841	35,542,329	2,931	96,760
50-99	1,344	96,422	2,896,765	21,006,569	—	57,732	—	—	2,337,435	12,476,963	67,201,071	6,624	282,802
100-199	1,384	198,790	7,300,214	46,406,962	—	127,354	—	—	6,129,295	26,557,401	136,426,641	13,967	802,704
200-299	715	174,241	7,069,396	43,691,962	—	119,897	—	—	5,520,378	22,098,360	115,702,333	12,056	768,131
300-399	409	140,914	5,771,409	35,745,365	—	98,177	—	—	4,256,591	16,660,008	87,856,816	8,952	638,447
400-499	201	89,384	3,671,203	23,397,229	—	64,100	—	—	2,740,915	9,145,040	62,219,361	5,307	435,738
500 or more	323	232,456	8,281,305	63,993,989	—	175,373	—	—	6,115,253	19,485,138	125,783,309	10,622	896,281
Psychiatric	488	89,595	749,473	27,831,592	—	76,349	—	—	3,194	214,806	7,504,590	2	0
Hospitals.	476	83,224	748,373	25,907,058	—	71,076	—	—	3,161	214,806	7,504,234	2	0
Institutions for mentally retarded	12	6,371	1,100	1,924,534	—	5,273	—	—	33	0	356	0	0
General	4,963	848,382	34,952,878	202,934,338	—	556,800	—	—	27,875,346	113,119,469	618,626,146	61,455	3,880,133
Hospitals.	4,937	845,450	34,923,850	202,215,627	—	554,832	—	—	27,860,858	113,050,025	617,213,682	61,455	3,880,133
Hospital units of institutions	26	2,932	29,028	718,711	—	1,968	—	—	14,488	69,444	1,412,464	0	0
TB and other respiratory diseases	4	259	829	47,201	—	129	—	—	0	0	2,257	6	0
Obstetrics and gynecology	14	1,858	88,506	439,682	—	1,204	—	—	62,691	137,341	1,492,775	510	47,588
Eye, ear, nose and throat	10	312	7,747	30,642	—	84	—	—	84,203	53,151	723,400	17	879
Rehabilitation	180	15,136	246,768	4,199,422	—	11,505	—	—	50,848	18,890	6,277,890	0	0
Orthopedic	23	1,359	45,578	251,322	—	690	—	—	89,386	37,216	626,815	0	0
Chronic Disease	19	6,264	21,049	1,970,290	—	5,397	—	—	7,405	30,458	314,109	0	0
All other	93	12,797	212,865	3,519,596	—	9,646	—	—	165,873	596,129	4,947,094	161	5,821
Federal	240	49,838	1,027,116	11,999,637	—	32,892	—	—	712,483	3,886,335	75,780,970	2,151	63,806
Psychiatric	11	4,153	27,772	1,228,187	—	3,365	—	—	3,145	0	1,518,989	0	0
General and other special	229	45,685	999,344	10,771,450	—	29,527	—	—	709,338	3,886,335	74,261,981	2,151	63,806
Nonfederal	5,554	926,124	35,298,577	229,224,448	—	628,912	—	—	27,626,463	110,321,125	564,734,106	60,000	3,870,615
Psychiatric	477	85,442	721,701	26,603,405	—	72,984	—	—	49	214,806	5,985,601	2	0
Hospitals.	465	79,071	720,601	24,678,871	—	67,711	—	—	16	214,806	5,985,245	2	0
Institutions for mentally retarded	12	6,371	1,100	1,924,534	—	5,273	—	—	33	0	356	0	0
TB and other respiratory diseases	4	259	829	47,201	—	129	—	—	0	0	2,257	6	0
Long-term general and other special	124	17,892	75,285	5,466,402	—	14,972	—	—	36,085	94,518	1,409,896	18	424
Short-term general and other special	4,949	822,531	34,500,762	197,107,440	322,970,965	540,827	885,994	5.7	27,590,329	110,011,801	557,336,352	59,974	3,870,191
Hospital units of institutions	22	1,878	22,482	417,341	—	1,142	—	—	13,654	60,063	932,140	0	0
Community Hospitals	4,927	820,653	34,478,280	196,690,099	322,970,965	539,685	885,994	5.7	27,576,675	109,951,738	556,404,212	59,974	3,870,191
6-24 Beds	321	5,629	161,716	666,858	2,175,292	1,826	5,994	4.1	187,026	1,053,994	5,929,797	468	10,297
25-49	931	33,200	1,062,147	5,313,229	12,766,654	14,595	35,082	5.0	996,859	5,851,427	29,726,357	2,748	90,518
50-99	1,072	76,882	2,471,386	15,874,178	32,032,806	43,583	87,938	6.4	2,224,072	11,669,278	53,342,237	6,226	262,390
100-199	1,190	171,625	6,826,388	38,569,069	68,744,851	105,877	188,624	5.6	5,935,695	25,708,579	117,573,082	13,786	786,784
200-299	625	152,682	6,799,664	37,122,247	59,840,770	101,900	164,198	5.5	5,352,273	21,513,390	102,423,950	11,888	753,559
300-399	358	123,399	5,606,593	30,625,907	47,302,622	84,133	129,872	5.5	4,171,451	16,337,980	79,092,441	8,929	634,624
400-499	174	77,145	3,592,594	19,862,987	29,959,771	54,418	82,078	5.5	2,720,297	9,056,989	57,841,206	5,307	435,738
500 or more	256	180,091	7,957,792	48,655,624	70,148,199	133,353	192,208	6.1	5,989,002	18,760,101	110,475,142	10,622	896,281
Nongovernment not-for-profit	3,025	582,179	25,424,613	142,590,945	235,342,664	391,293	645,650	5.6	20,845,177	78,266,830	416,909,994	43,241	2,820,159
Investor-owned (for profit)	766	108,422	4,365,425	23,276,060	33,944,458	63,924	93,197	5.3	3,366,792	13,505,713	45,214,667	7,467	496,988
State and Local Government	1,136	130,052	4,688,242	30,823,094	53,683,843	84,468	147,147	6.6	3,364,706	18,179,195	94,279,551	9,266	553,044

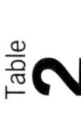

Table 2 (Continued)

CLASSIFICATION	FULL-TIME EQUIVALENT PERSONNEL					FULL-TIME EQUIVALENT TRAINEES			EXPENSES — LABOR				EXPENSES — TOTAL		
	Physicians and Dentists	Registered Nurses	Licensed Practical Nurses	Other Salaried Personnel	Total Personnel	Medical and Dental Residents	Other Trainees	Total Trainees	Payroll (in thousands)	Employee Benefits (in thousands)	Total (in thousands)	Percent of Total	Amount (in thousands)	Adjusted per Admission	Adjusted per Inpatient Day
UNITED STATES	99,829	1,073,468	155,863	3,281,046	4,610,206	88,536	8,602	97,138	$199,633,895	$46,296,856	$245,930,751	53.2	$462,221,560	—	—
6-24 Beds	1,129	7,179	2,297	29,365	39,970	32	57	89	$1,267,545	$346,553	$1,614,098	56.2	$2,873,817	—	—
25-49	4,253	33,818	10,296	128,477	176,844	187	85	272	$6,031,315	$1,390,061	$7,421,376	52.1	$14,249,089	—	—
50-99	6,997	79,459	21,943	278,420	386,819	900	226	1,126	$14,694,829	$3,386,185	$18,081,013	56.1	$32,202,657	—	—
100-199	16,998	195,517	34,423	612,492	859,430	6,994	729	7,723	$34,907,942	$8,274,405	$43,182,347	53.7	$80,475,524	—	—
200-299	15,649	199,240	26,710	584,894	826,493	7,936	1,144	9,080	$35,608,570	$8,369,118	$43,977,687	52.7	$83,410,349	—	—
300-399	11,664	167,032	21,409	492,013	692,118	11,870	1,229	13,099	$30,555,266	$6,982,119	$37,537,385	52.5	$71,512,522	—	—
400-499	11,592	113,737	11,807	332,375	469,511	13,715	2,363	16,078	$21,841,363	$5,102,788	$26,944,151	53.7	$50,191,230	—	—
500 or more	31,547	277,486	26,978	823,010	1,159,021	46,902	2,769	49,671	$54,727,066	$12,445,628	$67,172,694	52.8	$127,306,372	—	—
Psychiatric	4,988	26,324	10,192	162,922	204,426	531	282	813	$7,709,222	$2,247,297	$9,956,519	74.9	$13,292,996	—	—
Hospitals	4,886	25,883	9,850	151,442	192,061	531	275	806	$7,297,837	$2,142,735	$9,440,573	74.3	$12,707,956	—	—
Institutions for mentally retarded	102	441	342	11,480	12,365	0	7	7	$411,385	$104,562	$515,946	88.2	$585,040	—	—
General	91,912	1,021,041	139,122	3,012,493	4,264,673	86,935	7,998	94,933	$186,030,278	$42,653,769	$228,684,047	52.4	$436,250,965	—	—
Hospitals	91,643	1,020,099	138,629	3,008,142	4,258,513	86,928	7,994	94,922	$185,820,869	$42,591,228	$228,412,098	52.4	$435,849,684	—	—
Hospital units of institutions	269	942	598	4,351	6,160	7	4	11	$209,409	$62,540	$271,949	67.8	$401,281	—	—
TB and other respiratory diseases	0	119	89	467	675	0	0	0	$24,565	$6,349	$30,914	62.3	$49,633	—	—
Obstetrics and gynecology	178	2,709	314	6,832	10,033	42	0	42	$428,353	$94,087	$522,440	58.0	$901,521	—	—
Eye, ear, nose and throat	112	529	66	2,536	3,243	115	22	137	$124,453	$31,818	$156,271	46.2	$338,488	—	—
Rehabilitation	560	8,742	2,653	41,428	53,383	125	17	142	$2,042,585	$441,813	$2,484,398	59.1	$4,204,601	—	—
Orthopedic	355	1,662	221	6,009	8,247	53	1	54	$392,923	$92,440	$485,363	49.6	$979,242	—	—
Chronic Disease	282	1,748	947	9,656	12,633	17	16	33	$577,223	$189,717	$766,940	72.3	$1,060,578	—	—
All other	1,442	10,594	2,154	38,703	52,893	718	266	984	$2,304,293	$539,567	$2,843,859	55.3	$5,143,537	—	—
Federal	21,517	53,941	17,317	205,880	298,655	9,253	2,684	11,937	$14,650,188	$3,642,385	$18,292,573	61.6	$29,692,691	—	—
Psychiatric	462	1,714	775	8,714	11,665	16	33	49	$683,810	$166,639	$850,449	69.6	$1,222,233	—	—
General and other special	21,055	52,227	16,542	197,166	286,990	9,237	2,651	11,888	$13,966,378	$3,475,746	$17,442,124	61.3	$28,470,458	—	—
Nonfederal	78,312	1,019,527	138,546	3,075,166	4,311,551	79,283	5,918	85,201	$184,983,707	$42,654,471	$227,638,178	52.6	$432,528,869	—	—
Psychiatric	4,526	24,610	9,417	154,208	192,761	515	249	764	$7,025,412	$2,080,658	$9,106,070	75.4	$12,070,763	—	—
Hospitals	4,424	24,169	9,075	142,728	180,396	515	242	757	$6,614,027	$1,976,096	$8,590,124	74.8	$11,485,723	—	—
Institutions for mentally retarded	102	441	342	11,480	12,365	0	7	7	$411,385	$104,562	$515,946	88.2	$585,040	—	—
TB and other respiratory diseases	0	119	89	467	675	0	0	0	$24,565	$6,349	$30,914	62.3	$49,633	—	—
Long-term general and other special	819	6,038	2,706	36,185	45,748	47	206	253	$1,883,689	$490,560	$2,374,249	65.6	$3,617,144	—	—
Short-term general and other special	72,967	988,760	126,334	2,884,306	4,072,367	78,721	5,463	84,184	$176,050,040	$40,076,905	$216,126,945	51.9	$416,791,330	—	—
Hospital units of institutions	144	621	469	1,638	2,872	6	0	6	$88,561	$27,332	$115,893	57.9	$200,271	—	—
Community Hospitals	72,823	988,139	125,865	2,882,668	4,069,495	78,715	5,463	84,178	$175,961,479	$40,049,573	$216,011,053	51.9	$416,591,059	$7,354.60	$1,289.87
6-24 Beds	390	5,706	2,035	20,236	28,367	32	28	60	$938,481	$215,611	$1,154,093	51.6	$2,235,954	$4,135.32	$1,027.89
25-49	2,881	30,422	9,270	111,252	153,825	132	38	170	$5,292,448	$1,197,188	$6,489,636	51.5	$12,594,583	$4,847.57	$986.52
50-99	3,198	66,995	16,065	218,466	304,724	165	50	215	$11,342,604	$2,694,502	$14,037,106	53.7	$26,141,501	$5,197.17	$816.09
100-199	11,314	176,895	28,649	533,720	750,578	4,099	289	4,388	$30,347,011	$7,051,296	$37,398,307	52.4	$71,359,096	$5,934.93	$1,038.03
200-299	10,296	184,042	22,637	523,968	740,943	5,828	247	6,075	$31,843,887	$7,300,054	$39,143,941	51.8	$75,580,361	$6,951.35	$1,263.02
300-399	8,749	158,184	18,579	448,186	633,698	10,758	916	11,674	$27,672,704	$6,183,450	$33,856,154	51.2	$66,128,523	$7,634.87	$1,397.99
400-499	10,219	108,968	9,864	307,551	436,602	13,248	1,650	14,898	$20,179,892	$4,676,184	$24,856,077	52.4	$47,419,294	$8,762.13	$1,582.77
500 or more	25,776	256,927	18,766	719,289	1,020,758	44,453	2,245	46,698	$48,344,453	$10,731,287	$59,075,740	51.3	$115,131,748	$10,006.84	$1,641.26
Nongovernment not-for-profit	61,328	731,152	80,231	2,166,698	3,039,409	58,018	3,613	61,631	$133,106,102	$30,069,956	$163,176,058	52.2	$312,725,801	$7,457.84	$1,328.81
Investor-owned (for profit)	1,232	105,299	19,814	253,186	379,531	1,069	46	1,115	$15,587,588	$3,305,545	$18,893,133	47.1	$40,082,466	$6,161.44	$1,180.83
State and Local Government	10,263	151,688	25,820	462,784	650,555	19,628	1,804	21,432	$27,267,790	$6,674,072	$33,941,861	53.2	$63,782,792	$7,772.93	$1,188.12

Tables 3–6

TABLE **3**

TOTAL UNITED STATES

U.S. Registered Community Hospitals
(Nonfederal, short-term general and other special hospitals)

Overview 1998–2002

	2002	2001	2000	1999	1998
TOTAL U.S. Community Hospitals	4,927	4,908	4,915	4,956	5,015
Bed Size Category					
6-24	321	281	288	299	293
25-49	931	916	910	887	900
50-99	1,072	1,070	1,055	1,082	1,085
100-199	1,190	1,218	1,236	1,266	1,304
200-299	625	635	656	642	644
300-399	358	348	341	365	352
400-499	174	191	182	161	183
500 + ...	256	249	247	254	254
Location					
Hospitals Urban......................	2,749	2,741	2,740	2,767	2,816
Hospitals Rural	2,178	2,167	2,175	2,189	2,199
Control					
State and Local Government	1,136	1,156	1,163	1,197	1,218
Not for Profit	3,025	2,998	3,003	3,012	3,026
Investor owned	766	754	749	747	771
Physician Models					
Independent Practice Association........	771	770	831	874	966
Group Practice without Walls	193	195	211	198	232
Open Physician-Hospital Organization....	820	849	939	975	1,055
Closed Physician-Hospital Organization...	294	316	360	414	451
Management Service Organization.......	519	545	655	770	866
Integrated Salary Model	1,224	1,122	1,126	1,106	1,039
Equity Model	67	58	91	103	121
Foundation.........................	202	212	252	290	349
Insurance Products					
Health Maintenance Organization........	698	715	870	1,009	1,099
Preferred Provider Organization.........	923	873	1,028	1,156	1,303
Indemnity Fee for Service..............	265	247	286	303	387
Managed Care Contracts					
Health Maintenance Organization........	2,740	2,738	2,804	2,916	2,933
Preferred Provider Organization.........	3,218	3,217	3,233	3,310	3,291
Affiliations					
Hospitals in a System.................	2,261	2,260	2,217	2,238	2,176
Hospitals in a Network	1,343	1,341	1,327	1,310	1,380
Hospitals in a Group Purchasing Organization......................	3,495	3,495	3,344	3,080	2,778

TABLE 3

TOTAL UNITED STATES

U.S. Registered Community Hospitals
(Nonfederal, short-term general and other special hospitals)

Utilization, Personnel, Revenue and Expenses, Community Health Indicators 1998–2002

	2002	2001	2000	1999	1998
TOTAL FACILITY (Includes Hospital and Nursing Home Units)					
Utilization - Inpatient					
Beds	820,653	825,966	823,560	829,575	839,988
Admissions	34,478,280	33,813,589	33,089,467	32,359,042	31,811,673
Inpatient Days	196,690,099	194,106,316	192,420,368	191,884,270	191,430,450
Average Length of Stay	5.7	5.7	5.8	5.9	6.0
Inpatient Surgeries	10,105,010	9,779,583	9,729,336	9,539,593	9,735,705
Births	3,870,191	3,873,395	3,890,166	3,760,295	3,726,233
Utilization - Outpatient					
Emergency Outpatient Visits	109,951,738	105,957,778	103,144,030	99,484,462	94,771,405
Other Outpatient Visits	446,452,474	432,522,600	418,260,946	395,861,824	379,422,063
Total Outpatient Visits	556,404,212	538,480,378	521,404,976	495,346,286	474,193,468
Outpatient Surgeries	17,471,665	16,684,726	16,383,374	15,845,492	15,593,614
Personnel					
Full Time RNs	772,479	751,095	745,113	739,086	733,365
Full Time LPNs	104,058	104,534	101,683	106,739	109,882
Part Time RNs	431,274	413,832	424,801	397,950	392,622
Part Time LPNs	43,600	43,446	45,011	45,561	47,191
Total Full Time	3,489,190	3,428,159	3,332,232	3,297,689	3,294,274
Total Part Time	1,328,930	1,285,207	1,320,696	1,246,661	1,242,121
Revenue - Inpatient					
Gross Inpatient Revenue	$622,963,195,767	$544,087,612,104	$481,753,558,221	$436,802,516,912	$407,650,369,271
Revenue - Outpatient					
Gross Outpatient Revenue	$338,185,339,792	$289,605,612,366	$255,130,109,523	$224,677,472,092	$201,951,491,048
Revenue and Expenses - Totals					
(Includes Inpatient and Outpatient)					
Total Gross Revenue	$961,148,535,559	$833,693,224,470	$736,883,667,744	$661,439,989,004	$609,601,860,319
Deductions from Revenue	553,855,167,351	463,168,133,776	394,634,720,840	340,074,141,264	299,969,313,562
Net Patient Revenue	407,293,368,208	370,525,090,694	342,248,946,904	321,365,847,740	309,632,546,757
Other Operating Revenue	25,253,169,830	23,816,314,195	21,691,829,666	20,954,555,617	19,347,513,120
Other Nonoperating Revenue	3,333,738,368	6,353,280,081	9,649,649,680	9,207,219,318	9,322,323,105
Total Net Revenue	435,880,276,406	400,694,684,970	373,590,426,250	351,527,622,675	338,302,382,982
Total Expenses	416,591,058,927	383,734,757,143	356,563,789,627	335,197,410,905	318,833,870,519
HOSPITAL UNIT (Excludes Separate Nursing Home Units)					
Utilization - Inpatient					
Beds	749,058	753,592	746,918	746,638	758,186
Admissions	34,096,173	33,408,199	32,639,620	31,814,468	31,265,867
Inpatient Days	174,148,040	171,049,431	168,133,112	165,919,000	165,644,176
Average Length of Stay	5.1	5.1	5.2	5.2	5.3
Personnel					
Total Full Time	3,440,069	3,376,958	3,274,082	3,239,743	3,235,153
Total Part Time	1,304,545	1,259,927	1,291,840	1,218,813	1,213,426
Revenue and Expenses - Totals					
(Includes Inpatient and Outpatient)					
Total Net Revenue	$431,242,102,280	$396,133,790,471	$368,509,487,402	$346,323,409,701	$333,054,828,642
Total Expenses	412,517,083,689	380,087,229,391	353,070,652,573	331,217,766,222	314,709,758,455
COMMUNITY HEALTH INDICATORS PER 1000 POPULATION					
Total Population (in thousands)	288,369	284,797	281,422	272,691	270,248
Inpatient					
Beds	2.8	2.9	2.9	3.0	3.1
Admissions	119.6	118.7	117.6	118.7	117.7
Inpatient Days	682.1	681.6	683.7	703.7	708.4
Inpatient Surgeries	35.0	34.3	34.6	35.0	36.0
Births	13.4	13.6	13.8	13.8	13.8
Outpatient					
Emergency Outpatient Visits	381.3	372.0	366.5	364.8	350.7
Other Outpatient Visits	1,548.2	1,518.7	1,486.2	1,451.7	1,404.0
Total Outpatient Visits	1,929.5	1,890.8	1,852.8	1,816.5	1,754.7
Outpatient Surgeries	60.6	58.6	58.2	58.1	57.7
Expense per Capita (per person)	$1,444.6	$1,347.4	$1,267.0	$1,229.2	$1,179.8

TABLE **4**

BED SIZE CATEGORY 6-24

U.S. Registered Community Hospitals
(Nonfederal, short-term general and other special hospitals)

Overview 1998–2002

	2002	2001	2000	1999	1998
Total U.S. Community Hospitals in Bed Size Category 6-24	**321**	**281**	**288**	**299**	**293**
Location					
Hospitals Urban......................	66	56	57	64	59
Hospitals Rural	255	225	231	235	234
Control					
State and Local Government	146	135	143	151	155
Not for Profit	149	122	126	127	123
Investor owned	26	24	19	21	15
Physician Models					
Independent Practice Association........	42	36	31	25	26
Group Practice without Walls	14	10	12	9	12
Open Physician-Hospital Organization....	21	17	20	21	30
Closed Physician-Hospital Organization...	11	9	6	8	9
Management Service Organization.......	20	14	12	15	19
Integrated Salary Model	85	73	64	65	73
Equity Model	4	3	3	5	4
Foundation.........................	13	9	7	13	16
Insurance Products					
Health Maintenance Organization........	35	30	34	30	37
Preferred Provider Organization.........	53	35	42	40	48
Indemnity Fee for Service.............	18	11	10	5	12
Managed Care Contracts					
Health Maintenance Organization........	124	100	101	120	127
Preferred Provider Organization.........	181	160	164	175	174
Affiliations					
Hospitals in a System.................	92	73	72	64	67
Hospitals in a Network	97	79	77	67	66
Hospitals in a Group Purchasing Organization......................	212	192	178	169	162

Bed Size Categories

TABLE 4

BED SIZE CATEGORY 6-24

U.S. Registered Community Hospitals
(Nonfederal, short-term general and other special hospitals)

Utilization, Personnel, Revenue and Expenses 1998–2002

	2002	2001	2000	1999	1998
TOTAL FACILITY (Includes Hospital and Nursing Home Units)					
Utilization - Inpatient					
Beds	5,629	4,964	5,156	5,442	5,351
Admissions	161,716	140,467	140,735	145,418	138,676
Inpatient Days	666,858	566,345	601,199	651,124	643,241
Average Length of Stay	4.1	4.0	4.3	4.5	4.6
Inpatient Surgeries	26,172	23,655	21,084	22,445	24,994
Births	10,297	9,300	9,836	11,283	9,835
Utilization - Outpatient					
Emergency Outpatient Visits	1,053,994	796,297	743,260	676,879	720,202
Other Outpatient Visits	4,875,803	3,759,485	3,812,179	3,973,601	3,558,219
Total Outpatient Visits	5,929,797	4,555,782	4,555,439	4,650,480	4,278,421
Outpatient Surgeries	160,854	120,783	111,263	117,592	96,181
Personnel					
Full Time RNs	4,451	3,684	3,744	3,935	3,748
Full Time LPNs	1,677	1,468	1,363	1,469	1,516
Part Time RNs	2,498	2,069	2,443	2,369	2,182
Part Time LPNs	709	669	713	752	678
Total Full Time	23,058	18,993	18,944	20,593	18,869
Total Part Time	10,753	9,128	10,287	10,026	9,728
Revenue - Inpatient					
Gross Inpatient Revenue	$1,187,061,180	$865,976,268	$785,583,707	$803,992,451	$785,821,717
Revenue - Outpatient					
Gross Outpatient Revenue	$2,471,688,778	$1,560,963,930	$1,539,812,867	$1,377,204,771	$1,187,401,957
Revenue and Expenses - Totals					
(Includes Inpatient and Outpatient)					
Total Gross Revenue	$3,658,749,958	$2,426,940,198	$2,325,396,574	$2,181,197,222	$1,973,223,674
Deductions from Revenue	1,513,681,706	951,093,256	907,556,076	782,264,529	742,459,310
Net Patient Revenue	2,145,068,252	1,475,846,942	1,417,840,498	1,398,932,693	1,230,764,364
Other Operating Revenue	162,911,063	154,437,602	115,552,533	170,916,578	139,388,003
Other Nonoperating Revenue	28,315,990	33,912,311	38,248,611	87,134,276	43,645,742
Total Net Revenue	2,336,295,305	1,664,196,855	1,571,641,642	1,656,983,547	1,413,798,109
Total Expenses	2,235,953,879	1,613,936,534	1,549,776,034	1,658,451,372	1,382,369,992
HOSPITAL UNIT (Excludes Separate Nursing Home Units)					
Utilization - Inpatient					
Beds	5,470	4,864	5,063	5,352	5,246
Admissions	161,090	140,181	140,230	144,893	137,990
Inpatient Days	619,452	528,596	568,533	623,695	611,534
Average Length of Stay	3.8	3.8	4.1	4.3	4.4
Personnel					
Total Full Time	22,960	18,929	18,716	20,537	18,808
Total Part Time	10,689	9,066	10,074	9,985	9,684
Revenue and Expenses - Totals					
(Includes Inpatient and Outpatient)					
Total Net Revenue	$2,324,685,737	$1,654,040,740	$1,564,960,209	$1,650,222,760	$1,404,198,000
Total Expenses	2,230,173,614	1,608,501,142	1,543,940,406	1,653,276,803	1,376,587,586

Bed Size Categories

TABLE 4

BED SIZE CATEGORY 25-49

U.S. Registered Community Hospitals
(Nonfederal, short-term general and other special hospitals)

Overview 1998–2002

	2002	2001	2000	1999	1998
Total U.S. Community Hospitals in Bed Size Category 25-49	**931**	**916**	**910**	**887**	**900**
Location					
Hospitals Urban.......................	220	214	201	192	201
Hospitals Rural	711	702	709	695	699
Control					
State and Local Government	363	374	375	374	391
Not for Profit	461	442	440	423	411
Investor owned	107	100	95	90	98
Physician Models					
Independent Practice Association........	128	113	106	114	124
Group Practice without Walls	27	35	29	17	30
Open Physician-Hospital Organization....	87	83	102	96	118
Closed Physician-Hospital Organization...	33	33	39	40	39
Management Service Organization.......	56	53	62	64	75
Integrated Salary Model	212	200	183	169	139
Equity Model	6	4	10	9	12
Foundation.........................	19	23	26	31	36
Insurance Products					
Health Maintenance Organization........	78	87	89	110	115
Preferred Provider Organization.........	152	133	143	153	173
Indemnity Fee for Service.............	41	45	45	48	58
Managed Care Contracts					
Health Maintenance Organization........	421	416	406	436	439
Preferred Provider Organization.........	578	557	561	571	569
Affiliations					
Hospitals in a System.................	276	275	270	274	248
Hospitals in a Network	221	219	216	208	220
Hospitals in a Group Purchasing Organization......................	643	639	612	584	532

TABLE 4

BED SIZE CATEGORY 25-49

U.S. Registered Community Hospitals
(Nonfederal, short-term general and other special hospitals)

Utilization, Personnel, Revenue and Expenses 1998–2002

	2002	2001	2000	1999	1998
TOTAL FACILITY (Includes Hospital and Nursing Home Units)					
Utilization - Inpatient					
Beds	33,200	33,263	33,333	32,816	33,510
Admissions	1,062,147	1,030,375	994,641	959,482	964,802
Inpatient Days	5,313,229	5,159,467	5,031,151	4,957,792	5,034,160
Average Length of Stay	5.0	5.0	5.1	5.2	5.2
Inpatient Surgeries	224,701	205,619	206,859	197,717	209,849
Births	90,518	87,770	88,275	84,491	91,733
Utilization - Outpatient					
Emergency Outpatient Visits	5,851,427	5,346,064	5,195,946	5,055,140	4,945,356
Other Outpatient Visits	23,874,930	22,594,571	21,811,383	18,814,467	17,748,273
Total Outpatient Visits	29,726,357	27,940,635	27,007,329	23,869,607	22,693,629
Outpatient Surgeries	772,158	747,613	676,172	610,784	608,488
Personnel					
Full Time RNs	23,627	22,343	22,830	21,305	21,992
Full Time LPNs	7,654	7,400	7,333	6,978	7,214
Part Time RNs	13,569	13,038	14,072	13,333	13,828
Part Time LPNs	3,221	3,132	3,424	3,191	3,112
Total Full Time	126,569	120,976	116,462	110,210	110,258
Total Part Time	54,844	51,639	54,820	50,931	53,108
Revenue - Inpatient					
Gross Inpatient Revenue	$9,424,112,207	$7,883,987,594	$7,196,766,831	$6,561,005,229	$6,129,218,618
Revenue - Outpatient					
Gross Outpatient Revenue	$12,499,434,007	$10,608,878,116	$9,410,834,420	$7,991,583,099	$7,236,681,368
Revenue and Expenses - Totals					
(Includes Inpatient and Outpatient)					
Total Gross Revenue	$21,923,546,214	$18,492,865,710	$16,607,601,251	$14,552,588,328	$13,365,899,986
Deductions from Revenue	10,327,317,002	8,222,555,507	7,231,526,571	6,067,585,675	5,164,085,375
Net Patient Revenue	11,596,229,212	10,270,310,203	9,376,074,680	8,485,002,653	8,201,814,611
Other Operating Revenue	1,245,298,074	1,134,586,636	959,276,038	826,240,928	744,101,510
Other Nonoperating Revenue	135,373,750	212,155,156	312,430,036	217,293,330	222,857,115
Total Net Revenue	12,976,901,036	11,617,051,995	10,647,780,754	9,528,536,911	9,168,773,236
Total Expenses	12,594,583,292	11,381,539,275	10,391,935,057	9,283,978,476	8,835,814,359
HOSPITAL UNIT (Excludes Separate Nursing Home Units)					
Utilization - Inpatient					
Beds	31,025	31,189	31,299	30,763	31,513
Admissions	1,056,128	1,023,053	987,780	952,964	957,140
Inpatient Days	4,637,216	4,511,675	4,419,903	4,319,613	4,416,725
Average Length of Stay	4.4	4.4	4.5	4.5	4.6
Personnel					
Total Full Time	124,998	119,566	115,277	109,069	109,094
Total Part Time	54,116	50,898	54,115	50,264	52,363
Revenue and Expenses - Totals					
(Includes Inpatient and Outpatient)					
Total Net Revenue	$12,864,807,992	$11,521,210,710	$10,559,902,580	$9,428,841,798	$9,077,370,329
Total Expenses	12,509,264,997	11,315,045,682	10,335,837,413	9,223,711,698	8,767,241,151

TABLE 4

BED SIZE CATEGORY 50-99

U.S. Registered Community Hospitals
(Nonfederal, short-term general and other special hospitals)

Overview 1998–2002

	2002	2001	2000	1999	1998
Total U.S. Community Hospitals in Bed Size Category 50-99	**1,072**	**1,070**	**1,055**	**1,082**	**1,085**
Location					
Hospitals Urban.	417	407	400	414	419
Hospitals Rural	655	663	655	668	666
Control					
State and Local Government	273	278	279	285	281
Not for Profit	590	593	581	584	606
Investor owned	209	199	195	213	198
Physician Models					
Independent Practice Association.	137	138	153	158	168
Group Practice without Walls	34	37	38	36	38
Open Physician-Hospital Organization. . . .	162	158	168	177	189
Closed Physician-Hospital Organization. . .	45	45	54	61	62
Management Service Organization.	64	70	85	114	130
Integrated Salary Model	221	196	191	195	178
Equity Model	9	3	9	14	16
Foundation.	34	29	49	50	59
Insurance Products					
Health Maintenance Organization.	108	105	121	154	182
Preferred Provider Organization	170	149	178	226	250
Indemnity Fee for Service.	55	42	54	61	73
Managed Care Contracts					
Health Maintenance Organization.	499	509	511	541	529
Preferred Provider Organization	649	660	644	662	640
Affiliations					
Hospitals in a System.	433	435	405	431	414
Hospitals in a Network	260	267	264	269	264
Hospitals in a Group Purchasing Organization.	753	751	697	637	559

TABLE 4

BED SIZE CATEGORY 50-99

U.S. Registered Community Hospitals
(Nonfederal, short-term general and other special hospitals)

Utilization, Personnel, Revenue and Expenses 1998–2002

	2002	2001	2000	1999	1998
TOTAL FACILITY (Includes Hospital and Nursing Home Units)					
Utilization - Inpatient					
Beds	76,882	76,924	75,865	78,121	78,035
Admissions	2,471,386	2,421,938	2,354,896	2,316,862	2,264,836
Inpatient Days	15,874,178	15,461,340	15,195,600	15,548,467	15,564,337
Average Length of Stay	6.4	6.4	6.5	6.7	6.9
Inpatient Surgeries	610,705	588,354	580,886	568,696	655,043
Births	262,390	262,605	276,308	266,469	257,485
Utilization - Outpatient					
Emergency Outpatient Visits	11,669,278	11,093,357	10,601,048	10,292,153	9,781,573
Other Outpatient Visits	41,672,959	40,237,990	38,783,686	35,863,458	32,379,666
Total Outpatient Visits	53,342,237	51,331,347	49,384,734	46,155,611	42,161,239
Outpatient Surgeries	1,613,367	1,485,774	1,448,514	1,385,596	1,465,553
Personnel					
Full Time RNs	51,193	49,209	48,531	48,609	49,048
Full Time LPNs	13,012	12,956	12,749	13,349	12,965
Part Time RNs	31,630	29,477	31,250	30,651	29,470
Part Time LPNs	6,137	5,747	6,141	6,460	6,149
Total Full Time	247,846	244,068	233,169	233,659	233,003
Total Part Time	114,178	110,165	115,307	110,546	107,517
Revenue - Inpatient					
Gross Inpatient Revenue	$28,405,320,827	$24,513,608,917	$22,750,944,141	$21,097,563,298	$20,094,829,572
Revenue - Outpatient					
Gross Outpatient Revenue	$25,936,635,813	$22,106,129,277	$19,990,370,027	$17,597,291,726	$15,882,964,599
Revenue and Expenses - Totals					
(Includes Inpatient and Outpatient)					
Total Gross Revenue	$54,341,956,640	$46,619,738,194	$42,741,314,168	$38,694,855,024	$35,977,794,171
Deductions from Revenue	28,088,461,303	23,028,290,004	21,022,033,394	18,058,805,944	16,276,818,923
Net Patient Revenue	26,253,495,337	23,591,448,190	21,719,280,774	20,636,049,080	19,700,975,248
Other Operating Revenue	1,036,671,212	1,028,923,986	992,807,456	1,007,752,277	1,023,064,020
Other Nonoperating Revenue	260,065,744	683,658,777	657,785,910	448,107,493	496,150,441
Total Net Revenue	27,550,232,293	25,304,030,953	23,369,874,140	22,091,908,850	21,220,189,709
Total Expenses	26,141,500,525	24,030,935,779	22,322,022,731	20,967,397,999	20,021,471,000
HOSPITAL UNIT (Excludes Separate Nursing Home Units)					
Utilization - Inpatient					
Beds	64,086	64,717	63,189	65,129	65,288
Admissions	2,431,740	2,384,021	2,315,942	2,269,013	2,217,188
Inpatient Days	11,846,603	11,602,606	11,205,030	11,512,534	11,522,253
Average Length of Stay	4.9	4.9	4.8	5.1	5.2
Personnel					
Total Full Time	240,319	237,000	224,763	226,412	225,267
Total Part Time	109,200	105,562	110,426	106,029	102,640
Revenue and Expenses - Totals					
(Includes Inpatient and Outpatient)					
Total Net Revenue	$26,950,192,407	$24,745,283,010	$22,858,172,678	$21,542,991,451	$20,672,497,709
Total Expenses	25,675,955,624	23,602,034,845	21,923,794,277	20,558,590,538	19,608,707,134

Bed Size Categories

TABLE 4

BED SIZE CATEGORY 100-199

U.S. Registered Community Hospitals
(Nonfederal, short-term general and other special hospitals)

Overview 1998–2002

	2002	2001	2000	1999	1998
Total U.S. Community Hospitals in Bed Size Category 100-199	1,190	1,218	1,236	1,266	1,304
Location					
Hospitals Urban	766	783	795	816	848
Hospitals Rural	424	435	441	450	456
Control					
State and Local Government	181	198	196	214	212
Not for Profit	750	757	769	791	807
Investor owned	259	263	271	261	285
Physician Models					
Independent Practice Association.	193	198	229	222	268
Group Practice without Walls	48	50	55	50	64
Open Physician-Hospital Organization. . . .	220	242	274	294	316
Closed Physician-Hospital Organization. . .	78	82	87	100	130
Management Service Organization.	130	143	178	213	260
Integrated Salary Model	261	241	265	269	244
Equity Model	15	16	26	21	36
Foundation	43	46	60	66	90
Insurance Products					
Health Maintenance Organization.	150	151	196	243	269
Preferred Provider Organization	196	208	247	286	332
Indemnity Fee for Service.	53	51	59	79	104
Managed Care Contracts					
Health Maintenance Organization.	691	706	752	776	803
Preferred Provider Organization	776	805	820	849	870
Affiliations					
Hospitals in a System	573	580	591	606	609
Hospitals in a Network	313	325	315	315	349
Hospitals in a Group Purchasing Organization.	837	858	850	763	688

TABLE 4

BED SIZE CATEGORY 100-199

U.S. Registered Community Hospitals
(Nonfederal, short-term general and other special hospitals)

Utilization, Personnel, Revenue and Expenses 1998–2002

	2002	2001	2000	1999	1998
TOTAL FACILITY (Includes Hospital and Nursing Home Units)					
Utilization - Inpatient					
Beds	171,625	174,024	175,778	181,115	186,118
Admissions	6,826,388	6,777,542	6,734,707	6,683,621	6,656,196
Inpatient Days	38,569,069	38,508,731	38,624,802	39,220,552	39,597,014
Average Length of Stay	5.6	5.7	5.7	5.9	5.9
Inpatient Surgeries	1,975,373	1,907,604	1,857,378	1,855,847	1,934,998
Births	786,784	804,377	811,163	799,904	796,861
Utilization - Outpatient					
Emergency Outpatient Visits	25,708,579	25,605,993	25,135,121	24,700,172	23,518,323
Other Outpatient Visits	91,864,503	89,314,524	89,047,867	85,635,833	84,447,896
Total Outpatient Visits	117,573,082	114,920,517	114,182,988	110,336,005	107,966,219
Outpatient Surgeries	3,960,322	3,897,374	3,921,040	3,798,060	3,752,191
Personnel					
Full Time RNs	133,870	132,993	134,882	135,087	138,368
Full Time LPNs	23,445	23,871	23,104	24,310	25,706
Part Time RNs	86,030	84,269	89,261	87,233	87,516
Part Time LPNs	10,416	10,859	11,416	11,576	12,281
Total Full Time	617,804	612,894	601,589	607,315	618,784
Total Part Time	274,304	270,898	285,929	281,113	283,392
Revenue - Inpatient					
Gross Inpatient Revenue	$101,757,585,465	$88,826,998,928	$81,494,205,969	$73,304,767,289	$69,886,029,365
Revenue - Outpatient					
Gross Outpatient Revenue	$67,393,901,996	$59,081,658,626	$55,132,963,490	$48,727,503,116	$45,110,976,826
Revenue and Expenses - Totals **(Includes Inpatient and Outpatient)**					
Total Gross Revenue	$169,151,487,461	$147,908,657,554	$136,627,169,459	$122,032,270,405	$114,997,006,191
Deductions from Revenue	97,607,890,820	81,506,420,194	73,520,588,504	61,736,298,969	55,600,577,182
Net Patient Revenue	71,543,596,641	66,402,237,360	63,106,580,955	60,295,971,436	59,396,429,009
Other Operating Revenue	2,890,345,556	2,813,935,425	2,769,788,344	2,772,654,915	2,473,809,438
Other Nonoperating Revenue	793,439,831	1,064,678,719	1,377,282,079	1,366,384,506	1,472,900,513
Total Net Revenue	75,227,382,028	70,280,851,504	67,253,651,378	64,435,010,857	63,343,138,960
Total Expenses	71,359,095,546	66,360,396,087	63,358,364,315	60,794,792,716	59,398,078,592
HOSPITAL UNIT (Excludes Separate Nursing Home Units)					
Utilization - Inpatient					
Beds	150,384	152,541	153,990	156,820	162,427
Admissions	6,725,794	6,672,956	6,618,001	6,539,049	6,515,996
Inpatient Days	31,911,182	31,662,149	31,797,892	31,621,341	32,112,825
Average Length of Stay	4.7	4.7	4.8	4.8	4.9
Personnel					
Total Full Time	604,557	599,785	587,721	591,911	603,547
Total Part Time	266,592	263,165	277,067	272,228	274,306
Revenue and Expenses - Totals **(Includes Inpatient and Outpatient)**					
Total Net Revenue	$74,065,919,906	$69,200,831,169	$66,041,517,516	$63,158,997,513	$62,054,937,859
Total Expenses	70,382,713,681	65,492,148,426	62,568,627,003	59,804,230,111	58,459,560,010

TABLE 4

BED SIZE CATEGORY 200-299

U.S. Registered Community Hospitals
(Nonfederal, short-term general and other special hospitals)

Overview 1998–2002

	2002	2001	2000	1999	1998
Total U.S. Community Hospitals in Bed Size Category 200-299	**625**	**635**	**656**	**642**	**644**
Location					
Hospitals Urban......................	529	526	551	534	531
Hospitals Rural	96	109	105	108	113
Control					
State and Local Government	69	69	71	71	75
Not for Profit	462	467	488	480	467
Investor owned	94	99	97	91	102
Physician Models					
Independent Practice Association........	90	103	127	136	150
Group Practice without Walls	27	24	31	36	34
Open Physician-Hospital Organization....	140	143	171	178	187
Closed Physician-Hospital Organization...	45	56	61	71	78
Management Service Organization.......	86	92	118	152	156
Integrated Salary Model	159	154	167	151	147
Equity Model	11	10	20	23	18
Foundation.........................	29	34	43	49	58
Insurance Products					
Health Maintenance Organization........	105	113	151	146	153
Preferred Provider Organization........	125	123	154	160	180
Indemnity Fee for Service..............	43	41	46	42	49
Managed Care Contracts					
Health Maintenance Organization........	422	424	454	456	456
Preferred Provider Organization........	442	435	460	466	456
Affiliations					
Hospitals in a System.................	352	356	359	350	336
Hospitals in a Network	179	173	195	189	201
Hospitals in a Group Purchasing Organization.....................	462	459	461	418	357

TABLE 4 BED SIZE CATEGORY 200-299

U.S. Registered Community Hospitals
(Nonfederal, short-term general and other special hospitals)

Utilization, Personnel, Revenue and Expenses 1998–2002

	2002	2001	2000	1999	1998
TOTAL FACILITY (Includes Hospital and Nursing Home Units)					
Utilization - Inpatient					
Beds	152,682	154,420	159,807	155,831	156,978
Admissions	6,799,664	6,630,307	6,702,478	6,389,172	6,229,541
Inpatient Days	37,122,247	36,923,111	37,942,444	36,493,064	36,054,092
Average Length of Stay	5.5	5.6	5.7	5.7	5.8
Inpatient Surgeries	1,957,651	1,910,132	1,992,966	1,883,032	1,870,471
Births	753,559	733,456	788,352	755,274	719,232
Utilization - Outpatient					
Emergency Outpatient Visits	21,513,390	20,309,391	20,436,782	19,533,629	18,569,295
Other Outpatient Visits	80,910,560	79,286,800	78,811,142	71,343,993	66,924,481
Total Outpatient Visits	102,423,950	99,596,191	99,247,924	90,877,622	85,493,776
Outpatient Surgeries	3,394,622	3,265,812	3,358,516	3,163,861	3,117,508
Personnel					
Full Time RNs	141,467	136,338	137,548	132,812	132,749
Full Time LPNs	18,402	18,036	18,703	20,192	19,581
Part Time RNs	85,147	80,856	86,744	80,212	75,972
Part Time LPNs	8,442	8,752	9,181	9,349	8,931
Total Full Time	616,865	600,028	614,344	588,843	578,790
Total Part Time	260,312	247,526	265,162	249,790	238,607
Revenue - Inpatient					
Gross Inpatient Revenue	$119,690,492,836	$103,904,499,291	$92,657,723,538	$84,461,242,677	$78,694,263,284
Revenue - Outpatient					
Gross Outpatient Revenue	$64,425,216,711	$54,235,790,743	$47,912,514,899	$42,225,301,889	$38,024,413,991
Revenue and Expenses - Totals **(Includes Inpatient and Outpatient)**					
Total Gross Revenue	$184,115,709,547	$158,140,290,034	$140,570,238,437	$126,686,544,566	$116,718,677,275
Deductions from Revenue	108,902,937,426	90,371,126,069	75,560,084,371	67,487,466,289	60,181,099,208
Net Patient Revenue	75,212,772,121	67,769,163,965	65,010,154,066	59,199,078,277	56,537,578,067
Other Operating Revenue	3,204,222,444	3,278,654,426	3,511,441,863	3,261,463,827	2,942,181,355
Other Nonoperating Revenue	836,318,819	1,301,236,089	1,789,700,386	2,038,058,222	1,778,094,925
Total Net Revenue	79,253,313,384	72,349,054,480	70,311,296,315	64,498,600,326	61,257,854,347
Total Expenses	75,580,360,702	68,913,526,440	67,057,555,091	61,099,993,147	57,117,140,326
HOSPITAL UNIT (Excludes Separate Nursing Home Units)					
Utilization - Inpatient					
Beds	140,310	141,629	145,501	140,318	142,027
Admissions	6,706,901	6,530,211	6,592,395	6,261,091	6,094,572
Inpatient Days	33,216,134	32,784,136	33,230,080	31,689,032	31,359,766
Average Length of Stay	5.0	5.0	5.0	5.1	5.1
Personnel					
Total Full Time	608,134	591,000	602,872	577,378	567,747
Total Part Time	256,082	242,702	259,423	244,444	233,387
Revenue and Expenses - Totals **(Includes Inpatient and Outpatient)**					
Total Net Revenue	$78,446,952,108	$71,458,934,077	$69,473,697,175	$63,481,487,264	$60,166,099,815
Total Expenses	74,919,598,886	68,260,569,539	66,366,724,426	60,356,593,743	56,355,723,184

Bed Size Categories

TABLE 4

BED SIZE CATEGORY 300-399

U.S. Registered Community Hospitals
(Nonfederal, short-term general and other special hospitals)

Overview 1998–2002

	2002	2001	2000	1999	1998
Total U.S. Community Hospitals in Bed Size Category 300-399	358	348	341	365	352
Location					
Hospitals Urban	328	324	314	339	330
Hospitals Rural	30	24	27	26	22
Control					
State and Local Government	41	38	38	43	44
Not for Profit	270	269	255	274	262
Investor owned	47	41	48	48	46
Physician Models					
Independent Practice Association.	81	76	68	89	87
Group Practice without Walls	14	11	11	15	17
Open Physician-Hospital Organization. . . .	89	100	94	96	90
Closed Physician-Hospital Organization. . .	38	40	49	62	48
Management Service Organization.	65	72	79	93	93
Integrated Salary Model	108	96	90	103	106
Equity Model	6	9	5	13	10
Foundation	20	29	27	33	30
Insurance Products					
Health Maintenance Organization.	80	83	94	128	117
Preferred Provider Organization	88	87	96	121	124
Indemnity Fee for Service.	19	24	30	33	38
Managed Care Contracts					
Health Maintenance Organization.	257	251	237	261	239
Preferred Provider Organization	263	262	243	262	245
Affiliations					
Hospitals in a System	242	233	218	222	207
Hospitals in a Network	122	118	101	107	105
Hospitals in a Group Purchasing Organization.	270	263	235	229	206

TABLE **4**

BED SIZE CATEGORY 300-399

U.S. Registered Community Hospitals
(Nonfederal, short-term general and other special hospitals)

Utilization, Personnel, Revenue and Expenses 1998–2002

	2002	2001	2000	1999	1998
TOTAL FACILITY (Includes Hospital and Nursing Home Units)					
Utilization - Inpatient					
Beds	123,399	119,753	117,220	126,259	120,512
Admissions	5,606,593	5,328,441	5,135,313	5,419,172	5,021,409
Inpatient Days	30,625,907	28,949,110	28,175,816	30,446,266	28,467,524
Average Length of Stay	5.5	5.4	5.5	5.6	5.7
Inpatient Surgeries	1,670,246	1,575,266	1,548,365	1,633,543	1,563,495
Births	634,624	628,124	608,029	635,465	636,698
Utilization - Outpatient					
Emergency Outpatient Visits	16,337,980	15,412,370	14,679,081	14,883,092	13,300,137
Other Outpatient Visits	62,754,461	59,829,649	58,764,729	60,965,514	53,769,976
Total Outpatient Visits	79,092,441	75,242,019	73,443,810	75,848,606	67,070,113
Outpatient Surgeries	2,501,205	2,398,395	2,380,845	2,453,087	2,236,446
Personnel					
Full Time RNs	124,773	119,926	115,123	122,695	114,813
Full Time LPNs	15,634	14,521	12,961	13,849	15,245
Part Time RNs	66,826	63,220	64,123	65,952	64,009
Part Time LPNs	5,895	5,187	5,663	5,658	6,048
Total Full Time	546,123	523,968	501,162	532,328	495,732
Total Part Time	198,483	192,906	195,777	194,111	189,580
Revenue - Inpatient					
Gross Inpatient Revenue	$104,931,029,759	$90,736,055,640	$79,128,945,312	$76,331,193,232	$67,252,272,100
Revenue - Outpatient					
Gross Outpatient Revenue	$52,506,396,042	$43,966,846,914	$37,931,362,986	$36,396,156,547	$30,498,257,999
Revenue and Expenses - Totals					
(Includes Inpatient and Outpatient)					
Total Gross Revenue	$157,437,425,801	$134,702,902,554	$117,060,308,298	$112,727,349,779	$97,750,530,099
Deductions from Revenue	92,566,575,914	77,014,066,878	63,980,293,228	58,693,834,397	49,183,505,560
Net Patient Revenue	64,870,849,887	57,688,835,676	53,080,015,070	54,033,515,382	48,567,024,539
Other Operating Revenue	3,898,682,632	3,334,900,779	2,688,378,669	2,807,882,430	2,741,344,421
Other Nonoperating Revenue	518,357,079	858,386,079	1,305,643,872	1,555,611,944	1,466,462,294
Total Net Revenue	69,287,889,598	61,882,122,534	57,074,037,611	58,397,009,756	52,774,831,254
Total Expenses	66,128,522,671	59,027,238,261	54,273,518,296	55,544,241,173	49,618,989,358
HOSPITAL UNIT (Excludes Separate Nursing Home Units)					
Utilization - Inpatient					
Beds	116,100	112,537	110,180	117,501	113,215
Admissions	5,547,159	5,269,008	5,074,369	5,343,133	4,955,760
Inpatient Days	28,315,464	26,728,772	25,970,657	27,715,550	26,145,252
Average Length of Stay	5.1	5.1	5.1	5.2	5.3
Personnel					
Total Full Time	539,889	517,844	494,730	525,524	489,156
Total Part Time	195,895	190,500	193,029	190,991	186,491
Revenue and Expenses - Totals					
(Includes Inpatient and Outpatient)					
Total Net Revenue	$68,590,373,760	$61,250,007,293	$56,555,661,812	$57,738,046,612	$52,200,823,573
Total Expenses	65,561,221,517	58,607,498,709	53,867,071,704	55,030,932,464	49,147,092,391

TABLE **4**

BED SIZE CATEGORY 400-499

U.S. Registered Community Hospitals
(Nonfederal, short-term general and other special hospitals)

Overview 1998–2002

	2002	2001	2000	1999	1998
Total U.S. Community Hospitals in Bed Size Category 400-499	174	191	182	161	183
Location					
Hospitals Urban.	170	186	178	157	177
Hospitals Rural	4	5	4	4	6
Control					
State and Local Government	27	27	25	19	18
Not for Profit	139	153	147	132	152
Investor owned	8	11	10	10	13
Physician Models					
Independent Practice Association.	34	38	41	45	58
Group Practice without Walls	6	5	9	11	12
Open Physician-Hospital Organization. . . .	37	36	41	38	46
Closed Physician-Hospital Organization. . .	19	20	22	24	32
Management Service Organization.	34	37	41	42	53
Integrated Salary Model	63	59	61	53	49
Equity Model	5	3	5	5	8
Foundation	17	17	13	17	25
Insurance Products					
Health Maintenance Organization.	54	60	69	70	88
Preferred Provider Organization	54	53	63	55	74
Indemnity Fee for Service.	17	11	16	11	19
Managed Care Contracts					
Health Maintenance Organization.	131	137	138	121	143
Preferred Provider Organization	135	143	139	125	144
Affiliations					
Hospitals in a System	110	122	118	104	119
Hospitals in a Network	52	66	62	52	71
Hospitals in a Group Purchasing Organization.	127	141	131	107	115

TABLE 4

BED SIZE CATEGORY 400-499

U.S. Registered Community Hospitals
(Nonfederal, short-term general and other special hospitals)

Utilization, Personnel, Revenue and Expenses 1998–2002

	2002	2001	2000	1999	1998
TOTAL FACILITY (Includes Hospital and Nursing Home Units)					
Utilization - Inpatient					
Beds	77,145	84,745	80,763	71,580	81,247
Admissions	3,592,594	3,778,746	3,616,530	3,045,448	3,390,232
Inpatient Days	19,862,987	21,312,743	20,509,972	17,853,905	19,958,559
Average Length of Stay	5.5	5.6	5.7	5.9	5.9
Inpatient Surgeries	1,126,781	1,143,813	1,102,058	904,289	1,119,239
Births	435,738	462,372	439,821	357,548	402,499
Utilization - Outpatient					
Emergency Outpatient Visits	9,056,989	9,345,972	9,488,926	7,263,184	7,730,076
Other Outpatient Visits	48,784,217	50,233,673	42,716,283	36,604,300	41,292,412
Total Outpatient Visits	57,841,206	59,579,645	52,205,209	43,867,484	49,022,488
Outpatient Surgeries	1,593,516	1,642,696	1,578,111	1,366,726	1,453,863
Personnel					
Full Time RNs	84,885	87,244	82,895	72,380	79,795
Full Time LPNs	8,147	9,335	8,237	8,563	10,051
Part Time RNs	48,158	50,157	49,484	35,968	42,276
Part Time LPNs	3,431	3,334	3,052	3,315	4,452
Total Full Time	384,050	398,066	367,265	320,457	364,877
Total Part Time	134,897	140,706	139,517	106,306	127,806
Revenue - Inpatient					
Gross Inpatient Revenue	$76,255,983,382	$70,893,560,813	$59,609,190,161	$47,414,569,510	$50,002,475,994
Revenue - Outpatient					
Gross Outpatient Revenue	$36,410,066,420	$32,818,521,002	$28,221,840,088	$20,680,259,396	$21,386,610,279
Revenue and Expenses - Totals					
(Includes Inpatient and Outpatient)					
Total Gross Revenue	$112,666,049,802	$103,712,081,815	$87,831,030,249	$68,094,828,906	$71,389,086,273
Deductions from Revenue	66,486,965,120	58,861,160,338	48,605,733,601	36,254,726,963	36,658,972,721
Net Patient Revenue	46,179,084,682	44,850,921,477	39,225,296,648	31,840,101,943	34,730,113,552
Other Operating Revenue	3,352,108,431	3,212,320,490	2,780,992,924	2,533,086,920	2,511,192,215
Other Nonoperating Revenue	335,957,588	906,755,338	1,176,559,766	923,857,533	1,223,480,642
Total Net Revenue	49,867,150,701	48,969,997,305	43,182,849,338	35,297,046,396	38,464,786,409
Total Expenses	47,419,293,980	47,321,475,681	41,299,819,174	33,866,308,713	36,442,105,640
HOSPITAL UNIT (Excludes Separate Nursing Home Units)					
Utilization - Inpatient					
Beds	73,121	79,957	76,238	65,996	75,110
Admissions	3,561,076	3,739,662	3,573,245	2,995,719	3,341,213
Inpatient Days	18,643,835	19,847,882	19,084,886	16,114,892	18,132,991
Average Length of Stay	5.2	5.3	5.3	5.4	5.4
Personnel					
Total Full Time	381,097	394,265	362,720	316,695	358,783
Total Part Time	133,611	139,265	137,566	104,747	125,398
Revenue and Expenses - Totals					
(Includes Inpatient and Outpatient)					
Total Net Revenue	$49,559,582,082	$48,644,983,381	$42,890,966,938	$34,714,064,245	$38,014,252,666
Total Expenses	47,151,005,398	46,998,302,690	41,054,265,159	33,528,138,196	36,064,400,098

Bed Size Categories

Table 4

BED SIZE CATEGORY 500 +

U.S. Registered Community Hospitals
(Nonfederal, short-term general and other special hospitals)

Overview 1998–2002

	2002	2001	2000	1999	1998
Total U.S. Community Hospitals in Bed Size Category 500 + ...	256	249	247	254	254
Location					
Hospitals Urban......................	253	245	244	251	251
Hospitals Rural	3	4	3	3	3
Control					
State and Local Government	36	37	36	40	42
Not for Profit	204	195	197	201	198
Investor owned	16	17	14	13	14
Physician Models					
Independent Practice Association........	66	68	76	85	85
Group Practice without Walls	23	23	26	24	25
Open Physician-Hospital Organization....	64	70	69	75	79
Closed Physician-Hospital Organization...	25	31	42	48	53
Management Service Organization.......	64	64	80	77	80
Integrated Salary Model	115	103	105	101	103
Equity Model	11	10	13	13	17
Foundation..........................	27	25	27	31	35
Insurance Products					
Health Maintenance Organization........	88	86	116	128	138
Preferred Provider Organization.........	85	85	105	115	122
Indemnity Fee for Service.............	19	22	26	24	34
Managed Care Contracts					
Health Maintenance Organization........	195	195	205	205	197
Preferred Provider Organization.........	194	195	202	200	193
Affiliations					
Hospitals in a System.................	183	186	184	187	176
Hospitals in a Network	99	94	97	103	104
Hospitals in a Group Purchasing Organization......................	191	192	180	173	159

Bed Size Categories

TABLE **4**

BED SIZE CATEGORY 500 +

U.S. Registered Community Hospitals
(Nonfederal, short-term general and other special hospitals)

Utilization, Personnel, Revenue and Expenses 1998–2002

	2002	2001	2000	1999	1998
TOTAL FACILITY (Includes Hospital and Nursing Home Units)					
Utilization - Inpatient					
Beds	180,091	177,873	175,638	178,411	178,237
Admissions	7,957,792	7,705,773	7,410,167	7,399,867	7,145,981
Inpatient Days	48,655,624	47,225,469	46,339,384	46,713,100	46,111,523
Average Length of Stay...........	6.1	6.1	6.3	6.3	6.5
Inpatient Surgeries..............	2,513,381	2,425,140	2,419,740	2,474,024	2,357,616
Births........................	896,281	885,391	868,382	849,861	811,890
Utilization - Outpatient					
Emergency Outpatient Visits.......	18,760,101	18,048,334	16,863,866	17,080,213	16,206,443
Other Outpatient Visits...........	91,715,041	87,265,908	84,513,677	82,660,658	79,301,140
Total Outpatient Visits	110,475,142	105,314,242	101,377,543	99,740,871	95,507,583
Outpatient Surgeries	3,475,621	3,126,279	2,908,913	2,949,786	2,863,384
Personnel					
Full Time RNs	208,213	199,358	199,560	202,263	192,852
Full Time LPNs	16,087	16,947	17,233	18,029	17,604
Part Time RNs..................	97,416	90,746	87,424	82,232	77,369
Part Time LPNs	5,349	5,766	5,421	5,260	5,540
Total Full Time..................	926,875	909,166	879,297	884,284	873,961
Total Part Time	281,159	262,239	253,897	243,838	232,383
Revenue - Inpatient					
Gross Inpatient Revenue..........	$181,311,610,111	$156,462,924,653	$138,130,198,562	$126,828,183,226	$114,805,458,621
Revenue - Outpatient					
Gross Outpatient Revenue	$76,542,000,025	$65,226,823,758	$54,990,410,746	$49,682,171,548	$42,624,184,029
Revenue and Expenses - Totals					
(Includes Inpatient and Outpatient)					
Total Gross Revenue.............	$257,853,610,136	$221,689,748,411	$193,120,609,308	$176,470,354,774	$157,429,642,650
Deductions from Revenue.........	148,361,338,060	123,213,421,530	103,806,905,095	90,993,158,498	76,161,795,283
Net Patient Revenue	109,492,272,076	98,476,326,881	89,313,704,213	85,477,196,276	81,267,847,367
Other Operating Revenue	9,462,930,418	8,858,554,851	7,873,591,839	7,574,557,742	6,772,432,158
Other Nonoperating Revenue	425,909,567	1,292,497,612	2,991,999,020	2,570,772,014	2,618,731,433
Total Net Revenue...............	119,381,112,061	108,627,379,344	100,179,295,072	95,622,526,032	90,659,010,958
Total Expenses.................	115,131,748,332	105,085,709,086	96,310,798,929	91,982,247,309	86,017,901,252
HOSPITAL UNIT (Excludes Separate Nursing Home Units)					
Utilization - Inpatient					
Beds	168,562	166,158	161,458	164,759	163,360
Admissions	7,906,285	7,649,107	7,337,658	7,308,606	7,046,008
Inpatient Days	44,958,154	43,383,615	41,856,131	42,322,343	41,342,830
Average Length of Stay...........	5.7	5.7	5.7	5.8	5.9
Personnel					
Total Full Time..................	918,115	898,569	867,283	872,217	862,751
Total Part Time	278,360	258,769	250,140	240,125	229,157
Revenue and Expenses - Totals					
(Includes Inpatient and Outpatient)					
Total Net Revenue...............	$118,439,588,288	$107,658,500,091	$98,564,608,494	$94,608,758,058	$89,464,648,691
Total Expenses.................	114,087,149,972	104,203,128,358	95,410,392,185	91,062,292,669	84,930,446,901

Census Divisions

Census Division 1

New England
Connecticut, Maine, Massachusetts, New Hampshire, Rhode Island, Vermont

Census Division 2

Middle Atlantic
New Jersey, New York, Pennsylvania

Census Division 3

South Atlantic
Delaware, District of Columbia, Florida, Georgia, Maryland, North Carolina, South Carolina, Virginia, West Virginia

Census Division 4

East North Central
Illinois, Indiana, Michigan, Ohio, Wisconsin

Census Division 5

East South Central
Alabama, Kentucky, Mississippi, Tennessee

Census Division 6

West North Central
Iowa, Kansas, Minnesota, Missouri, Nebraska, North Dakota, South Dakota

Census Division 7

West South Central
Arkansas, Louisiana, Oklahoma, Texas

Census Division 8

Mountain
Arizona, Colorado, Idaho, Montana, Nevada, New Mexico, Utah, Wyoming

Census Division 9

Pacific
Alaska, California, Hawaii, Oregon, Washington

U.S. Census Divisions

TABLE **5**

U.S. CENSUS DIVISION 1: NEW ENGLAND

U.S. Registered Community Hospitals
(Nonfederal, short-term general and other special hospitals)

Overview 1998–2002

	2002	2001	2000	1999	1998
Total U.S. Community Hospitals in Census Division 1, New England	203	205	205	204	207
Bed Size Category					
6-24	8	3	4	5	5
25-49	32	39	38	35	36
50-99	46	44	44	46	50
100-199	58	60	61	62	62
200-299	30	28	26	25	28
300-399	15	16	17	16	11
400-499	1	2	2	2	3
500 + ...	13	13	13	13	12
Location					
Hospitals Urban.	126	128	128	127	130
Hospitals Rural	77	77	77	77	77
Control					
State and Local Government	7	8	8	9	9
Not for Profit	185	186	185	184	187
Investor owned	11	11	12	11	11
Physician Models					
Independent Practice Association	58	57	52	61	57
Group Practice without Walls.	16	18	15	18	18
Open Physician-Hospital Organization	66	71	71	78	76
Closed Physician-Hospital Organization	18	20	21	21	22
Management Service Organization	33	36	36	48	47
Integrated Salary Model	73	71	67	71	64
Equity Model	6	4	4	4	5
Foundation.	13	15	13	18	19
Insurance Products					
Health Maintenance Organization	23	28	31	37	49
Preferred Provider Organization.	22	19	18	22	37
Indemnity Fee for Service	5	5	5	5	11
Managed Care Contracts					
Health Maintenance Organization	156	163	161	169	170
Preferred Provider Organization.	143	149	148	151	153
Affiliations					
Hospitals in a System.	110	107	99	109	96
Hospitals in a Network	60	61	66	60	53
Hospitals in a Group Purchasing Organization. .	161	164	155	153	144

U.S. Census Divisions

TABLE 5

U.S. CENSUS DIVISION 1: NEW ENGLAND

U.S. Registered Community Hospitals
(Nonfederal, short-term general and other special hospitals)

Utilization, Personnel, Revenue and Expenses, Community Health Indicators 1998–2002

	2002	2001	2000	1999	1998
TOTAL FACILITY (Includes Hospital and Nursing Home Units)					
Utilization - Inpatient					
Beds	34,324	35,385	34,944	34,915	34,303
Admissions	1,580,396	1,567,000	1,519,012	1,500,667	1,488,810
Inpatient Days	9,120,976	9,144,828	8,917,327	8,771,404	8,500,264
Average Length of Stay	5.8	5.8	5.9	5.8	5.7
Inpatient Surgeries	459,541	444,897	448,066	447,135	448,843
Births	168,792	169,198	170,638	169,142	167,926
Utilization - Outpatient					
Emergency Outpatient Visits	6,233,520	5,973,441	5,916,202	5,784,739	5,371,671
Other Outpatient Visits	29,869,397	29,179,090	26,862,517	25,245,873	24,883,550
Total Outpatient Visits	36,102,917	35,152,531	32,778,719	31,030,612	30,255,221
Outpatient Surgeries	1,004,499	987,409	956,844	903,825	868,615
Personnel					
Full Time RNs	33,504	34,016	32,203	30,186	29,955
Full Time LPNs	2,408	2,390	2,391	2,078	2,302
Part Time RNs	33,457	33,183	33,845	33,145	32,958
Part Time LPNs	2,160	2,219	2,321	2,272	2,352
Total Full Time	186,629	186,757	173,630	165,298	164,720
Total Part Time	105,969	105,157	107,014	105,196	103,830
Revenue - Inpatient					
Gross Inpatient Revenue	$25,243,211,994	$23,006,462,654	$21,145,777,686	$19,052,712,630	$17,981,275,871
Revenue - Outpatient					
Gross Outpatient Revenue	$20,277,289,066	$17,354,624,925	$15,014,223,925	$13,647,875,340	$12,012,290,460
Revenue and Expenses - Totals					
(Includes Inpatient and Outpatient)					
Total Gross Revenue	$45,520,501,060	$40,361,087,579	$36,160,001,611	$32,700,587,970	$29,993,566,331
Deductions from Revenue	22,938,130,804	19,755,206,105	17,289,206,287	15,008,365,053	12,978,565,939
Net Patient Revenue	22,582,370,256	20,605,881,474	18,870,795,324	17,692,222,917	17,015,000,392
Other Operating Revenue	2,275,478,442	2,061,229,915	1,644,812,612	1,737,545,613	1,802,476,446
Other Nonoperating Revenue	69,173,336	256,835,969	706,498,132	665,388,606	654,758,408
Total Net Revenue	24,927,022,034	22,923,947,358	21,222,106,068	20,095,157,136	19,472,235,246
Total Expenses	24,762,701,274	22,650,945,919	20,923,125,622	19,745,944,243	19,006,482,876
HOSPITAL UNIT (Excludes Separate Nursing Home Units)					
Utilization - Inpatient					
Beds	32,069	32,730	32,263	32,117	32,505
Admissions	1,563,633	1,550,961	1,498,475	1,477,023	1,473,480
Inpatient Days	8,350,064	8,190,799	8,007,120	7,885,831	7,942,077
Average Length of Stay	5.3	5.3	5.3	5.3	5.4
Personnel					
Total Full Time	185,430	184,640	171,537	163,198	163,025
Total Part Time	104,927	103,487	105,170	103,333	102,503
Revenue and Expenses - Totals					
(Includes Inpatient and Outpatient)					
Total Net Revenue	$24,763,704,581	$22,729,636,795	$21,051,443,144	$19,894,763,328	$19,279,686,014
Total Expenses	24,599,025,809	22,469,904,390	20,769,362,219	19,578,964,509	18,859,372,118
COMMUNITY HEALTH INDICATORS PER 1000 POPULATION					
Total Population (in thousands)	14,144	14,022	13,923	13,496	13,429
Inpatient					
Beds	2.4	2.5	2.5	2.6	2.6
Admissions	111.7	111.8	109.1	111.2	110.9
Inpatient Days	644.9	652.2	640.5	649.9	633.0
Inpatient Surgeries	32.5	31.7	32.2	33.1	33.4
Births	11.9	12.1	12.3	12.5	12.5
Outpatient					
Emergency Outpatient Visits	440.7	426.0	424.9	428.6	400.0
Other Outpatient Visits	2,111.8	2,080.9	1,929.4	1,870.6	1,853.0
Total Outpatient Visits	2,552.5	2,506.9	2,354.4	2,299.3	2,253.0
Outpatient Surgeries	71.0	70.4	68.7	67.0	64.7
Expense per Capita (per person)	$1,750.7	$1,615.4	$1,502.8	$1,463.1	$1,415.4

TABLE 5

U.S. CENSUS DIVISION 2: MIDDLE ATLANTIC

U.S. Registered Community Hospitals
(Nonfederal, short-term general and other special hospitals)

Overview 1998–2002

	2002	2001	2000	1999	1998
Total U.S. Community Hospitals in Census					
Division 2, Middle Atlantic	493	495	502	509	517
Bed Size Category					
6-24	8	7	8	7	7
25-49	21	22	20	25	23
50-99	64	61	64	59	60
100-199	148	145	152	151	158
200-299	103	111	112	116	110
300-399	55	52	47	52	55
400-499	40	42	46	41	44
500 + ...	54	55	53	58	60
Location					
Hospitals Urban..........................	412	415	423	428	436
Hospitals Rural	81	80	79	81	81
Control					
State and Local Government...............	30	29	28	28	28
Not for Profit	441	444	453	461	470
Investor owned	22	22	21	20	19
Physician Models					
Independent Practice Association	99	98	120	126	136
Group Practice without Walls...............	21	20	26	20	22
Open Physician-Hospital Organization	76	81	104	101	120
Closed Physician-Hospital Organization	26	25	33	44	48
Management Service Organization	64	72	89	96	100
Integrated Salary Model....................	118	99	112	93	100
Equity Model.............................	9	6	14	13	11
Foundation...............................	11	9	14	17	28
Insurance Products					
Health Maintenance Organization	82	70	97	101	125
Preferred Provider Organization..............	79	79	98	97	123
Indemnity Fee for Service	17	17	15	15	21
Managed Care Contracts					
Health Maintenance Organization	317	330	351	351	354
Preferred Provider Organization..............	300	315	332	321	316
Affiliations					
Hospitals in a System.....................	235	236	248	220	224
Hospitals in a Network....................	152	148	155	146	160
Hospitals in a Group Purchasing Organization..	350	350	334	289	287

TABLE 5

U.S. CENSUS DIVISION 2: MIDDLE ATLANTIC

U.S. Registered Community Hospitals
(Nonfederal, short-term general and other special hospitals)

Utilization, Personnel, Revenue and Expenses, Community Health Indicators 1998–2002

	2002	2001	2000	1999	1998
TOTAL FACILITY (Includes Hospital and Nursing Home Units)					
Utilization - Inpatient					
Beds	130,198	134,007	134,044	136,493	139,603
Admissions	5,356,471	5,303,235	5,285,812	5,230,020	5,199,574
Inpatient Days	34,925,191	35,582,339	35,972,872	36,152,830	36,893,769
Average Length of Stay	6.5	6.7	6.8	6.9	7.1
Inpatient Surgeries	1,540,104	1,530,873	1,570,780	1,573,521	1,615,322
Births	503,700	502,368	504,630	506,591	497,211
Utilization - Outpatient					
Emergency Outpatient Visits	15,474,182	15,262,789	14,855,507	14,638,689	14,081,408
Other Outpatient Visits	79,593,390	80,890,968	79,672,796	76,499,179	75,468,918
Total Outpatient Visits	95,067,572	96,153,757	94,528,303	91,137,868	89,550,326
Outpatient Surgeries	2,779,831	2,688,679	2,673,923	2,560,005	2,597,905
Personnel					
Full Time RNs	124,834	125,764	125,727	124,392	123,604
Full Time LPNs	14,200	14,431	14,326	14,634	14,860
Part Time RNs	58,048	55,226	57,785	56,507	56,071
Part Time LPNs	5,567	5,408	5,704	5,939	6,170
Total Full Time	591,456	587,752	580,514	578,915	579,154
Total Part Time	182,720	179,456	182,798	179,758	178,219
Revenue - Inpatient					
Gross Inpatient Revenue	$114,499,007,759	$102,755,097,357	$88,555,896,320	$79,559,155,616	$75,599,548,059
Revenue - Outpatient					
Gross Outpatient Revenue	$53,178,962,709	$45,742,770,658	$39,791,596,044	$35,350,638,604	$32,012,687,719
Revenue and Expenses - Totals					
(Includes Inpatient and Outpatient)					
Total Gross Revenue	$167,677,970,468	$148,497,868,015	$128,347,492,364	$114,909,794,220	$107,612,235,778
Deductions from Revenue	101,832,776,300	87,693,668,174	71,418,197,617	61,003,893,361	54,696,994,230
Net Patient Revenue	65,845,194,168	60,804,199,841	56,929,294,747	53,905,900,859	52,915,241,548
Other Operating Revenue	4,945,663,508	4,858,174,712	4,373,128,371	4,158,957,000	3,768,576,982
Other Nonoperating Revenue	473,985,594	879,603,162	1,200,687,387	1,229,111,646	1,553,981,165
Total Net Revenue	71,264,843,270	66,541,977,715	62,503,110,505	59,293,969,505	58,237,799,695
Total Expenses	70,060,852,900	65,738,326,638	61,666,014,763	58,864,243,581	57,242,223,412
HOSPITAL UNIT (Excludes Separate Nursing Home Units)					
Utilization - Inpatient					
Beds	118,462	122,977	121,947	123,387	126,707
Admissions	5,305,173	5,251,290	5,228,518	5,165,103	5,140,274
Inpatient Days	30,977,155	31,838,056	31,790,693	31,784,098	32,589,512
Average Length of Stay	5.8	6.1	6.1	6.2	6.3
Personnel					
Total Full Time	582,279	579,127	569,721	570,193	570,505
Total Part Time	178,921	175,863	178,618	176,154	174,551
Revenue and Expenses - Totals					
(Includes Inpatient and Outpatient)					
Total Net Revenue	$70,357,276,445	$65,632,075,736	$61,678,553,426	$58,381,802,745	$57,275,786,421
Total Expenses	69,170,940,306	65,050,830,005	61,035,255,854	58,149,232,081	56,519,715,726
COMMUNITY HEALTH INDICATORS PER 1000 POPULATION					
Total Population (in thousands)	40,083	39,783	39,672	38,334	38,257
Inpatient					
Beds	3.2	3.4	3.4	3.6	3.6
Admissions	133.6	133.3	133.2	136.4	135.9
Inpatient Days	871.3	894.4	906.8	943.1	964.4
Inpatient Surgeries	38.4	38.5	39.6	41.0	42.2
Births	12.6	12.6	12.7	13.2	13.0
Outpatient					
Emergency Outpatient Visits	386.1	383.7	374.5	381.9	368.1
Other Outpatient Visits	1,985.7	2,033.3	2,008.3	1,995.6	1,972.7
Total Outpatient Visits	2,371.8	2,417.0	2,382.8	2,377.5	2,340.8
Outpatient Surgeries	69.4	67.6	67.4	66.8	67.9
Expense per Capita (per person)	$1,747.9	$1,652.4	$1,554.4	$1,535.6	$1,496.3

TABLE 5

U.S. CENSUS DIVISION 3: SOUTH ATLANTIC

U.S. Registered Community Hospitals
(Nonfederal, short-term general and other special hospitals)

Overview 1998–2002

	2002	2001	2000	1999	1998
Total U.S. Community Hospitals in Census Division 3, South Atlantic	**731**	**730**	**739**	**749**	**761**
Bed Size Category					
6-24	21	14	17	15	19
25-49	97	101	104	100	98
50-99	135	134	128	131	130
100-199	200	201	212	225	232
200-299	116	121	122	119	125
300-399	73	66	66	76	70
400-499	30	34	35	29	33
500 + ...	59	59	55	54	54
Location					
Hospitals Urban.........................	442	442	449	456	466
Hospitals Rural	289	288	290	293	295
Control					
State and Local Government................	138	142	145	152	154
Not for Profit	407	398	400	404	407
Investor owned	186	190	194	193	200
Physician Models					
Independent Practice Association	54	69	82	90	99
Group Practice without Walls...............	11	16	23	25	35
Open Physician-Hospital Organization	119	127	136	149	162
Closed Physician-Hospital Organization	39	47	59	68	85
Management Service Organization	64	73	95	114	136
Integrated Salary Model....................	175	158	162	157	139
Equity Model	15	9	20	23	23
Foundation..............................	20	17	18	27	35
Insurance Products					
Health Maintenance Organization	85	97	122	145	144
Preferred Provider Organization..............	136	137	158	193	212
Indemnity Fee for Service	39	37	48	47	56
Managed Care Contracts					
Health Maintenance Organization	391	385	407	412	419
Preferred Provider Organization..............	475	462	476	492	507
Affiliations					
Hospitals in a System.....................	353	361	363	368	336
Hospitals in a Network....................	228	228	224	235	243
Hospitals in a Group Purchasing Organization..	471	460	447	438	393

Table 5

U.S. CENSUS DIVISION 3: SOUTH ATLANTIC

U.S. Registered Community Hospitals
(Nonfederal, short-term general and other special hospitals)

Utilization, Personnel, Revenue and Expenses, Community Health Indicators 1998–2002

	2002	2001	2000	1999	1998
TOTAL FACILITY (Includes Hospital and Nursing Home Units)					
Utilization - Inpatient					
Beds	152,236	152,052	150,851	151,812	153,488
Admissions	6,587,288	6,453,744	6,262,051	6,069,521	5,921,407
Inpatient Days	37,509,493	36,338,028	35,935,189	35,729,929	35,386,749
Average Length of Stay	5.7	5.6	5.7	5.9	6.0
Inpatient Surgeries	2,024,048	1,975,208	1,890,490	1,838,331	1,839,043
Births	695,805	694,845	682,848	644,602	640,494
Utilization - Outpatient					
Emergency Outpatient Visits	21,281,267	20,100,193	19,803,910	18,439,689	17,836,356
Other Outpatient Visits	61,195,587	58,426,774	56,939,217	52,499,260	49,944,907
Total Outpatient Visits	82,476,854	78,526,967	76,743,127	70,938,949	67,781,263
Outpatient Surgeries	3,403,716	3,193,345	3,038,185	2,975,263	2,848,232
Personnel					
Full Time RNs	154,257	149,286	148,599	145,609	144,810
Full Time LPNs	19,491	19,553	19,172	20,456	19,985
Part Time RNs	68,654	66,294	66,561	58,528	55,727
Part Time LPNs	6,084	5,903	6,265	6,674	6,521
Total Full Time	646,894	632,576	616,500	600,721	601,954
Total Part Time	196,385	189,909	197,464	180,821	173,116
Revenue - Inpatient					
Gross Inpatient Revenue	$109,659,179,223	$94,782,493,433	$86,421,077,582	$77,252,538,734	$72,017,626,254
Revenue - Outpatient					
Gross Outpatient Revenue	$59,025,023,880	$49,302,316,636	$44,278,693,852	$38,501,572,608	$34,478,992,937
Revenue and Expenses - Totals					
(Includes Inpatient and Outpatient)					
Total Gross Revenue	$168,684,203,103	$144,084,810,069	$130,699,771,434	$115,754,111,342	$106,496,619,191
Deductions from Revenue	95,540,558,726	77,834,582,485	69,108,825,847	58,573,353,779	51,565,031,185
Net Patient Revenue	73,143,644,377	66,250,227,584	61,590,945,587	57,180,757,563	54,931,588,006
Other Operating Revenue	3,729,711,113	3,560,755,143	3,203,398,523	3,141,920,126	2,740,968,270
Other Nonoperating Revenue	271,679,355	1,030,898,593	1,593,464,950	1,555,718,488	1,534,174,491
Total Net Revenue	77,145,034,845	70,841,881,320	66,387,809,060	61,878,396,177	59,206,730,767
Total Expenses	73,497,910,915	66,532,756,720	62,074,155,739	57,070,729,065	54,248,588,217
HOSPITAL UNIT (Excludes Separate Nursing Home Units)					
Utilization - Inpatient					
Beds	139,408	139,864	137,102	137,364	139,020
Admissions	6,530,617	6,395,710	6,192,854	5,997,119	5,847,237
Inpatient Days	33,321,870	32,356,811	31,455,354	30,973,296	30,748,971
Average Length of Stay	5.1	5.1	5.1	5.2	5.3
Personnel					
Total Full Time	636,583	622,774	605,040	589,107	590,779
Total Part Time	192,884	186,585	193,201	176,916	169,483
Revenue and Expenses - Totals					
(Includes Inpatient and Outpatient)					
Total Net Revenue	$76,360,437,261	$70,107,007,948	$64,887,088,976	$61,054,258,380	$58,320,553,086
Total Expenses	72,794,408,670	65,904,113,552	61,442,541,205	56,365,852,982	53,515,276,584
COMMUNITY HEALTH INDICATORS PER 1000 POPULATION					
Total Population (in thousands)	53,633	52,763	51,769	49,560	48,927
Inpatient					
Beds	2.8	2.9	2.9	3.1	3.1
Admissions	122.8	122.3	121.0	122.5	121.0
Inpatient Days	699.4	688.7	694.1	720.9	723.3
Inpatient Surgeries	37.7	37.4	36.5	37.1	37.6
Births	13.0	13.2	13.2	13.0	13.1
Outpatient					
Emergency Outpatient Visits	396.8	381.0	382.5	372.1	364.6
Other Outpatient Visits	1,141.0	1,107.4	1,099.9	1,059.3	1,020.8
Total Outpatient Visits	1,537.8	1,488.3	1,482.4	1,431.4	1,385.4
Outpatient Surgeries	63.5	60.5	58.7	60.0	58.2
Expense per Capita (per person)	$1,370.4	$1,261.0	$1,199.1	$1,151.5	$1,108.8

U.S. Census Divisions

TABLE 5

U.S. CENSUS DIVISION 4: EAST NORTH CENTRAL

U.S. Registered Community Hospitals
(Nonfederal, short-term general and other special hospitals)

Overview 1998–2002

	2002	2001	2000	1999	1998
Total U.S. Community Hospitals in Census Division 4, East North Central	737	734	732	744	760
Bed Size Category					
6-24	28	22	22	27	25
25-49	121	114	108	107	106
50-99	173	178	171	180	181
100-199	189	193	200	200	205
200-299	101	100	104	103	110
300-399	59	58	56	54	57
400-499	26	30	29	30	34
500 + ...	40	39	42	43	42
Location					
Hospitals Urban.	444	440	443	448	465
Hospitals Rural	293	294	289	296	295
Control					
State and Local Government.	113	114	112	119	122
Not for Profit	592	592	591	596	600
Investor owned	32	28	29	29	38
Physician Models					
Independent Practice Association	102	108	111	110	125
Group Practice without Walls.	43	47	41	36	37
Open Physician-Hospital Organization	189	195	206	203	214
Closed Physician-Hospital Organization	72	74	82	88	89
Management Service Organization	106	120	136	141	153
Integrated Salary Model.	235	229	244	247	233
Equity Model	12	16	18	18	18
Foundation.	33	38	41	43	55
Insurance Products					
Health Maintenance Organization	142	154	179	199	212
Preferred Provider Organization.	164	165	207	225	238
Indemnity Fee for Service	43	46	62	58	63
Managed Care Contracts					
Health Maintenance Organization	503	515	530	545	557
Preferred Provider Organization.	554	565	575	602	604
Affiliations					
Hospitals in a System.	353	362	355	361	353
Hospitals in a Network	223	225	218	211	219
Hospitals in a Group Purchasing Organization. .	592	593	593	550	463

U.S. Census Divisions

TABLE 5

U.S. CENSUS DIVISION 4: EAST NORTH CENTRAL

U.S. Registered Community Hospitals
(Nonfederal, short-term general and other special hospitals)

Utilization, Personnel, Revenue and Expenses, Community Health Indicators 1998–2002

	2002	2001	2000	1999	1998
TOTAL FACILITY (Includes Hospital and Nursing Home Units)					
Utilization - Inpatient					
Beds	129,716	130,407	131,722	133,061	137,667
Admissions	5,549,822	5,418,071	5,299,180	5,188,356	5,184,548
Inpatient Days	29,754,022	29,208,239	29,197,099	29,318,858	29,828,809
Average Length of Stay	5.4	5.4	5.5	5.7	5.8
Inpatient Surgeries	1,588,289	1,532,612	1,536,652	1,471,103	1,507,364
Births	594,899	600,441	607,172	593,698	597,087
Utilization - Outpatient					
Emergency Outpatient Visits	18,125,078	17,712,357	17,307,818	16,699,402	16,553,952
Other Outpatient Visits	88,307,662	87,341,487	84,498,586	78,099,894	75,159,642
Total Outpatient Visits	106,432,740	105,053,844	101,806,404	94,799,296	91,713,594
Outpatient Surgeries	3,101,230	2,952,188	2,876,537	2,818,860	2,772,289
Personnel					
Full Time RNs	120,224	118,745	120,794	121,346	121,550
Full Time LPNs	12,113	12,747	12,183	12,823	13,436
Part Time RNs	91,896	88,913	86,191	81,180	82,308
Part Time LPNs	7,846	8,117	7,573	7,764	8,116
Total Full Time	573,239	568,559	560,718	554,898	562,730
Total Part Time	288,607	277,406	267,821	258,605	260,915
Revenue - Inpatient					
Gross Inpatient Revenue	$87,407,038,737	$77,251,473,672	$69,620,488,497	$63,685,574,779	$61,824,762,835
Revenue - Outpatient					
Gross Outpatient Revenue	$59,494,801,802	$51,950,625,736	$45,806,914,434	$40,204,948,871	$36,725,357,346
Revenue and Expenses - Totals (Includes Inpatient and Outpatient)					
Total Gross Revenue	$146,901,840,539	$129,202,099,408	$115,427,402,931	$103,890,523,650	$98,550,120,181
Deductions from Revenue	77,136,739,719	65,676,992,538	56,498,399,187	48,691,629,504	44,146,428,562
Net Patient Revenue	69,765,100,820	63,525,106,870	58,929,003,744	55,198,894,146	54,403,691,619
Other Operating Revenue	3,815,440,330	3,607,534,822	3,175,250,858	3,010,491,498	3,056,945,596
Other Nonoperating Revenue	293,313,105	917,722,672	2,618,184,368	2,339,165,296	2,184,116,633
Total Net Revenue	73,873,854,255	68,050,364,364	64,722,438,970	60,548,550,940	59,644,753,848
Total Expenses	71,241,901,629	65,691,365,693	60,750,436,230	57,553,715,808	55,835,095,439
HOSPITAL UNIT (Excludes Separate Nursing Home Units)					
Utilization - Inpatient					
Beds	120,239	119,618	119,146	119,021	124,140
Admissions	5,486,852	5,346,426	5,218,146	5,091,228	5,093,302
Inpatient Days	26,833,806	25,943,340	25,392,256	25,194,957	25,619,752
Average Length of Stay	4.9	4.9	4.9	4.9	5.0
Personnel					
Total Full Time	567,494	561,829	551,564	545,069	552,820
Total Part Time	284,867	273,564	262,824	253,308	255,483
Revenue and Expenses - Totals (Includes Inpatient and Outpatient)					
Total Net Revenue	$73,267,139,602	$67,427,818,977	$64,122,423,465	$59,695,796,166	$58,792,191,305
Total Expenses	70,722,664,220	65,195,547,192	60,219,162,173	56,849,086,779	55,104,048,550
COMMUNITY HEALTH INDICATORS PER 1000 POPULATION					
Total Population (in thousands)	45,673	45,363	45,155	44,442	44,257
Inpatient					
Beds	2.8	2.9	2.9	3.0	3.1
Admissions	121.5	119.4	117.4	116.7	117.1
Inpatient Days	651.5	643.9	646.6	659.7	674.0
Inpatient Surgeries	34.8	33.8	34.0	33.1	34.1
Births	13.0	13.2	13.4	13.4	13.5
Outpatient					
Emergency Outpatient Visits	396.8	390.5	383.3	375.8	374.0
Other Outpatient Visits	1,933.5	1,925.4	1,871.3	1,757.3	1,698.2
Total Outpatient Visits	2,330.3	2,315.8	2,254.6	2,133.1	2,072.3
Outpatient Surgeries	67.9	65.1	63.7	63.4	62.6
Expense per Capita (per person)	$1,559.8	$1,448.1	$1,345.4	$1,295.0	$1,261.6

U.S. Census Divisions

TABLE 5

U.S. CENSUS DIVISION 5: EAST SOUTH
CENTRAL

U.S. Registered Community Hospitals
(Nonfederal, short-term general and other special hospitals)

Overview 1998–2002

	2002	2001	2000	1999	1998
Total U.S. Community Hospitals in Census Division 5, East South Central	426	429	429	431	434
Bed Size Category					
6-24	15	8	8	7	7
25-49	83	81	79	77	71
50-99	118	118	120	131	140
100-199	113	125	126	120	122
200-299	41	42	45	44	42
300-399	23	21	21	24	21
400-499	12	16	12	8	13
500 + ...	21	18	18	20	18
Location					
Hospitals Urban.	168	169	167	168	169
Hospitals Rural	258	260	262	263	265
Control					
State and Local Government.	118	125	127	130	134
Not for Profit	197	196	194	197	198
Investor owned	111	108	108	104	102
Physician Models					
Independent Practice Association	50	39	47	54	59
Group Practice without Walls.	17	8	16	13	16
Open Physician-Hospital Organization	58	58	56	68	79
Closed Physician-Hospital Organization	15	12	16	20	17
Management Service Organization	53	48	53	61	65
Integrated Salary Model.	81	69	62	58	54
Equity Model	2	5	6	7	10
Foundation.	28	28	33	29	26
Insurance Products					
Health Maintenance Organization	56	54	60	73	76
Preferred Provider Organization.	130	113	103	132	138
Indemnity Fee for Service	32	30	26	32	35
Managed Care Contracts					
Health Maintenance Organization	184	169	150	166	169
Preferred Provider Organization.	244	244	183	200	202
Affiliations					
Hospitals in a System.	186	203	174	192	189
Hospitals in a Network	99	96	81	86	93
Hospitals in a Group Purchasing Organization. .	222	219	190	190	166

TABLE 5

U.S. CENSUS DIVISION 5: EAST SOUTH CENTRAL

U.S. Registered Community Hospitals
(Nonfederal, short-term general and other special hospitals)

Utilization, Personnel, Revenue and Expenses, Community Health Indicators 1998–2002

	2002	2001	2000	1999	1998
TOTAL FACILITY (Includes Hospital and Nursing Home Units)					
Utilization - Inpatient					
Beds	64,591	65,898	65,356	65,106	65,925
Admissions	2,492,114	2,467,417	2,424,100	2,407,150	2,354,428
Inpatient Days	13,856,950	13,998,816	14,074,178	14,113,317	14,054,783
Average Length of Stay	5.6	5.7	5.8	5.9	6.0
Inpatient Surgeries	727,890	713,144	721,871	717,980	737,115
Births	224,418	227,383	225,101	226,028	219,666
Utilization - Outpatient					
Emergency Outpatient Visits	8,643,710	8,156,784	8,104,971	7,978,531	7,536,558
Other Outpatient Visits	23,996,038	21,946,093	22,539,023	20,776,140	19,280,003
Total Outpatient Visits	32,639,748	30,102,877	30,643,994	28,754,671	26,816,561
Outpatient Surgeries	1,226,607	1,213,146	1,188,571	1,137,417	1,092,446
Personnel					
Full Time RNs	55,716	53,990	55,378	56,988	56,281
Full Time LPNs	10,859	11,156	10,173	10,980	12,739
Part Time RNs	23,303	20,347	19,888	17,267	16,791
Part Time LPNs	3,233	2,953	2,788	2,706	3,296
Total Full Time	237,483	240,670	234,318	235,391	239,503
Total Part Time	70,708	61,263	63,007	54,327	55,290
Revenue - Inpatient					
Gross Inpatient Revenue	$37,236,405,608	$33,763,537,509	$30,460,414,643	$28,522,093,205	$26,782,314,962
Revenue - Outpatient					
Gross Outpatient Revenue	$21,335,998,517	$18,799,075,976	$16,791,511,923	$14,755,549,582	$13,281,422,038
Revenue and Expenses - Totals					
(Includes Inpatient and Outpatient)					
Total Gross Revenue	$58,572,404,125	$52,562,613,485	$47,251,926,566	$43,277,642,787	$40,063,737,000
Deductions from Revenue	33,820,962,603	29,633,078,052	26,118,962,696	23,230,987,570	20,499,152,910
Net Patient Revenue	24,751,441,522	22,929,535,433	21,132,963,870	20,046,655,217	19,564,584,090
Other Operating Revenue	1,112,863,364	1,079,038,669	1,196,170,102	1,213,648,825	966,961,293
Other Nonoperating Revenue	246,155,552	537,095,911	626,610,283	460,092,660	491,564,566
Total Net Revenue	26,110,460,438	24,545,670,013	22,955,744,255	21,720,396,702	21,023,109,949
Total Expenses	24,262,441,941	23,153,845,874	21,606,133,823	20,621,277,359	19,556,107,048
HOSPITAL UNIT (Excludes Separate Nursing Home Units)					
Utilization - Inpatient					
Beds	59,825	60,461	59,945	58,914	59,963
Admissions	2,464,015	2,440,081	2,396,395	2,374,559	2,327,111
Inpatient Days	12,297,077	12,160,748	12,269,882	12,083,301	12,124,969
Average Length of Stay	5.0	5.0	5.1	5.1	5.2
Personnel					
Total Full Time	233,711	236,531	230,035	229,862	234,564
Total Part Time	69,573	60,176	61,799	52,946	54,215
Revenue and Expenses - Totals					
(Includes Inpatient and Outpatient)					
Total Net Revenue	$25,813,696,396	$24,261,954,693	$22,629,453,822	$21,349,301,577	$20,725,426,356
Total Expenses	24,024,754,092	22,927,686,517	21,350,689,942	20,365,677,195	19,324,088,783
COMMUNITY HEALTH INDICATORS PER 1000 POPULATION					
Total Population (in thousands)	17,248	17,128	17,023	16,583	16,469
Inpatient					
Beds	3.7	3.8	3.8	3.9	4.0
Admissions	144.5	144.1	142.4	145.2	143.0
Inpatient Days	803.4	817.3	826.8	851.1	853.4
Inpatient Surgeries	42.2	41.6	42.4	43.3	44.8
Births	13.0	13.3	13.2	13.6	13.3
Outpatient					
Emergency Outpatient Visits	501.1	476.2	476.1	481.1	457.6
Other Outpatient Visits	1,391.2	1,281.3	1,324.0	1,252.9	1,170.7
Total Outpatient Visits	1,892.3	1,757.5	1,800.2	1,734.0	1,628.3
Outpatient Surgeries	71.1	70.8	69.8	68.6	66.3
Expense per Capita (per person)	$1,406.6	$1,351.8	$1,269.2	$1,243.5	$1,187.4

U.S. Census Divisions

TABLE **5**

U.S. CENSUS DIVISION 6: WEST NORTH CENTRAL

U.S. Registered Community Hospitals
(Nonfederal, short-term general and other special hospitals)

Overview 1998–2002

	2002	2001	2000	1999	1998
Total U.S. Community Hospitals in Census Division 6, West North Central.............	**679**	**673**	**673**	**672**	**681**
Bed Size Category					
6-24..................................	89	85	87	85	88
25-49.................................	192	188	186	183	188
50-99.................................	186	185	182	185	180
100-199...............................	111	112	113	116	121
200-299...............................	46	48	48	44	48
300-399...............................	22	22	25	31	25
400-499...............................	15	14	13	7	9
500 +.................................	18	19	19	21	22
Location					
Hospitals Urban.........................	180	181	176	175	178
Hospitals Rural	499	492	497	497	503
Control					
State and Local Government................	247	245	250	248	258
Not for Profit............................	404	402	403	402	396
Investor owned	28	26	20	22	27
Physician Models					
Independent Practice Association	96	95	95	83	95
Group Practice without Walls...............	18	22	24	23	32
Open Physician-Hospital Organization	86	97	99	103	113
Closed Physician-Hospital Organization	45	46	50	62	64
Management Service Organization	33	35	37	57	68
Integrated Salary Model....................	240	230	221	219	204
Equity Model............................	8	5	7	5	11
Foundation.............................	13	16	17	31	39
Insurance Products					
Health Maintenance Organization	84	90	119	139	140
Preferred Provider Organization.............	137	130	152	162	176
Indemnity Fee for Service	39	37	41	45	56
Managed Care Contracts					
Health Maintenance Organization	321	338	337	338	339
Preferred Provider Organization.............	485	501	508	491	483
Affiliations					
Hospitals in a System.....................	289	287	283	280	280
Hospitals in a Network....................	257	262	262	239	255
Hospitals in a Group Purchasing Organization..	551	577	570	527	483

TABLE 5

U.S. CENSUS DIVISION 6: WEST NORTH CENTRAL

U.S. Registered Community Hospitals
(Nonfederal, short-term general and other special hospitals)

Utilization, Personnel, Revenue and Expenses, Community Health Indicators 1998–2002

	2002	2001	2000	1999	1998
TOTAL FACILITY (Includes Hospital and Nursing Home Units)					
Utilization - Inpatient					
Beds	74,277	75,020	75,842	76,718	76,825
Admissions	2,509,141	2,481,753	2,411,096	2,346,771	2,305,119
Inpatient Days	16,581,836	16,650,444	16,570,765	16,752,113	16,798,552
Average Length of Stay	6.6	6.7	6.9	7.1	7.3
Inpatient Surgeries	720,434	702,686	686,916	685,775	689,445
Births	261,872	261,796	256,291	256,899	256,377
Utilization - Outpatient					
Emergency Outpatient Visits	7,108,385	6,937,436	6,666,448	6,682,798	5,911,276
Other Outpatient Visits	38,591,201	37,737,290	36,706,774	34,185,839	28,000,033
Total Outpatient Visits	45,699,586	44,674,726	43,373,222	40,868,637	33,911,309
Outpatient Surgeries	1,470,067	1,329,461	1,309,685	1,289,568	1,241,055
Personnel					
Full Time RNs	54,055	51,206	51,850	52,237	53,036
Full Time LPNs	8,391	8,162	8,099	8,358	8,990
Part Time RNs	49,543	49,074	46,048	45,113	42,035
Part Time LPNs	6,403	6,465	6,384	6,904	6,630
Total Full Time	255,451	247,196	241,470	240,530	242,835
Total Part Time	161,431	160,957	152,362	145,649	138,554
Revenue - Inpatient					
Gross Inpatient Revenue	$38,854,088,608	$34,125,326,110	$30,690,964,864	$27,978,962,967	$25,754,385,615
Revenue - Outpatient					
Gross Outpatient Revenue	$24,929,041,928	$21,796,597,517	$18,954,856,055	$16,696,279,258	$14,731,910,689
Revenue and Expenses - Totals					
(Includes Inpatient and Outpatient)					
Total Gross Revenue	$63,783,130,536	$55,921,923,627	$49,645,820,919	$44,675,242,225	$40,486,296,304
Deductions from Revenue	33,035,135,970	27,904,622,957	23,918,824,972	20,629,836,841	17,831,563,136
Net Patient Revenue	30,747,994,566	28,017,300,670	25,726,995,947	24,045,405,384	22,654,733,168
Other Operating Revenue	1,794,417,297	1,614,130,546	1,472,106,386	1,441,566,383	1,352,605,326
Other Nonoperating Revenue	239,434,505	447,993,850	654,168,860	576,521,233	753,864,537
Total Net Revenue	32,781,846,368	30,079,425,066	27,853,271,193	26,063,493,000	24,761,203,031
Total Expenses	31,131,081,814	28,645,889,268	26,440,620,590	24,629,816,297	22,971,405,642
HOSPITAL UNIT (Excludes Separate Nursing Home Units)					
Utilization - Inpatient					
Beds	60,750	60,574	60,766	61,370	60,236
Admissions	2,461,630	2,428,943	2,348,985	2,275,386	2,205,432
Inpatient Days	12,331,933	12,028,176	11,854,940	11,875,181	11,475,570
Average Length of Stay	5.0	5.0	5.0	5.2	5.2
Personnel					
Total Full Time	248,644	239,190	232,906	232,075	233,198
Total Part Time	154,831	153,653	144,687	138,530	130,520
Revenue and Expenses - Totals					
(Includes Inpatient and Outpatient)					
Total Net Revenue	$32,099,995,655	$29,384,362,820	$27,176,111,952	$25,386,846,064	$23,955,585,610
Total Expenses	30,539,871,194	28,042,574,090	25,851,000,854	24,051,512,537	22,296,721,901
COMMUNITY HEALTH INDICATORS PER 1000 POPULATION					
Total Population (in thousands)	19,469	19,324	19,238	18,800	18,693
Inpatient					
Beds	3.8	3.9	3.9	4.1	4.1
Admissions	128.9	128.4	125.3	124.8	123.3
Inpatient Days	851.7	861.6	861.4	891.1	898.7
Inpatient Surgeries	37.0	36.4	35.7	36.5	36.9
Births	13.5	13.5	13.3	13.7	13.7
Outpatient					
Emergency Outpatient Visits	365.1	359.0	346.5	355.5	316.2
Other Outpatient Visits	1,982.2	1,952.9	1,908.1	1,818.4	1,497.9
Total Outpatient Visits	2,347.3	2,311.9	2,254.6	2,173.8	1,814.1
Outpatient Surgeries	75.5	68.8	68.1	68.6	66.4
Expense per Capita (per person)	$1,599.0	$1,482.4	$1,374.4	$1,310.1	$1,228.9

U.S. Census Divisions

TABLE 5

U.S. CENSUS DIVISION 7: WEST SOUTH CENTRAL

U.S. Registered Community Hospitals
(Nonfederal, short-term general and other special hospitals)

Overview 1998–2002

	2002	2001	2000	1999	1998
Total U.S. Community Hospitals in Census Division 7, West South Central	**736**	**727**	**717**	**722**	**717**
Bed Size Category					
6-24	82	80	73	78	71
25-49	199	195	196	187	191
50-99	160	153	151	151	148
100-199	151	155	146	159	160
200-299	58	58	68	63	64
300-399	44	44	41	44	36
400-499	16	15	14	14	19
500 + ...	26	27	28	26	28
Location					
Hospitals Urban...........................	401	394	384	388	384
Hospitals Rural	335	333	333	334	333
Control					
State and Local Government...............	240	243	245	252	254
Not for Profit	287	276	271	265	257
Investor owned	209	208	201	205	206
Physician Models					
Independent Practice Association	124	117	124	137	145
Group Practice without Walls...............	28	25	30	26	32
Open Physician-Hospital Organization	152	151	181	176	189
Closed Physician-Hospital Organization	45	52	50	60	80
Management Service Organization	90	86	119	142	161
Integrated Salary Model....................	118	101	100	104	113
Equity Model	10	9	18	24	34
Foundation..............................	43	51	60	67	79
Insurance Products					
Health Maintenance Organization	99	104	129	160	169
Preferred Provider Organization..............	146	131	170	196	219
Indemnity Fee for Service	40	32	43	56	68
Managed Care Contracts					
Health Maintenance Organization	447	452	454	478	462
Preferred Provider Organization..............	541	550	553	578	547
Affiliations					
Hospitals in a System.....................	353	343	345	339	333
Hospitals in a Network....................	157	153	171	185	215
Hospitals in a Group Purchasing Organization..	553	547	521	417	378

TABLE 5

U.S. CENSUS DIVISION 7: WEST SOUTH CENTRAL

U.S. Registered Community Hospitals
(Nonfederal, short-term general and other special hospitals)

Utilization, Personnel, Revenue and Expenses, Community Health Indicators 1998–2002

	2002	2001	2000	1999	1998
TOTAL FACILITY (Includes Hospital and Nursing Home Units)					
Utilization - Inpatient					
Beds	95,764	95,071	94,317	94,732	95,291
Admissions	4,055,293	3,949,513	3,818,189	3,716,015	3,614,369
Inpatient Days	21,541,966	20,782,167	20,064,215	19,957,836	19,575,370
Average Length of Stay	5.3	5.3	5.3	5.4	5.4
Inpatient Surgeries	1,161,699	1,128,483	1,125,604	1,097,488	1,088,948
Births	510,996	509,537	503,994	483,514	470,142
Utilization - Outpatient					
Emergency Outpatient Visits	13,229,179	12,453,535	11,823,842	11,499,044	11,009,388
Other Outpatient Visits	40,646,350	38,124,472	36,704,726	34,854,535	35,091,925
Total Outpatient Visits	53,875,529	50,578,007	48,528,568	46,353,579	46,101,313
Outpatient Surgeries	1,714,003	1,661,253	1,659,492	1,647,551	1,566,478
Personnel					
Full Time RNs	90,845	86,746	85,534	85,777	84,100
Full Time LPNs	20,342	20,274	20,174	21,987	21,403
Part Time RNs	31,644	31,071	29,440	27,595	28,301
Part Time LPNs	5,984	6,264	5,767	5,806	5,741
Total Full Time	391,498	382,735	375,496	378,422	376,299
Total Part Time	103,037	100,545	94,690	91,406	96,359
Revenue - Inpatient					
Gross Inpatient Revenue	$71,476,469,794	$61,419,028,742	$53,960,636,392	$48,750,503,268	$44,816,152,292
Revenue - Outpatient					
Gross Outpatient Revenue	$36,305,540,752	$31,134,758,847	$26,985,710,323	$24,048,411,053	$21,841,270,539
Revenue and Expenses - Totals					
(Includes Inpatient and Outpatient)					
Total Gross Revenue	$107,782,010,546	$92,553,787,589	$80,946,346,715	$72,758,914,321	$66,657,422,831
Deductions from Revenue	64,781,749,664	54,100,450,992	46,520,754,796	39,647,718,729	34,734,533,296
Net Patient Revenue	43,000,260,882	38,453,336,597	34,425,591,919	33,111,195,592	31,922,889,535
Other Operating Revenue	3,420,018,355	3,072,362,313	2,917,928,679	2,836,835,943	2,549,861,558
Other Nonoperating Revenue	273,239,612	598,918,958	687,359,457	688,647,700	608,344,145
Total Net Revenue	46,693,518,849	42,124,617,868	38,030,880,055	36,636,679,235	35,081,095,238
Total Expenses	42,808,056,150	39,110,488,373	36,305,621,658	33,769,783,746	32,473,333,390
HOSPITAL UNIT (Excludes Separate Nursing Home Units)					
Utilization - Inpatient					
Beds	92,331	91,100	89,865	89,550	90,049
Admissions	4,019,877	3,903,804	3,757,331	3,641,325	3,532,413
Inpatient Days	20,607,960	19,699,547	18,867,455	18,527,824	18,133,098
Average Length of Stay	5.1	5.0	5.0	5.1	5.1
Personnel					
Total Full Time	388,745	379,354	371,015	374,262	371,204
Total Part Time	102,090	99,685	93,749	90,326	94,936
Revenue and Expenses - Totals					
(Includes Inpatient and Outpatient)					
Total Net Revenue	$46,432,845,269	$41,800,329,627	$37,720,612,218	$36,016,882,393	$34,572,654,887
Total Expenses	42,603,810,235	38,889,779,063	36,104,024,942	33,477,930,476	32,125,816,230
COMMUNITY HEALTH INDICATORS PER 1000 POPULATION					
Total Population (in thousands)	32,466	31,943	31,445	30,326	29,953
Inpatient					
Beds	2.9	3.0	3.0	3.1	3.2
Admissions	124.9	123.6	121.4	122.5	120.7
Inpatient Days	663.5	650.6	638.1	658.1	653.5
Inpatient Surgeries	35.8	35.3	35.8	36.2	36.4
Births	15.7	16.0	16.0	15.9	15.7
Outpatient					
Emergency Outpatient Visits	407.5	389.9	376.0	379.2	367.6
Other Outpatient Visits	1,252.0	1,193.5	1,167.3	1,149.3	1,171.6
Total Outpatient Visits	1,659.4	1,583.4	1,543.3	1,528.5	1,539.1
Outpatient Surgeries	52.8	52.0	52.8	54.3	52.3
Expense per Capita (per person)	$1,318.5	$1,224.4	$1,154.6	$1,113.6	$1,084.1

U.S. Census Divisions

TABLE 5

U.S. Registered Community Hospitals
(Nonfederal, short-term general and other special hospitals)

Overview 1998–2002

	2002	2001	2000	1999	1998
Total U.S. Community Hospitals in Census Division 8, Mountain.....................	**349**	**345**	**347**	**346**	**350**
Bed Size Category					
6-24	38	35	38	39	40
25-49	90	86	88	82	90
50-99	85	87	87	91	85
100-199	67	69	67	71	69
200-299	35	33	34	32	33
300-399	19	20	18	17	19
400-499	9	9	10	9	10
500 + ...	6	6	5	5	4
Location					
Hospitals Urban............................	143	140	136	136	137
Hospitals Rural	206	205	211	210	213
Control					
State and Local Government................	103	108	110	116	113
Not for Profit	180	175	176	175	181
Investor owned	66	62	61	55	56
Physician Models					
Independent Practice Association	46	45	60	67	78
Group Practice without Walls................	12	11	11	13	14
Open Physician-Hospital Organization	41	36	49	58	66
Closed Physician-Hospital Organization	17	15	22	23	16
Management Service Organization	20	20	26	33	45
Integrated Salary Model.....................	84	87	78	77	71
Equity Model	4	2	1	3	4
Foundation................................	8	9	13	16	20
Insurance Products					
Health Maintenance Organization	51	56	61	55	71
Preferred Provider Organization..............	51	55	70	57	79
Indemnity Fee for Service	27	27	31	25	47
Managed Care Contracts					
Health Maintenance Organization	146	143	154	172	165
Preferred Provider Organization..............	176	176	188	185	178
Affiliations					
Hospitals in a System......................	110	124	126	124	133
Hospitals in a Network.....................	87	88	85	80	76
Hospitals in a Group Purchasing Organization..	236	252	239	215	202

U.S. Census Divisions

TABLE 5

U.S. CENSUS DIVISION 8: MOUNTAIN

U.S. Registered Community Hospitals
(Nonfederal, short-term general and other special hospitals)

Utilization, Personnel, Revenue and Expenses, Community Health Indicators 1998–2002

	2002	2001	2000	1999	1998
TOTAL FACILITY (Includes Hospital and Nursing Home Units)					
Utilization - Inpatient					
Beds	42,499	42,116	41,536	41,168	40,825
Admissions	1,894,701	1,825,214	1,773,119	1,708,013	1,646,228
Inpatient Days	9,643,564	9,432,684	9,198,430	9,134,857	8,882,182
Average Length of Stay	5.1	5.2	5.2	5.3	5.4
Inpatient Surgeries	573,886	551,364	551,078	554,791	529,048
Births	292,890	277,576	273,536	264,003	253,440
Utilization - Outpatient					
Emergency Outpatient Visits	6,124,812	5,444,391	5,579,598	5,254,445	4,724,837
Other Outpatient Visits	23,424,496	22,599,897	21,879,555	21,342,609	20,300,196
Total Outpatient Visits	29,549,308	28,044,288	27,459,153	26,597,054	25,025,033
Outpatient Surgeries	868,934	813,341	838,426	849,404	784,044
Personnel					
Full Time RNs	42,583	38,561	38,435	37,953	36,847
Full Time LPNs	4,955	4,809	4,412	4,718	4,955
Part Time RNs	20,935	18,430	20,841	18,639	20,723
Part Time LPNs	2,112	1,965	2,185	1,990	2,426
Total Full Time	179,836	170,748	162,370	163,460	155,730
Total Part Time	65,555	60,208	65,617	59,319	64,597
Revenue - Inpatient					
Gross Inpatient Revenue	$33,651,462,085	$27,813,469,466	$25,420,640,854	$22,802,959,773	$20,124,462,635
Revenue - Outpatient					
Gross Outpatient Revenue	$17,572,433,747	$14,608,268,942	$13,088,918,718	$11,360,904,338	$10,209,844,005
Revenue and Expenses - Totals **(Includes Inpatient and Outpatient)**					
Total Gross Revenue	$51,223,895,832	$42,421,738,408	$38,509,559,572	$34,163,864,111	$30,334,306,640
Deductions from Revenue	29,266,253,620	23,195,132,956	20,763,767,673	17,542,214,999	14,865,885,966
Net Patient Revenue	21,957,642,212	19,226,605,452	17,745,791,899	16,621,649,112	15,468,420,674
Other Operating Revenue	1,082,083,144	1,165,866,873	914,977,655	857,114,840	791,106,156
Other Nonoperating Revenue	247,116,847	355,603,623	350,531,542	333,030,721	345,922,560
Total Net Revenue	23,286,842,203	20,748,075,948	19,011,301,096	17,811,794,673	16,605,449,390
Total Expenses	21,439,442,983	19,222,843,051	17,634,866,621	16,728,824,652	15,200,038,183
HOSPITAL UNIT (Excludes Separate Nursing Home Units)					
Utilization - Inpatient					
Beds	38,104	37,453	36,716	35,984	35,608
Admissions	1,878,936	1,804,483	1,750,242	1,659,661	1,613,954
Inpatient Days	8,282,586	7,973,579	7,691,884	7,569,524	7,278,010
Average Length of Stay	4.4	4.4	4.4	4.6	4.5
Personnel					
Total Full Time	176,918	167,386	159,111	160,221	152,142
Total Part Time	63,778	58,435	63,895	57,735	62,865
Revenue and Expenses - Totals **(Includes Inpatient and Outpatient)**					
Total Net Revenue	$23,087,760,662	$20,511,142,311	$18,801,244,040	$17,573,081,317	$16,327,873,454
Total Expenses	21,258,843,110	19,017,095,330	17,452,526,303	16,526,820,028	14,988,846,873
COMMUNITY HEALTH INDICATORS PER 1000 POPULATION					
Total Population (in thousands)	19,057	18,650	18,172	17,127	16,805
Inpatient					
Beds	2.2	2.3	2.3	2.4	2.4
Admissions	99.4	97.9	97.6	99.7	98.0
Inpatient Days	506.0	505.8	506.2	533.3	528.6
Inpatient Surgeries	30.1	29.6	30.3	32.4	31.5
Births	15.4	14.9	15.1	15.4	15.1
Outpatient					
Emergency Outpatient Visits	321.4	291.9	307.0	306.8	281.2
Other Outpatient Visits	1,229.2	1,211.8	1,204.0	1,246.1	1,208.0
Total Outpatient Visits	1,550.6	1,503.7	1,511.0	1,552.9	1,489.2
Outpatient Surgeries	45.6	43.6	46.1	49.6	46.7
Expense per Capita (per person)	$1,125.0	$1,030.7	$970.4	$976.7	$904.5

U.S. Census Divisions

TABLE 5

U.S. CENSUS DIVISION 9: PACIFIC

U.S. Registered Community Hospitals
(Nonfederal, short-term general and other special hospitals)

Overview 1998–2002

	2002	2001	2000	1999	1998
Total U.S. Community Hospitals in Census Division 9, Pacific	573	570	571	579	588
Bed Size Category					
6-24	32	27	31	36	31
25-49	96	90	91	91	97
50-99	105	110	108	108	111
100-199	153	158	159	162	175
200-299	95	94	97	96	84
300-399	48	49	50	51	58
400-499	25	29	21	21	18
500 +	19	13	14	14	14
Location					
Hospitals Urban	433	432	434	441	451
Hospitals Rural	140	138	137	138	137
Control					
State and Local Government	140	142	138	143	146
Not for Profit	332	329	330	328	330
Investor owned	101	99	103	108	112
Physician Models					
Independent Practice Association	142	142	140	146	172
Group Practice without Walls	27	28	25	24	26
Open Physician-Hospital Organization	33	33	37	39	36
Closed Physician-Hospital Organization	17	25	27	28	30
Management Service Organization	56	55	64	78	91
Integrated Salary Model	100	78	80	80	61
Equity Model	1	2	3	6	5
Foundation	33	29	43	42	48
Insurance Products					
Health Maintenance Organization	76	62	72	100	113
Preferred Provider Organization	58	44	52	72	81
Indemnity Fee for Service	23	16	15	20	30
Managed Care Contracts					
Health Maintenance Organization	275	243	260	285	298
Preferred Provider Organization	300	255	270	290	301
Affiliations					
Hospitals in a System	272	237	224	245	232
Hospitals in a Network	80	80	65	68	66
Hospitals in a Group Purchasing Organization	359	333	295	301	262

TABLE 5

U.S. CENSUS DIVISION 9: PACIFIC

U.S. Registered Community Hospitals
(Nonfederal, short-term general and other special hospitals)

Utilization, Personnel, Revenue and Expenses, Community Health Indicators 1998–2002

	2002	2001	2000	1999	1998
TOTAL FACILITY (Includes Hospital and Nursing Home Units)					
Utilization - Inpatient					
Beds	97,048	96,010	94,948	95,570	96,061
Admissions	4,453,054	4,347,642	4,296,908	4,192,529	4,097,190
Inpatient Days	23,756,101	22,968,771	22,490,293	21,953,126	21,509,972
Average Length of Stay...........	5.3	5.3	5.2	5.2	5.2
Inpatient Surgeries...............	1,309,119	1,200,316	1,197,879	1,153,469	1,280,577
Births..........................	616,819	630,251	665,956	615,818	623,890
Utilization - Outpatient					
Emergency Outpatient Visits	13,731,605	13,916,852	13,085,734	12,507,125	11,745,959
Other Outpatient Visits...........	60,828,353	56,276,529	52,457,752	52,358,495	51,292,889
Total Outpatient Visits	74,559,958	70,193,381	65,543,486	64,865,620	63,038,848
Outpatient Surgeries	1,902,778	1,845,904	1,841,711	1,663,599	1,822,550
Personnel					
Full Time RNs	96,461	92,781	86,593	84,598	83,182
Full Time LPNs	11,299	11,012	10,753	10,705	11,212
Part Time RNs..................	53,794	51,294	64,202	59,976	57,708
Part Time LPNs	4,211	4,152	6,024	5,506	5,939
Total Full Time	426,704	411,166	387,216	380,054	371,349
Total Part Time	154,518	150,306	189,923	171,580	171,241
Revenue - Inpatient					
Gross Inpatient Revenue..........	$104,936,331,959	$89,170,723,161	$75,477,661,383	$69,198,015,940	$62,749,840,748
Revenue - Outpatient					
Gross Outpatient Revenue	$46,066,247,391	$38,916,573,129	$34,417,684,249	$30,111,292,438	$26,657,715,315
Revenue and Expenses - Totals (Includes Inpatient and Outpatient)					
Total Gross Revenue.............	$151,002,579,350	$128,087,296,290	$109,895,345,632	$99,309,308,378	$89,407,556,063
Deductions from Revenue.........	95,502,859,945	77,374,399,517	62,997,781,765	55,746,141,428	48,651,158,338
Net Patient Revenue	55,499,719,405	50,712,896,773	46,897,563,867	43,563,166,950	40,756,397,725
Other Operating Revenue	3,077,494,277	2,797,221,202	2,794,056,480	2,556,475,389	2,318,011,493
Other Nonoperating Revenue	1,219,640,462	1,328,607,343	1,212,144,701	1,359,542,968	1,195,596,600
Total Net Revenue..............	59,796,854,144	54,838,725,318	50,903,765,048	47,479,185,307	44,270,005,818
Total Expenses.................	57,386,669,321	52,988,295,607	49,162,814,581	46,213,076,154	42,300,596,312
HOSPITAL UNIT (Excludes Separate Nursing Home Units)					
Utilization - Inpatient					
Beds	87,870	88,815	89,168	88,931	89,958
Admissions	4,385,440	4,286,501	4,248,674	4,133,064	4,032,664
Inpatient Days	21,145,589	20,858,375	20,803,528	20,024,988	19,732,217
Average Length of Stay...........	4.8	4.9	4.9	4.8	4.9
Personnel					
Total Full Time..................	420,265	406,127	383,153	375,756	366,916
Total Part Time	152,674	148,479	187,897	169,565	168,870
Revenue and Expenses - Totals (Includes Inpatient and Outpatient)					
Total Net Revenue..............	$59,059,246,409	$54,279,461,564	$50,442,556,359	$46,970,677,731	$43,805,071,509
Total Expenses.................	56,802,766,053	52,589,699,252	48,846,089,081	45,852,689,635	41,975,871,690
COMMUNITY HEALTH INDICATORS PER 1000 POPULATION					
Total Population (in thousands)	46,595	45,821	45,026	44,023	43,458
Inpatient					
Beds	2.1	2.1	2.1	2.2	2.2
Admissions	95.6	94.9	95.4	95.2	94.3
Inpatient Days	509.8	501.3	499.5	498.7	495.0
Inpatient Surgeries...............	28.1	26.2	26.6	26.2	29.5
Births..........................	13.2	13.8	14.8	14.0	14.4
Outpatient					
Emergency Outpatient Visits	294.7	303.7	290.6	284.1	270.3
Other Outpatient Visits...........	1,305.5	1,228.2	1,165.1	1,189.4	1,180.3
Total Outpatient Visits	1,600.2	1,531.9	1,455.7	1,473.5	1,450.6
Outpatient Surgeries	40.8	40.3	40.9	37.8	41.9
Expense per Capita (per person)....	$1,231.6	$1,156.4	$1,091.9	$1,049.8	$973.4

TABLE 6

ALABAMA

U.S. Registered Community Hospitals
(Nonfederal, short-term general and other special hospitals)

Overview 1998–2002

	2002	2001	2000	1999	1998
Total U.S. Community Hospitals in Alabama ...	106	107	108	109	110
Bed Size Category					
6-24	6	4	4	4	3
25-49	15	18	17	17	13
50-99	30	26	28	29	32
100-199	30	34	34	33	35
200-299	13	11	13	14	13
300-399	7	7	7	6	7
400-499	1	4	3	3	5
500 + ...	4	3	2	3	2
Location					
Hospitals Urban..........................	57	57	57	57	57
Hospitals Rural	49	50	51	52	53
Control					
State and Local Government................	36	40	40	43	44
Not for Profit	35	37	39	40	38
Investor owned	35	30	29	26	28
Physician Models					
Independent Practice Association	4	6	9	13	19
Group Practice without Walls...............	3	1	4	3	4
Open Physician-Hospital Organization	2	4	7	7	6
Closed Physician-Hospital Organization	0	1	1	2	2
Management Service Organization	8	8	9	15	17
Integrated Salary Model...................	9	8	11	10	9
Equity Model...........................	0	2	3	1	1
Foundation.............................	6	4	6	2	5
Insurance Products					
Health Maintenance Organization	2	3	14	19	18
Preferred Provider Organization.............	13	14	20	25	24
Indemnity Fee for Service	3	2	1	4	3
Managed Care Contracts					
Health Maintenance Organization	33	34	40	48	49
Preferred Provider Organization.............	42	46	56	60	61
Affiliations					
Hospitals in a System.....................	42	42	44	53	55
Hospitals in a Network....................	8	7	9	9	13
Hospitals in a Group Purchasing Organization..	49	52	58	59	52

TABLE 6

ALABAMA

U.S. Registered Community Hospitals
(Nonfederal, short-term general and other special hospitals)

Utilization, Personnel, Revenue and Expenses, Community Health Indicators 1998–2002

	2002	2001	2000	1999	1998
TOTAL FACILITY (Includes Hospital and Nursing Home Units)					
Utilization - Inpatient					
Beds	15,935	16,627	16,370	16,306	16,998
Admissions	676,337	684,923	680,395	670,059	644,283
Inpatient Days	3,244,123	3,570,273	3,585,804	3,603,498	3,639,125
Average Length of Stay..........	4.8	5.2	5.3	5.4	5.6
Inpatient Surgeries.............	198,225	190,655	198,439	196,715	213,314
Births.........................	55,677	55,794	57,501	57,787	55,025
Utilization - Outpatient					
Emergency Outpatient Visits.......	2,162,011	1,959,967	2,070,702	1,969,275	1,905,603
Other Outpatient Visits...........	7,883,504	5,826,096	5,893,511	5,866,213	4,857,719
Total Outpatient Visits	10,045,515	7,786,063	7,964,213	7,835,488	6,763,322
Outpatient Surgeries	319,658	293,428	287,725	279,495	276,581
Personnel					
Full Time RNs	15,328	14,825	14,551	14,642	14,317
Full Time LPNs	2,680	2,905	2,693	3,060	4,184
Part Time RNs................	5,382	4,799	4,782	4,285	5,078
Part Time LPNs	750	695	745	709	1,161
Total Full Time................	63,011	62,655	60,209	60,570	60,650
Total Part Time	14,924	13,575	13,408	12,302	15,698
Revenue - Inpatient					
Gross Inpatient Revenue..........	$10,908,904,536	$9,398,051,190	$8,966,154,419	$8,625,893,202	$8,129,325,907
Revenue - Outpatient					
Gross Outpatient Revenue	$5,203,241,240	$4,564,975,896	$4,271,722,359	$3,898,882,021	$3,638,475,901
Revenue and Expenses - Totals					
(Includes Inpatient and Outpatient)					
Total Gross Revenue.............	$16,112,145,776	$13,963,027,086	$13,237,876,778	$12,524,775,223	$11,767,801,808
Deductions from Revenue.........	10,194,892,253	8,380,028,417	8,048,660,850	7,494,355,021	6,852,791,684
Net Patient Revenue	5,917,253,523	5,582,998,669	5,189,215,928	5,030,420,202	4,915,010,124
Other Operating Revenue	343,884,634	281,472,509	392,404,366	440,819,124	247,784,982
Other Nonoperating Revenue	66,577,418	112,779,032	138,535,799	137,896,417	176,142,839
Total Net Revenue..............	6,327,715,575	5,977,250,210	5,720,156,093	5,609,135,743	5,338,937,945
Total Expenses.................	5,767,179,494	5,664,284,252	5,461,919,463	5,222,381,900	5,096,414,752
HOSPITAL UNIT (Excludes Separate Nursing Home Units)					
Utilization - Inpatient					
Beds	15,678	15,704	15,382	15,052	15,704
Admissions	672,860	681,266	676,250	665,857	640,217
Inpatient Days	3,178,161	3,274,368	3,264,746	3,183,661	3,194,922
Average Length of Stay..........	4.7	4.8	4.8	4.8	5.0
Personnel					
Total Full Time.................	62,861	62,162	59,546	59,630	59,730
Total Part Time	14,895	13,518	13,272	12,117	15,534
Revenue and Expenses - Totals					
(Includes Inpatient and Outpatient)					
Total Net Revenue..............	$6,315,357,773	$5,942,050,549	$5,695,856,842	$5,567,541,618	$5,288,429,187
Total Expenses.................	5,754,090,214	5,626,134,980	5,439,545,167	5,185,831,549	5,050,868,793
COMMUNITY HEALTH INDICATORS PER 1000 POPULATION					
Total Population (in thousands)	4,487	4,464	4,447	4,370	4,351
Inpatient					
Beds	3.6	3.7	3.7	3.7	3.9
Admissions	150.7	153.4	153.0	153.3	148.1
Inpatient Days	723.1	799.7	806.3	824.6	836.4
Inpatient Surgeries.............	44.2	42.7	44.6	45.0	49.0
Births.........................	12.4	12.5	12.9	13.2	12.6
Outpatient					
Emergency Outpatient Visits.......	481.9	439.0	465.6	450.6	438.0
Other Outpatient Visits...........	1,757.2	1,305.0	1,325.2	1,342.4	1,116.5
Total Outpatient Visits	2,239.0	1,744.1	1,790.9	1,793.1	1,554.4
Outpatient Surgeries	71.2	65.7	64.7	64.0	63.6
Expense per Capita (per person)....	$1,285.4	$1,268.8	$1,228.2	$1,195.1	$1,171.3

TABLE 6

ALASKA

U.S. Registered Community Hospitals
(Nonfederal, short-term general and other special hospitals)

Overview 1998–2002

	2002	2001	2000	1999	1998
Total U.S. Community Hospitals in Alaska	19	19	18	17	17
Bed Size Category					
6-24	5	5	4	5	5
25-49	6	6	7	6	6
50-99	4	4	3	3	3
100-199	3	2	2	1	2
200-299	0	1	1	1	0
300-399	1	1	1	1	1
400-499	0	0	0	0	0
500 + ...	0	0	0	0	0
Location					
Hospitals Urban	3	3	3	2	2
Hospitals Rural	16	16	15	15	15
Control					
State and Local Government	7	8	7	7	8
Not for Profit	11	10	10	9	8
Investor owned	1	1	1	1	1
Physician Models					
Independent Practice Association.	3	3	5	2	1
Group Practice without Walls	3	3	4	2	2
Open Physician-Hospital Organization. . . .	3	3	4	2	1
Closed Physician-Hospital Organization. . .	0	0	1	0	0
Management Service Organization.	0	1	2	2	2
Integrated Salary Model	5	3	3	2	2
Equity Model	0	0	1	0	0
Foundation	0	0	1	0	0
Insurance Products					
Health Maintenance Organization.	0	0	0	0	0
Preferred Provider Organization	1	0	1	1	2
Indemnity Fee for Service.	0	0	1	1	1
Managed Care Contracts					
Health Maintenance Organization.	0	0	0	0	0
Preferred Provider Organization	6	3	7	5	4
Affiliations					
Hospitals in a System	7	4	6	7	5
Hospitals in a Network	2	1	0	0	0
Hospitals in a Group Purchasing Organization.	11	9	12	13	10

TABLE 6

ALASKA

U.S. Registered Community Hospitals
(Nonfederal, short-term general and other special hospitals)

Utilization, Personnel, Revenue and Expenses, Community Health Indicators 1998–2002

	2002	2001	2000	1999	1998
TOTAL FACILITY (Includes Hospital and Nursing Home Units)					
Utilization - Inpatient					
Beds	1,378	1,442	1,417	1,250	1,240
Admissions	47,560	49,065	46,887	40,785	41,294
Inpatient Days	300,060	303,092	293,707	246,872	378,357
Average Length of Stay...........	6.3	6.2	6.3	6.1	9.2
Inpatient Surgeries..............	22,359	15,888	15,196	12,762	10,914
Births.........................	7,596	7,448	7,728	6,618	6,790
Utilization - Outpatient					
Emergency Outpatient Visits	254,592	205,595	187,226	164,113	160,519
Other Outpatient Visits...........	1,083,024	1,182,031	1,083,881	868,170	878,092
Total Outpatient Visits	1,337,616	1,387,626	1,271,107	1,032,283	1,038,611
Outpatient Surgeries	35,136	37,849	34,678	25,640	20,070
Personnel					
Full Time RNs	1,734	1,504	1,466	1,052	998
Full Time LPNs	144	189	200	86	171
Part Time RNs	752	956	768	832	855
Part Time LPNs	58	97	61	60	97
Total Full Time.................	7,447	6,544	5,763	4,154	5,106
Total Part Time	2,221	2,907	2,340	2,216	2,487
Revenue - Inpatient					
Gross Inpatient Revenue..........	$960,861,590	$875,560,013	$741,246,222	$625,651,216	$616,562,865
Revenue - Outpatient					
Gross Outpatient Revenue	$665,750,510	$579,556,236	$452,257,752	$372,382,270	$373,071,577
Revenue and Expenses - Totals **(Includes Inpatient and Outpatient)**					
Total Gross Revenue.............	$1,626,612,100	$1,455,116,249	$1,193,503,974	$998,033,486	$989,634,442
Deductions from Revenue.........	755,063,643	624,227,686	460,734,350	383,654,287	363,552,966
Net Patient Revenue	871,548,457	830,888,563	732,769,624	614,379,199	626,081,476
Other Operating Revenue	40,119,994	72,758,253	34,360,208	29,498,177	29,106,660
Other Nonoperating Revenue	53,664,515	19,704,156	17,142,523	15,285,517	14,512,051
Total Net Revenue..............	965,332,966	923,350,972	784,272,355	659,162,893	669,700,187
Total Expenses.................	942,611,948	918,694,601	741,993,877	591,317,689	590,184,996
HOSPITAL UNIT (Excludes Separate Nursing Home Units)					
Utilization - Inpatient					
Beds	1,146	1,282	1,199	1,047	1,055
Admissions	47,038	48,661	46,246	40,167	40,891
Inpatient Days	228,355	252,692	227,379	182,521	319,789
Average Length of Stay...........	4.9	5.2	4.9	4.5	7.8
Personnel					
Total Full Time.................	7,261	6,404	5,619	4,021	4,975
Total Part Time	2,099	2,820	2,220	2,093	2,364
Revenue and Expenses - Totals **(Includes Inpatient and Outpatient)**					
Total Net Revenue..............	$938,542,659	$902,447,973	$759,807,432	$637,789,467	$651,330,722
Total Expenses.................	923,049,072	902,546,954	727,117,622	577,708,366	577,187,974
COMMUNITY HEALTH INDICATORS PER 1000 POPULATION					
Total Population (in thousands)	644	635	627	620	615
Inpatient					
Beds	2.1	2.3	2.3	2.0	2.0
Admissions	73.9	77.3	74.8	65.8	67.1
Inpatient Days	466.1	477.4	468.5	398.5	615.0
Inpatient Surgeries..............	34.7	25.0	24.2	20.6	17.7
Births.........................	11.8	11.7	12.3	10.7	11.0
Outpatient					
Emergency Outpatient Visits	395.5	323.8	298.6	264.9	260.9
Other Outpatient Visits...........	1,682.3	1,861.8	1,728.9	1,401.4	1,427.3
Total Outpatient Visits	2,077.7	2,185.6	2,027.5	1,666.3	1,688.2
Outpatient Surgeries	54.6	59.6	55.3	41.4	32.6
Expense per Capita (per person)....	$1,464.2	$1,447.0	$1,183.5	$954.5	$959.3

States

TABLE 6

ARIZONA

U.S. Registered Community Hospitals
(Nonfederal, short-term general and other special hospitals)

Overview 1998–2002

	2002	2001	2000	1999	1998
Total U.S. Community Hospitals in					
Arizona	61	61	61	61	64
Bed Size Category					
6-24	3	1	2	3	3
25-49	10	10	9	8	10
50-99	11	12	13	14	14
100-199	14	16	17	16	15
200-299	13	12	10	12	12
300-399	4	5	5	3	5
400-499	3	2	2	2	3
500 + ...	3	3	3	3	2
Location					
Hospitals Urban.....................	46	46	46	45	48
Hospitals Rural	15	15	15	16	16
Control					
State and Local Government	5	4	5	6	5
Not for Profit	37	37	37	40	43
Investor owned	19	20	19	15	16
Physician Models					
Independent Practice Association........	5	4	8	12	17
Group Practice without Walls	2	4	2	2	3
Open Physician-Hospital Organization....	4	3	5	12	15
Closed Physician-Hospital Organization...	3	4	6	8	8
Management Service Organization.......	1	3	5	10	8
Integrated Salary Model	7	10	8	12	8
Equity Model	0	0	0	1	2
Foundation........................	0	0	0	3	5
Insurance Products					
Health Maintenance Organization........	7	6	6	8	13
Preferred Provider Organization.........	3	3	5	4	11
Indemnity Fee for Service.............	2	1	2	2	7
Managed Care Contracts					
Health Maintenance Organization........	27	28	33	33	35
Preferred Provider Organization.........	29	30	34	31	33
Affiliations					
Hospitals in a System.................	22	25	25	30	29
Hospitals in a Network	11	7	5	7	8
Hospitals in a Group Purchasing					
Organization.......................	33	38	32	28	25

States

TABLE 6

ARIZONA

U.S. Registered Community Hospitals
(Nonfederal, short-term general and other special hospitals)

Utilization, Personnel, Revenue and Expenses, Community Health Indicators 1998–2002

	2002	2001	2000	1999	1998
TOTAL FACILITY (Includes Hospital and Nursing Home Units)					
Utilization - Inpatient					
Beds	10,930	10,732	10,864	10,576	10,857
Admissions	591,094	562,824	538,704	511,084	495,155
Inpatient Days	2,544,370	2,520,301	2,501,003	2,383,512	2,407,367
Average Length of Stay...........	4.3	4.5	4.6	4.7	4.9
Inpatient Surgeries..............	150,482	159,691	160,251	156,688	150,682
Births........................	85,418	80,408	77,851	74,255	73,470
Utilization - Outpatient					
Emergency Outpatient Visits.......	1,559,078	1,401,509	1,520,393	1,340,258	1,179,377
Other Outpatient Visits...........	3,577,803	3,670,119	3,779,713	3,602,695	3,404,523
Total Outpatient Visits	5,136,881	5,071,628	5,300,106	4,942,953	4,583,900
Outpatient Surgeries	208,797	197,227	212,829	200,933	184,461
Personnel					
Full Time RNs	11,156	10,027	10,777	10,564	9,379
Full Time LPNs	1,115	1,130	1,087	1,074	1,089
Part Time RNs..................	5,226	4,596	5,489	4,490	5,384
Part Time LPNs	388	339	483	342	490
Total Full Time.................	45,502	43,534	44,168	45,637	39,692
Total Part Time	15,229	13,146	16,142	12,958	16,233
Revenue - Inpatient					
Gross Inpatient Revenue..........	$10,826,730,126	$9,022,219,011	$9,060,359,014	$7,422,253,864	$6,671,768,461
Revenue - Outpatient					
Gross Outpatient Revenue	$4,770,650,607	$3,772,046,879	$3,805,828,209	$2,988,190,051	$2,751,942,554
Revenue and Expenses - Totals **(Includes Inpatient and Outpatient)**					
Total Gross Revenue.............	$15,597,380,733	$12,794,265,890	$12,866,187,223	$10,410,443,915	$9,423,711,015
Deductions from Revenue........	9,857,162,745	7,796,688,881	7,953,167,237	6,128,351,767	5,261,902,297
Net Patient Revenue	5,740,217,988	4,997,577,009	4,913,019,986	4,282,092,148	4,161,808,718
Other Operating Revenue	225,138,375	208,436,718	181,210,600	216,768,538	218,272,428
Other Nonoperating Revenue	34,008,928	50,890,354	82,678,089	92,131,062	86,281,497
Total Net Revenue..............	5,999,365,291	5,256,904,081	5,176,908,675	4,590,991,748	4,466,362,643
Total Expenses.................	5,647,682,344	4,986,268,299	4,797,810,319	4,496,686,959	4,146,260,978
HOSPITAL UNIT (Excludes Separate Nursing Home Units)					
Utilization - Inpatient					
Beds	10,653	10,325	10,205	9,687	9,879
Admissions	587,452	556,648	529,994	480,299	481,335
Inpatient Days	2,449,864	2,377,612	2,296,954	2,130,184	2,131,761
Average Length of Stay...........	4.2	4.3	4.3	4.4	4.4
Personnel					
Total Full Time..................	45,138	42,966	43,521	44,926	39,061
Total Part Time	15,130	13,025	15,952	12,773	16,056
Revenue and Expenses - Totals **(Includes Inpatient and Outpatient)**					
Total Net Revenue...............	$5,976,493,274	$5,225,561,891	$5,127,715,363	$4,525,282,814	$4,392,952,619
Total Expenses..................	5,623,701,779	4,951,790,513	4,752,834,132	4,438,540,156	4,083,472,789
COMMUNITY HEALTH INDICATORS PER 1000 POPULATION					
Total Population (in thousands)	5,456	5,307	5,131	4,778	4,667
Inpatient					
Beds	2.0	2.0	2.1	2.2	2.3
Admissions	108.3	106.0	105.0	107.0	106.1
Inpatient Days	466.3	474.9	487.5	498.8	515.8
Inpatient Surgeries..............	27.6	30.1	31.2	32.8	32.3
Births........................	15.7	15.2	15.2	15.5	15.7
Outpatient					
Emergency Outpatient Visits.......	285.7	264.1	296.3	280.5	252.7
Other Outpatient Visits...........	655.7	691.5	736.7	754.0	729.4
Total Outpatient Visits	941.4	955.6	1,033.0	1,034.5	982.1
Outpatient Surgeries	38.3	37.2	41.5	42.1	39.5
Expense per Capita (per person)....	$1,035.0	$939.5	$935.1	$941.1	$888.4

States

TABLE 6

ARKANSAS

U.S. Registered Community Hospitals
(Nonfederal, short-term general and other special hospitals)

Overview 1998–2002

	2002	2001	2000	1999	1998
Total U.S. Community Hospitals in Arkansas............................	87	83	83	83	82
Bed Size Category					
6-24	6	8	5	4	3
25-49	20	17	18	17	18
50-99	28	26	28	29	26
100-199	21	19	18	19	22
200-299	5	6	8	7	7
300-399	5	5	3	4	3
400-499	0	0	0	0	0
500 + ...	2	2	3	3	3
Location					
Hospitals Urban.......................	31	28	28	28	27
Hospitals Rural	56	55	55	55	55
Control					
State and Local Government	15	15	15	16	15
Not for Profit	51	49	49	48	48
Investor owned	21	19	19	19	19
Physician Models					
Independent Practice Association........	18	12	11	7	10
Group Practice without Walls	6	4	4	4	1
Open Physician-Hospital Organization....	29	24	30	24	22
Closed Physician-Hospital Organization...	9	6	7	9	12
Management Service Organization.......	18	12	10	15	16
Integrated Salary Model	15	11	10	7	9
Equity Model	2	0	1	0	0
Foundation..........................	10	11	13	14	15
Insurance Products					
Health Maintenance Organization........	21	17	18	14	15
Preferred Provider Organization.........	30	22	24	19	22
Indemnity Fee for Service..............	8	3	7	6	7
Managed Care Contracts					
Health Maintenance Organization........	48	47	48	36	32
Preferred Provider Organization.........	73	69	68	54	49
Affiliations					
Hospitals in a System..................	46	38	39	32	30
Hospitals in a Network	28	24	25	18	20
Hospitals in a Group Purchasing Organization.......................	79	74	70	51	40

TABLE 6

ARKANSAS

U.S. Registered Community Hospitals
(Nonfederal, short-term general and other special hospitals)

Utilization, Personnel, Revenue and Expenses, Community Health Indicators 1998–2002

	2002	2001	2000	1999	1998
TOTAL FACILITY (Includes Hospital and Nursing Home Units)					
Utilization - Inpatient					
Beds	9,942	9,535	9,784	10,051	9,876
Admissions	383,509	371,080	368,287	375,297	358,068
Inpatient Days	2,110,323	2,034,589	2,092,183	2,195,965	2,108,469
Average Length of Stay...........	5.5	5.5	5.7	5.9	5.9
Inpatient Surgeries...............	119,478	109,244	111,178	104,278	98,224
Births.........................	38,191	36,863	37,723	36,561	34,702
Utilization - Outpatient					
Emergency Outpatient Visits.......	1,224,053	1,152,995	1,170,079	1,073,440	931,213
Other Outpatient Visits...........	3,614,451	3,340,779	3,237,000	2,882,432	3,236,970
Total Outpatient Visits	4,838,504	4,493,774	4,407,079	3,955,872	4,168,183
Outpatient Surgeries	159,314	151,651	154,713	154,726	147,547
Personnel					
Full Time RNs	8,417	8,359	8,817	9,235	8,418
Full Time LPNs	2,717	2,742	2,956	3,088	2,682
Part Time RNs..................	3,744	3,461	3,192	3,186	2,668
Part Time LPNs.................	969	976	879	888	645
Total Full Time.................	36,967	35,358	36,051	38,857	37,029
Total Part Time	11,843	11,629	11,110	10,349	10,143
Revenue - Inpatient					
Gross Inpatient Revenue..........	$5,484,336,913	$4,758,131,946	$4,388,134,177	$3,950,394,296	$3,586,801,167
Revenue - Outpatient					
Gross Outpatient Revenue	$3,139,609,992	$2,687,321,039	$2,451,987,458	$2,145,741,679	$1,995,030,902
Revenue and Expenses - Totals					
(Includes Inpatient and Outpatient)					
Total Gross Revenue.............	$8,623,946,905	$7,445,452,985	$6,840,121,635	$6,096,135,975	$5,581,832,069
Deductions from Revenue........	4,920,059,934	4,144,999,443	3,722,444,602	3,162,771,954	2,722,206,991
Net Patient Revenue	3,703,886,971	3,300,453,542	3,117,677,033	2,933,364,021	2,859,625,078
Other Operating Revenue	134,834,877	103,461,117	95,650,547	95,687,603	103,252,406
Other Nonoperating Revenue	34,677,549	42,618,122	48,896,908	42,627,476	49,083,754
Total Net Revenue..............	3,873,399,397	3,446,532,781	3,262,224,488	3,071,679,100	3,011,961,238
Total Expenses.................	3,612,279,530	3,249,943,830	3,176,562,841	2,972,492,256	2,802,389,937
HOSPITAL UNIT (Excludes Separate Nursing Home Units)					
Utilization - Inpatient					
Beds	9,388	9,041	9,018	9,372	9,188
Admissions	380,945	368,569	364,432	371,400	353,300
Inpatient Days	1,935,371	1,875,344	1,855,365	1,967,250	1,881,151
Average Length of Stay...........	5.1	5.1	5.1	5.3	5.3
Personnel					
Total Full Time.................	36,629	35,066	35,476	38,481	36,506
Total Part Time	11,717	11,549	10,979	10,282	10,023
Revenue and Expenses - Totals					
(Includes Inpatient and Outpatient)					
Total Net Revenue..............	$3,850,828,585	$3,427,559,010	$3,241,028,997	$3,048,845,221	$2,983,447,352
Total Expenses.................	3,598,316,687	3,238,102,085	3,158,262,454	2,951,957,813	2,780,940,022
COMMUNITY HEALTH INDICATORS PER 1000 POPULATION					
Total Population (in thousands)	2,710	2,692	2,673	2,551	2,538
Inpatient					
Beds	3.7	3.5	3.7	3.9	3.9
Admissions	141.5	137.8	137.8	147.1	141.1
Inpatient Days	778.7	755.8	782.6	860.7	830.7
Inpatient Surgeries..............	44.1	40.6	41.6	40.9	38.7
Births.........................	14.1	13.7	14.1	14.3	13.7
Outpatient					
Emergency Outpatient Visits.......	451.7	428.3	437.7	420.7	366.9
Other Outpatient Visits...........	1,333.7	1,241.0	1,210.8	1,129.8	1,275.3
Total Outpatient Visits	1,785.4	1,669.3	1,648.5	1,550.5	1,642.2
Outpatient Surgeries	58.8	56.3	57.9	60.6	58.1
Expense per Capita (per person)....	$1,332.9	$1,207.2	$1,188.2	$1,165.1	$1,104.1

States

TABLE 6

CALIFORNIA

U.S. Registered Community Hospitals
(Nonfederal, short-term general and other special hospitals)

Overview 1998–2002

	2002	2001	2000	1999	1998
Total U.S. Community Hospitals in California	383	384	389	395	405
Bed Size Category					
6-24	10	10	14	16	14
25-49	47	39	38	38	43
50-99	63	67	72	74	77
100-199	114	121	123	121	130
200-299	74	74	73	76	68
300-399	38	38	40	40	45
400-499	20	24	17	18	16
500 +	17	11	12	12	12
Location					
Hospitals Urban	343	344	348	354	364
Hospitals Rural	40	40	41	41	41
Control					
State and Local Government	74	75	71	73	76
Not for Profit	217	220	224	222	226
Investor owned	92	89	94	100	103
Physician Models					
Independent Practice Association	107	100	98	109	135
Group Practice without Walls	18	17	19	18	20
Open Physician-Hospital Organization	14	10	13	11	14
Closed Physician-Hospital Organization	11	17	20	18	21
Management Service Organization	43	39	48	60	74
Integrated Salary Model	35	27	30	35	26
Equity Model	1	1	0	3	3
Foundation	30	24	37	37	44
Insurance Products					
Health Maintenance Organization	50	40	50	64	78
Preferred Provider Organization	29	21	26	36	49
Indemnity Fee for Service	18	10	8	11	20
Managed Care Contracts					
Health Maintenance Organization	180	153	172	187	211
Preferred Provider Organization	184	155	170	185	210
Affiliations					
Hospitals in a System	191	158	153	170	169
Hospitals in a Network	42	37	31	32	33
Hospitals in a Group Purchasing Organization	219	199	172	173	152

TABLE 6

CALIFORNIA

U.S. Registered Community Hospitals
(Nonfederal, short-term general and other special hospitals)

Utilization, Personnel, Revenue and Expenses, Community Health Indicators 1998–2002

	2002	2001	2000	1999	1998
TOTAL FACILITY (Includes Hospital and Nursing Home Units)					
Utilization - Inpatient					
Beds	74,343	73,291	72,707	73,672	74,482
Admissions	3,430,241	3,332,839	3,315,316	3,244,086	3,170,435
Inpatient Days	18,591,536	17,835,799	17,481,600	17,150,813	16,658,170
Average Length of Stay	5.4	5.4	5.3	5.3	5.3
Inpatient Surgeries	978,223	882,138	884,506	843,269	989,428
Births	475,383	493,383	528,444	480,910	488,930
Utilization - Outpatient					
Emergency Outpatient Visits	10,111,529	10,262,726	9,704,390	9,294,157	8,717,395
Other Outpatient Visits	43,221,919	38,284,808	35,240,037	35,484,904	36,312,939
Total Outpatient Visits	53,333,448	48,547,534	44,944,427	44,779,061	45,030,334
Outpatient Surgeries	1,342,641	1,270,674	1,331,626	1,181,547	1,348,773
Personnel					
Full Time RNs	74,071	69,584	63,988	65,955	63,560
Full Time LPNs	9,138	8,885	8,535	8,855	9,032
Part Time RNs	32,758	32,774	45,077	40,309	40,093
Part Time LPNs	2,607	3,008	4,430	3,840	4,395
Total Full Time	319,738	304,856	288,372	291,859	281,708
Total Part Time	92,674	97,102	133,503	115,347	118,499
Revenue - Inpatient					
Gross Inpatient Revenue	$89,111,302,638	$75,039,514,757	$62,888,212,691	$57,872,210,168	$52,606,987,346
Revenue - Outpatient					
Gross Outpatient Revenue	$34,457,820,473	$29,444,438,788	$26,342,290,083	$22,979,554,909	$20,697,199,456
Revenue and Expenses - Totals					
(Includes Inpatient and Outpatient)					
Total Gross Revenue	$123,569,123,111	$104,483,953,545	$89,230,502,774	$80,851,765,077	$73,304,186,802
Deductions from Revenue	82,589,461,723	66,687,816,045	54,071,554,980	48,233,268,070	42,424,919,273
Net Patient Revenue	40,979,661,388	37,796,137,500	35,158,947,794	32,618,497,007	30,879,267,529
Other Operating Revenue	2,256,752,569	1,977,991,741	2,111,614,257	1,920,808,322	1,758,564,441
Other Nonoperating Revenue	1,114,663,017	1,133,993,257	931,691,027	1,113,488,295	930,586,609
Total Net Revenue	44,351,076,974	40,908,122,498	38,202,253,078	35,652,793,624	33,568,418,579
Total Expenses	42,504,560,362	39,559,376,603	37,075,150,430	34,970,489,094	32,167,200,150
HOSPITAL UNIT (Excludes Separate Nursing Home Units)					
Utilization - Inpatient					
Beds	67,012	67,949	69,021	69,254	70,008
Admissions	3,370,381	3,282,183	3,276,996	3,197,409	3,115,912
Inpatient Days	16,560,872	16,282,337	16,393,006	15,871,206	15,371,332
Average Length of Stay	4.9	5.0	5.0	5.0	4.9
Personnel					
Total Full Time	314,423	301,146	285,607	289,021	278,659
Total Part Time	91,515	95,942	132,111	114,039	116,817
Revenue and Expenses - Totals					
(Includes Inpatient and Outpatient)					
Total Net Revenue	$43,726,173,992	$40,457,487,441	$37,843,321,779	$35,260,844,072	$33,192,772,385
Total Expenses	42,020,741,045	39,259,239,984	36,841,630,156	34,701,831,498	31,918,474,511
COMMUNITY HEALTH INDICATORS PER 1000 POPULATION					
Total Population (in thousands)	35,116	34,501	33,872	33,145	32,683
Inpatient					
Beds	2.1	2.1	2.1	2.2	2.3
Admissions	97.7	96.6	97.9	97.9	97.0
Inpatient Days	529.4	517.0	516.1	517.4	509.7
Inpatient Surgeries	27.9	25.6	26.1	25.4	30.3
Births	13.5	14.3	15.6	14.5	15.0
Outpatient					
Emergency Outpatient Visits	287.9	297.5	286.5	280.4	266.7
Other Outpatient Visits	1,230.8	1,109.7	1,040.4	1,070.6	1,111.1
Total Outpatient Visits	1,518.8	1,407.1	1,326.9	1,351.0	1,377.8
Outpatient Surgeries	38.2	36.8	39.3	35.6	41.3
Expense per Capita (per person)	$1,210.4	$1,146.6	$1,094.6	$1,055.1	$984.2

States

TABLE 6

COLORADO

U.S. Registered Community Hospitals
(Nonfederal, short-term general and other special hospitals)

Overview 1998–2002

	2002	2001	2000	1999	1998
Total U.S. Community Hospitals in					
Colorado	68	66	69	67	69
Bed Size Category					
6-24	7	7	9	8	9
25-49	17	16	17	16	19
50-99	16	16	16	16	13
100-199	8	8	8	9	10
200-299	9	7	8	6	6
300-399	8	8	6	8	8
400-499	3	3	5	4	4
500 + ...	0	1	0	0	0
Location					
Hospitals Urban.....................	32	31	32	32	33
Hospitals Rural	36	35	37	35	36
Control					
State and Local Government	27	26	28	27	27
Not for Profit	32	32	32	32	32
Investor owned	9	8	9	8	10
Physician Models					
Independent Practice Association........	8	8	7	9	15
Group Practice without Walls	4	1	2	3	4
Open Physician-Hospital Organization....	12	8	14	16	14
Closed Physician-Hospital Organization...	5	3	8	4	3
Management Service Organization.......	7	6	7	7	16
Integrated Salary Model	22	18	16	17	17
Equity Model	2	0	1	1	1
Foundation.........................	4	4	5	4	4
Insurance Products					
Health Maintenance Organization........	7	8	11	11	12
Preferred Provider Organization.........	9	8	13	13	15
Indemnity Fee for Service.............	3	2	4	4	12
Managed Care Contracts					
Health Maintenance Organization........	41	38	45	51	48
Preferred Provider Organization.........	41	39	46	48	43
Affiliations					
Hospitals in a System................	22	22	26	19	22
Hospitals in a Network	18	20	21	17	22
Hospitals in a Group Purchasing					
Organization......................	46	46	50	46	38

States

TABLE 6

COLORADO

U.S. Registered Community Hospitals
(Nonfederal, short-term general and other special hospitals)

Utilization, Personnel, Revenue and Expenses, Community Health Indicators 1998–2002

	2002	2001	2000	1999	1998
TOTAL FACILITY (Includes Hospital and Nursing Home Units)					
Utilization - Inpatient					
Beds	9,575	9,442	9,391	9,349	9,179
Admissions	426,560	413,605	397,026	383,283	373,257
Inpatient Days	2,172,074	2,111,549	1,986,526	1,947,693	1,875,297
Average Length of Stay.	5.1	5.1	5.0	5.1	5.0
Inpatient Surgeries	129,569	124,570	125,630	121,742	132,188
Births	65,284	61,708	61,859	54,800	54,806
Utilization - Outpatient					
Emergency Outpatient Visits	1,501,013	1,380,740	1,377,130	1,324,504	1,176,404
Other Outpatient Visits.	5,511,485	5,531,785	5,335,591	5,115,007	4,869,311
Total Outpatient Visits	7,012,498	6,912,525	6,712,721	6,439,511	6,045,715
Outpatient Surgeries	185,162	201,029	219,396	207,411	192,979
Personnel					
Full Time RNs	10,881	10,136	9,656	9,417	9,609
Full Time LPNs	960	824	694	820	957
Part Time RNs	4,522	4,179	4,346	4,221	4,656
Part Time LPNs	298	280	283	317	390
Total Full Time	44,913	43,027	39,556	39,830	40,766
Total Part Time	13,444	12,781	13,204	12,649	14,345
Revenue - Inpatient					
Gross Inpatient Revenue	$8,494,295,044	$7,227,257,609	$5,902,881,921	$5,465,908,323	$4,873,956,748
Revenue - Outpatient					
Gross Outpatient Revenue	$4,938,808,685	$4,189,489,714	$3,614,340,221	$3,052,304,763	$2,621,444,182
Revenue and Expenses - Totals					
(Includes Inpatient and Outpatient)					
Total Gross Revenue	$13,433,103,729	$11,416,747,323	$9,517,222,142	$8,518,213,086	$7,495,400,930
Deductions from Revenue	7,638,320,935	6,439,372,017	4,994,563,358	4,429,949,594	3,602,908,633
Net Patient Revenue	5,794,782,794	4,977,375,306	4,522,658,784	4,088,263,492	3,892,492,297
Other Operating Revenue	250,396,757	479,100,659	321,544,924	244,779,945	191,236,964
Other Nonoperating Revenue	97,026,733	141,537,462	106,349,090	99,153,654	79,577,825
Total Net Revenue	6,142,206,284	5,598,013,427	4,950,552,798	4,432,197,091	4,163,307,086
Total Expenses.	5,472,452,136	4,948,616,302	4,453,861,107	4,188,116,091	3,797,350,129
HOSPITAL UNIT (Excludes Separate Nursing Home Units)					
Utilization - Inpatient					
Beds	8,890	8,661	8,715	8,695	8,532
Admissions	423,839	410,743	394,223	379,249	369,151
Inpatient Days	1,966,328	1,867,438	1,767,350	1,749,055	1,672,531
Average Length of Stay.	4.6	4.5	4.5	4.6	4.5
Personnel					
Total Full Time	44,448	42,445	39,056	39,356	40,168
Total Part Time	13,270	12,595	12,997	12,429	14,113
Revenue and Expenses - Totals					
(Includes Inpatient and Outpatient)					
Total Net Revenue	$6,107,394,817	$5,547,464,684	$4,922,342,002	$4,401,477,273	$4,130,522,694
Total Expenses.	5,440,791,541	4,910,277,563	4,425,039,103	4,161,145,943	3,772,942,264
COMMUNITY HEALTH INDICATORS PER 1000 POPULATION					
Total Population (in thousands)	4,507	4,418	4,301	4,056	3,969
Inpatient					
Beds	2.1	2.1	2.2	2.3	2.3
Admissions	94.7	93.6	92.3	94.5	94.0
Inpatient Days	482.0	478.0	461.8	480.2	472.5
Inpatient Surgeries	28.8	28.2	29.2	30.0	33.3
Births	14.5	14.0	14.4	13.5	13.8
Outpatient					
Emergency Outpatient Visits	333.1	312.5	320.2	326.5	296.4
Other Outpatient Visits.	1,223.0	1,252.2	1,240.5	1,261.1	1,226.8
Total Outpatient Visits	1,556.1	1,564.7	1,560.6	1,587.6	1,523.2
Outpatient Surgeries	41.1	45.5	51.0	51.1	48.6
Expense per Capita (per person). . . .	$1,214.3	$1,120.2	$1,035.5	$1,032.5	$956.8

TABLE 6

CONNECTICUT

U.S. Registered Community Hospitals
(Nonfederal, short-term general and other special hospitals)

Overview 1998–2002

	2002	2001	2000	1999	1998
Total U.S. Community Hospitals in					
Connecticut.........................	35	35	35	35	33
Bed Size Category					
6-24	0	0	0	0	0
25-49	0	1	1	0	0
50-99	10	10	10	10	10
100-199	11	9	11	11	11
200-299	5	6	4	7	7
300-399	5	4	4	2	1
400-499	0	1	1	1	1
500 + ...	4	4	4	4	3
Location					
Hospitals Urban......................	29	29	29	29	27
Hospitals Rural	6	6	6	6	6
Control					
State and Local Government	1	1	1	2	2
Not for Profit	34	34	33	33	31
Investor owned	0	0	1	0	0
Physician Models					
Independent Practice Association........	10	12	12	15	16
Group Practice without Walls	1	2	3	5	3
Open Physician-Hospital Organization....	13	13	14	17	14
Closed Physician-Hospital Organization...	0	2	2	4	3
Management Service Organization.......	6	7	8	10	14
Integrated Salary Model	6	5	5	8	8
Equity Model	0	0	0	0	1
Foundation.........................	0	2	2	1	1
Insurance Products					
Health Maintenance Organization........	2	9	12	15	18
Preferred Provider Organization.........	5	7	7	7	11
Indemnity Fee for Service..............	0	0	0	0	0
Managed Care Contracts					
Health Maintenance Organization........	25	28	32	32	31
Preferred Provider Organization.........	24	27	30	29	28
Affiliations					
Hospitals in a System.................	18	16	17	18	17
Hospitals in a Network	10	11	15	12	10
Hospitals in a Group Purchasing					
Organization.......................	27	29	32	31	24

TABLE 6

CONNECTICUT

U.S. Registered Community Hospitals
(Nonfederal, short-term general and other special hospitals)

Utilization, Personnel, Revenue and Expenses, Community Health Indicators 1998–2002

	2002	2001	2000	1999	1998
TOTAL FACILITY (Includes Hospital and Nursing Home Units)					
Utilization - Inpatient					
Beds	7,714	8,041	7,719	7,872	6,949
Admissions	375,686	360,007	348,780	337,821	330,091
Inpatient Days	2,239,055	2,184,918	2,114,362	2,070,480	1,758,052
Average Length of Stay	6.0	6.1	6.1	6.1	5.3
Inpatient Surgeries	108,975	102,924	101,548	105,211	105,163
Births	42,607	42,694	42,839	43,063	42,915
Utilization - Outpatient					
Emergency Outpatient Visits	1,392,274	1,328,651	1,323,999	1,344,816	1,164,247
Other Outpatient Visits	5,249,471	5,160,775	5,409,523	5,473,361	5,334,173
Total Outpatient Visits	6,641,745	6,489,426	6,733,522	6,818,177	6,498,420
Outpatient Surgeries	190,334	192,473	192,522	185,381	179,562
Personnel					
Full Time RNs	7,275	6,817	6,784	6,597	6,664
Full Time LPNs	403	323	360	331	345
Part Time RNs	6,952	6,866	5,413	5,727	5,378
Part Time LPNs	431	397	321	363	415
Total Full Time	36,424	35,996	34,079	33,264	33,281
Total Part Time	22,010	22,275	19,311	19,557	18,364
Revenue - Inpatient					
Gross Inpatient Revenue	$6,057,484,644	$5,235,105,389	$4,793,838,712	$4,607,260,826	$4,282,299,864
Revenue - Outpatient					
Gross Outpatient Revenue	$3,680,120,901	$3,092,163,110	$2,787,895,246	$2,554,529,729	$2,215,490,372
Revenue and Expenses - Totals					
(Includes Inpatient and Outpatient)					
Total Gross Revenue	$9,737,605,545	$8,327,268,499	$7,581,733,958	$7,161,790,555	$6,497,790,236
Deductions from Revenue	4,688,468,374	3,787,142,271	3,417,644,028	3,082,461,893	2,620,865,505
Net Patient Revenue	5,049,137,171	4,540,126,228	4,164,089,930	4,079,328,662	3,876,924,731
Other Operating Revenue	190,947,384	187,046,158	180,038,222	235,827,532	221,385,804
Other Nonoperating Revenue	37,644,997	89,196,050	139,597,475	130,391,249	131,068,417
Total Net Revenue	5,277,729,552	4,816,368,436	4,483,725,627	4,445,547,443	4,229,378,952
Total Expenses	5,243,316,266	4,718,315,413	4,396,429,072	4,339,548,425	4,060,531,565
HOSPITAL UNIT (Excludes Separate Nursing Home Units)					
Utilization - Inpatient					
Beds	7,228	7,262	6,854	7,007	6,845
Admissions	374,638	358,242	347,414	336,878	329,790
Inpatient Days	2,036,015	1,863,319	1,795,186	1,781,174	1,721,983
Average Length of Stay	5.4	5.2	5.2	5.3	5.2
Personnel					
Total Full Time	36,321	35,093	33,092	32,782	33,200
Total Part Time	21,930	21,647	18,570	19,062	18,306
Revenue and Expenses - Totals					
(Includes Inpatient and Outpatient)					
Total Net Revenue	$5,229,759,070	$4,750,389,473	$4,425,572,619	$4,401,579,596	$4,214,483,042
Total Expenses	5,183,998,846	4,644,731,988	4,334,999,636	4,295,663,582	4,051,497,724
COMMUNITY HEALTH INDICATORS PER 1000 POPULATION					
Total Population (in thousands)	3,461	3,425	3,406	3,282	3,273
Inpatient					
Beds	2.2	2.3	2.3	2.4	2.1
Admissions	108.6	105.1	102.4	102.9	100.9
Inpatient Days	647.0	637.9	620.9	630.9	537.2
Inpatient Surgeries	31.5	30.1	29.8	32.1	32.1
Births	12.3	12.5	12.6	13.1	13.1
Outpatient					
Emergency Outpatient Visits	402.3	387.9	388.8	409.8	355.8
Other Outpatient Visits	1,517.0	1,506.8	1,588.4	1,667.7	1,630.0
Total Outpatient Visits	1,919.3	1,894.7	1,977.2	2,077.4	1,985.7
Outpatient Surgeries	55.0	56.2	56.5	56.5	54.9
Expense per Capita (per person)	$1,515.2	$1,377.6	$1,291.0	$1,322.2	$1,240.8

States

TABLE **6**

DELAWARE

U.S. Registered Community Hospitals
(Nonfederal, short-term general and other special hospitals)

Overview 1998–2002

	2002	2001	2000	1999	1998
Total U.S. Community Hospitals in Delaware	6	5	5	6	6
Bed Size Category					
6-24	0	0	0	0	0
25-49	0	0	0	0	0
50-99	0	0	0	0	0
100-199	2	1	0	1	1
200-299	2	2	3	3	3
300-399	1	1	1	1	1
400-499	0	0	0	0	0
500 +	1	1	1	1	1
Location					
Hospitals Urban	4	3	3	4	4
Hospitals Rural	2	2	2	2	2
Control					
State and Local Government	0	0	0	0	0
Not for Profit	6	5	5	6	6
Investor owned	0	0	0	0	0
Physician Models					
Independent Practice Association	0	0	1	1	1
Group Practice without Walls	0	0	0	0	0
Open Physician-Hospital Organization	1	1	1	2	2
Closed Physician-Hospital Organization	0	0	1	1	1
Management Service Organization	0	0	0	0	0
Integrated Salary Model	4	2	3	2	2
Equity Model	0	0	0	0	0
Foundation	0	0	0	1	1
Insurance Products					
Health Maintenance Organization	1	1	1	1	2
Preferred Provider Organization	1	0	0	0	0
Indemnity Fee for Service	1	0	0	0	0
Managed Care Contracts					
Health Maintenance Organization	5	4	3	6	6
Preferred Provider Organization	5	4	3	6	6
Affiliations					
Hospitals in a System	3	3	2	4	4
Hospitals in a Network	0	0	0	0	0
Hospitals in a Group Purchasing Organization	6	5	4	6	4

States

TABLE 6

DELAWARE

U.S. Registered Community Hospitals
(Nonfederal, short-term general and other special hospitals)

Utilization, Personnel, Revenue and Expenses, Community Health Indicators 1998–2002

	2002	2001	2000	1999	1998
TOTAL FACILITY (Includes Hospital and Nursing Home Units)					
Utilization - Inpatient					
Beds	2,014	1,853	1,839	2,000	1,977
Admissions	93,275	83,047	83,318	87,200	84,319
Inpatient Days	546,058	502,238	505,422	492,551	508,870
Average Length of Stay	5.9	6.0	6.1	5.6	6.0
Inpatient Surgeries	29,696	24,321	25,878	27,295	27,420
Births	11,350	11,286	11,375	10,896	10,775
Utilization - Outpatient					
Emergency Outpatient Visits	305,634	268,517	286,231	285,276	267,369
Other Outpatient Visits	1,642,184	1,216,401	1,175,657	1,062,037	1,028,481
Total Outpatient Visits	1,947,818	1,484,918	1,461,888	1,347,313	1,295,850
Outpatient Surgeries	66,987	57,342	52,972	66,234	61,375
Personnel					
Full Time RNs	2,609	2,058	2,179	2,455	2,042
Full Time LPNs	198	171	174	173	163
Part Time RNs	1,671	1,522	1,433	1,347	1,061
Part Time LPNs	86	77	74	84	79
Total Full Time	12,044	9,465	9,412	8,772	8,775
Total Part Time	4,759	3,936	3,798	3,933	3,234
Revenue - Inpatient					
Gross Inpatient Revenue	$1,257,109,446	$934,270,274	$899,982,681	$931,058,817	$866,020,507
Revenue - Outpatient					
Gross Outpatient Revenue	$697,074,088	$543,554,090	$465,864,889	$474,399,061	$454,760,376
Revenue and Expenses - Totals (Includes Inpatient and Outpatient)					
Total Gross Revenue	$1,954,183,534	$1,477,824,364	$1,365,847,570	$1,405,457,878	$1,320,780,883
Deductions from Revenue	821,168,346	535,555,319	484,935,362	489,660,170	412,465,075
Net Patient Revenue	1,133,015,188	942,269,045	880,912,208	915,797,708	908,315,808
Other Operating Revenue	81,264,100	64,471,002	120,518,768	102,355,170	88,643,163
Other Nonoperating Revenue	-14,105,872	-6,015,492	39,475,261	43,155,449	39,565,691
Total Net Revenue	1,200,173,416	1,000,724,555	1,040,906,237	1,061,308,327	1,036,524,662
Total Expenses	1,201,883,266	1,049,014,326	1,020,468,822	990,513,404	962,105,695
HOSPITAL UNIT (Excludes Separate Nursing Home Units)					
Utilization - Inpatient					
Beds	1,686	1,561	1,561	1,786	1,699
Admissions	91,880	81,719	82,238	85,787	83,107
Inpatient Days	440,860	395,736	405,399	421,774	416,541
Average Length of Stay	4.8	4.8	4.9	4.9	5.0
Personnel					
Total Full Time	11,753	9,181	9,194	8,625	8,516
Total Part Time	4,630	3,806	3,736	3,846	3,139
Revenue and Expenses - Totals (Includes Inpatient and Outpatient)					
Total Net Revenue	$1,174,652,121	$978,200,536	$1,003,754,485	$1,042,456,545	$1,019,156,844
Total Expenses	1,174,014,509	1,023,947,668	1,004,383,808	968,889,580	945,393,771
COMMUNITY HEALTH INDICATORS PER 1000 POPULATION					
Total Population (in thousands)	807	796	784	754	744
Inpatient					
Beds	2.5	2.3	2.3	2.7	2.7
Admissions	115.5	104.3	106.3	115.7	113.3
Inpatient Days	676.3	630.8	645.0	653.7	683.9
Inpatient Surgeries	36.8	30.5	33.0	36.2	36.9
Births	14.1	14.2	14.5	14.5	14.5
Outpatient					
Emergency Outpatient Visits	378.5	337.3	365.3	378.6	359.3
Other Outpatient Visits	2,034.0	1,527.8	1,500.3	1,409.4	1,382.2
Total Outpatient Visits	2,412.5	1,865.1	1,865.6	1,788.0	1,741.6
Outpatient Surgeries	83.0	72.0	67.6	87.9	82.5
Expense per Capita (per person)	$1,488.6	$1,317.6	$1,302.3	$1,314.5	$1,293.0

States

TABLE 6

DISTRICT OF COLUMBIA

U.S. Registered Community Hospitals
(Nonfederal, short-term general and other special hospitals)

Overview 1998–2002

	2002	2001	2000	1999	1998
Total U.S. Community Hospitals in District of Columbia	10	10	11	12	12
Bed Size Category					
6-24	0	0	0	0	0
25-49	0	0	0	0	0
50-99	0	0	1	1	1
100-199	3	3	3	3	3
200-299	1	2	3	4	4
300-399	4	3	2	2	2
400-499	0	0	0	0	0
500 + ...	2	2	2	2	2
Location					
Hospitals Urban......................	10	10	11	12	12
Hospitals Rural	0	0	0	0	0
Control					
State and Local Government	0	0	0	1	1
Not for Profit	7	7	8	8	9
Investor owned	3	3	3	3	2
Physician Models					
Independent Practice Association........	1	0	0	2	2
Group Practice without Walls	0	1	1	0	1
Open Physician-Hospital Organization....	1	1	2	1	1
Closed Physician-Hospital Organization...	2	2	2	3	2
Management Service Organization.......	1	1	2	3	3
Integrated Salary Model	4	5	4	5	6
Equity Model	0	0	0	0	0
Foundation..........................	0	0	0	0	0
Insurance Products					
Health Maintenance Organization........	3	4	4	5	5
Preferred Provider Organization.........	1	1	2	0	1
Indemnity Fee for Service..............	0	0	1	0	0
Managed Care Contracts					
Health Maintenance Organization........	8	8	7	9	11
Preferred Provider Organization.........	6	7	7	6	9
Affiliations					
Hospitals in a System.................	5	6	4	5	5
Hospitals in a Network	0	2	2	1	1
Hospitals in a Group Purchasing Organization......................	7	7	7	8	9

TABLE 6

DISTRICT OF COLUMBIA

U.S. Registered Community Hospitals
(Nonfederal, short-term general and other special hospitals)

Utilization, Personnel, Revenue and Expenses, Community Health Indicators 1998–2002

	2002	2001	2000	1999	1998
TOTAL FACILITY (Includes Hospital and Nursing Home Units)					
Utilization - Inpatient					
Beds	3,352	3,372	3,339	3,541	3,552
Admissions	137,172	131,906	129,056	138,408	140,293
Inpatient Days	936,124	903,469	901,167	984,094	977,258
Average Length of Stay	6.8	6.8	7.0	7.1	7.0
Inpatient Surgeries	43,815	42,789	58,333	61,982	47,272
Births	13,843	12,583	11,439	11,824	15,211
Utilization - Outpatient					
Emergency Outpatient Visits	352,942	337,851	284,075	330,143	354,334
Other Outpatient Visits	1,173,119	1,081,197	1,047,332	1,053,206	1,101,426
Total Outpatient Visits	1,526,061	1,419,048	1,331,407	1,383,349	1,455,760
Outpatient Surgeries	62,102	55,491	74,848	95,860	62,753
Personnel					
Full Time RNs	3,700	3,731	4,041	4,249	3,940
Full Time LPNs	285	261	286	324	237
Part Time RNs	1,835	1,695	1,908	1,328	1,852
Part Time LPNs	75	64	93	99	66
Total Full Time	18,939	18,187	18,519	17,209	17,756
Total Part Time	5,321	4,877	5,266	4,514	4,937
Revenue - Inpatient					
Gross Inpatient Revenue	$3,403,763,454	$3,109,126,002	$2,730,685,206	$2,761,995,772	$2,704,578,426
Revenue - Outpatient					
Gross Outpatient Revenue	$1,443,430,513	$1,192,439,734	$963,364,001	$972,983,386	$853,089,506
Revenue and Expenses - Totals					
(Includes Inpatient and Outpatient)					
Total Gross Revenue	$4,847,193,967	$4,301,565,736	$3,694,049,207	$3,734,979,158	$3,557,667,932
Deductions from Revenue	2,709,835,364	2,344,359,123	1,987,583,335	2,036,092,141	1,956,975,216
Net Patient Revenue	2,137,358,603	1,957,206,613	1,706,465,872	1,698,887,017	1,600,692,716
Other Operating Revenue	153,122,453	151,214,377	111,158,200	144,298,148	181,047,807
Other Nonoperating Revenue	-14,807,356	42,742,302	53,069,156	97,579,393	82,508,594
Total Net Revenue	2,275,673,700	2,151,163,292	1,870,693,228	1,940,764,558	1,864,249,117
Total Expenses	2,313,103,242	2,157,226,423	1,845,801,885	1,971,499,970	1,819,975,151
HOSPITAL UNIT (Excludes Separate Nursing Home Units)					
Utilization - Inpatient					
Beds	3,052	3,080	3,056	3,256	3,199
Admissions	135,377	130,307	127,615	136,998	139,094
Inpatient Days	833,747	804,586	803,418	880,583	858,824
Average Length of Stay	6.2	6.2	6.3	6.4	6.2
Personnel					
Total Full Time	18,654	17,880	18,235	16,977	17,403
Total Part Time	5,234	4,755	5,163	4,409	4,747
Revenue and Expenses - Totals					
(Includes Inpatient and Outpatient)					
Total Net Revenue	$2,244,040,209	$2,119,026,870	$1,846,118,330	$1,910,666,848	$1,828,063,922
Total Expenses	2,282,999,519	2,130,816,375	1,824,373,545	1,946,444,149	1,804,493,901
COMMUNITY HEALTH INDICATORS PER 1000 POPULATION					
Total Population (in thousands)	571	572	572	519	521
Inpatient					
Beds	5.9	5.9	5.8	6.8	6.8
Admissions	240.3	230.7	225.6	266.7	269.1
Inpatient Days	1,639.7	1,580.0	1,575.3	1,896.1	1,874.2
Inpatient Surgeries	76.7	74.8	102.0	119.4	90.7
Births	24.2	22.0	20.0	22.8	29.2
Outpatient					
Emergency Outpatient Visits	618.2	590.8	496.6	636.1	679.5
Other Outpatient Visits	2,054.9	1,890.8	1,830.8	2,029.3	2,112.3
Total Outpatient Visits	2,673.1	2,481.6	2,327.4	2,665.4	2,791.9
Outpatient Surgeries	108.8	97.0	130.8	184.7	120.3
Expense per Capita (per person)	$4,051.7	$3,772.5	$3,226.6	$3,798.7	$3,490.4

States

TABLE 6

FLORIDA

U.S. Registered Community Hospitals
(Nonfederal, short-term general and other special hospitals)

Overview 1998–2002

	2002	2001	2000	1999	1998
Total U.S. Community Hospitals in					
Florida	**202**	**202**	**202**	**203**	**204**
Bed Size Category					
6-24	3	2	2	3	5
25-49	21	21	22	20	15
50-99	29	30	27	32	29
100-199	50	51	53	52	57
200-299	38	37	38	37	41
300-399	27	24	24	24	23
400-499	11	14	14	13	13
500 + ...	23	23	22	22	21
Location					
Hospitals Urban.....................	170	170	171	172	173
Hospitals Rural	32	32	31	31	31
Control					
State and Local Government	20	20	19	24	21
Not for Profit	86	87	88	86	90
Investor owned	96	95	95	93	93
Physician Models					
Independent Practice Association........	9	22	22	21	27
Group Practice without Walls	2	6	7	7	10
Open Physician-Hospital Organization....	16	20	24	23	29
Closed Physician-Hospital Organization...	7	7	13	18	22
Management Service Organization.......	13	16	27	30	37
Integrated Salary Model	27	30	29	31	30
Equity Model	1	1	2	3	1
Foundation	1	1	2	4	4
Insurance Products					
Health Maintenance Organization........	16	20	25	30	30
Preferred Provider Organization.........	17	19	22	34	38
Indemnity Fee for Service.............	8	8	10	3	7
Managed Care Contracts					
Health Maintenance Organization........	93	90	94	97	103
Preferred Provider Organization.........	98	97	96	96	106
Affiliations					
Hospitals in a System.................	90	88	88	91	84
Hospitals in a Network	36	31	31	38	29
Hospitals in a Group Purchasing					
Organization......................	110	98	93	89	73

States

TABLE 6   **FLORIDA**

U.S. Registered Community Hospitals
(Nonfederal, short-term general and other special hospitals)

Utilization, Personnel, Revenue and Expenses, Community Health Indicators 1998–2002

	2002	2001	2000	1999	1998
TOTAL FACILITY (Includes Hospital and Nursing Home Units)					
Utilization - Inpatient					
Beds	51,201	51,762	51,170	49,434	49,231
Admissions	2,315,230	2,207,147	2,119,052	2,020,073	1,947,024
Inpatient Days	12,303,559	11,521,025	11,345,469	11,135,544	10,839,718
Average Length of Stay	5.3	5.2	5.4	5.5	5.6
Inpatient Surgeries	688,383	660,330	614,345	570,283	597,151
Births	208,996	204,753	193,344	180,857	180,131
Utilization - Outpatient					
Emergency Outpatient Visits	6,623,448	5,879,596	6,041,546	5,488,609	5,285,638
Other Outpatient Visits	15,866,843	14,891,198	15,752,042	14,210,881	14,160,604
Total Outpatient Visits	22,490,291	20,770,794	21,793,588	19,699,490	19,446,242
Outpatient Surgeries	912,233	857,272	816,677	803,554	825,987
Personnel					
Full Time RNs	49,218	48,277	47,635	45,140	44,510
Full Time LPNs	6,111	6,224	6,258	6,898	6,345
Part Time RNs	16,534	14,235	17,432	15,741	14,439
Part Time LPNs	1,615	1,550	1,799	1,894	1,614
Total Full Time	203,256	198,925	193,653	186,175	186,555
Total Part Time	49,095	40,983	52,267	48,474	43,501
Revenue - Inpatient					
Gross Inpatient Revenue	$46,105,920,999	$38,526,016,053	$36,166,618,934	$30,772,909,076	$28,063,792,535
Revenue - Outpatient					
Gross Outpatient Revenue	$21,541,764,183	$17,579,375,385	$16,339,412,601	$14,207,698,162	$12,690,404,737
Revenue and Expenses - Totals					
(Includes Inpatient and Outpatient)					
Total Gross Revenue	$67,647,685,182	$56,105,391,438	$52,506,031,535	$44,980,607,238	$40,754,197,272
Deductions from Revenue	44,385,926,589	35,545,733,610	33,270,201,252	27,234,827,859	23,887,698,462
Net Patient Revenue	23,261,758,593	20,559,657,828	19,235,830,283	17,745,779,379	16,866,498,810
Other Operating Revenue	1,443,094,405	1,232,856,710	1,060,248,158	993,711,653	915,677,497
Other Nonoperating Revenue	113,856,010	287,972,889	516,162,789	438,224,356	404,349,404
Total Net Revenue	24,818,709,008	22,080,487,427	20,812,241,230	19,177,715,388	18,186,525,711
Total Expenses	23,194,124,932	20,475,866,330	19,289,627,098	17,522,447,345	16,741,873,851
HOSPITAL UNIT (Excludes Separate Nursing Home Units)					
Utilization - Inpatient					
Beds	49,786	49,865	48,979	47,342	46,735
Admissions	2,304,044	2,193,104	2,098,216	1,999,574	1,923,396
Inpatient Days	11,864,811	10,918,750	10,688,767	10,464,347	10,058,943
Average Length of Stay	5.1	5.0	5.1	5.2	5.2
Personnel					
Total Full Time	201,890	197,587	191,191	183,992	184,283
Total Part Time	48,872	40,716	51,396	47,889	42,974
Revenue and Expenses - Totals					
(Includes Inpatient and Outpatient)					
Total Net Revenue	$24,696,657,727	$21,928,434,635	$20,649,613,293	$18,999,058,161	$17,971,784,870
Total Expenses	23,082,690,334	20,345,809,450	19,160,212,008	17,374,197,783	16,582,856,855
COMMUNITY HEALTH INDICATORS PER 1000 POPULATION					
Total Population (in thousands)	16,713	16,397	15,982	15,111	14,908
Inpatient					
Beds	3.1	3.2	3.2	3.3	3.3
Admissions	138.5	134.6	132.6	133.7	130.6
Inpatient Days	736.2	702.7	709.9	736.9	727.1
Inpatient Surgeries	41.2	40.3	38.4	37.7	40.1
Births	12.5	12.5	12.1	12.0	12.1
Outpatient					
Emergency Outpatient Visits	396.3	358.6	378.0	363.2	354.5
Other Outpatient Visits	949.4	908.2	985.6	940.4	949.9
Total Outpatient Visits	1,345.7	1,266.8	1,363.6	1,303.6	1,304.4
Outpatient Surgeries	54.6	52.3	51.1	53.2	55.4
Expense per Capita (per person)	$1,387.8	$1,248.8	$1,206.9	$1,159.6	$1,123.0

States

TABLE **6**

GEORGIA

U.S. Registered Community Hospitals
(Nonfederal, short-term general and other special hospitals)

Overview 1998–2002

	2002	2001	2000	1999	1998
Total U.S. Community Hospitals in					
Georgia	146	147	151	154	156
Bed Size Category					
6-24	7	4	5	4	5
25-49	30	34	36	36	36
50-99	25	28	28	23	24
100-199	42	42	43	51	49
200-299	15	13	14	14	16
300-399	12	10	11	14	13
400-499	10	9	9	9	10
500 + ...	5	7	5	3	3
Location					
Hospitals Urban......................	63	64	67	68	68
Hospitals Rural	83	83	84	86	88
Control					
State and Local Government	52	53	56	55	60
Not for Profit	64	62	62	63	58
Investor owned	30	32	33	36	38
Physician Models					
Independent Practice Association........	15	16	18	16	15
Group Practice without Walls	1	2	4	2	3
Open Physician-Hospital Organization....	22	22	21	21	21
Closed Physician-Hospital Organization...	18	24	25	16	19
Management Service Organization.......	14	17	17	15	16
Integrated Salary Model	25	18	26	14	10
Equity Model	2	2	2	1	2
Foundation.........................	5	4	4	3	2
Insurance Products					
Health Maintenance Organization........	9	14	16	20	18
Preferred Provider Organization.........	39	41	36	43	42
Indemnity Fee for Service..............	9	10	9	8	11
Managed Care Contracts					
Health Maintenance Organization........	56	58	65	60	56
Preferred Provider Organization.........	99	98	103	111	102
Affiliations					
Hospitals in a System................	66	73	75	76	60
Hospitals in a Network	62	69	61	58	54
Hospitals in a Group Purchasing					
Organization......................	103	109	103	98	79

States

TABLE 6

GEORGIA

U.S. Registered Community Hospitals
(Nonfederal, short-term general and other special hospitals)

Utilization, Personnel, Revenue and Expenses, Community Health Indicators 1998–2002

	2002	2001	2000	1999	1998
TOTAL FACILITY (Includes Hospital and Nursing Home Units)					
Utilization - Inpatient					
Beds	24,500	24,113	23,875	24,784	25,236
Admissions	885,142	903,663	862,797	824,376	821,895
Inpatient Days	5,774,911	5,484,805	5,479,389	5,625,261	5,471,839
Average Length of Stay	6.5	6.1	6.4	6.8	6.7
Inpatient Surgeries	288,573	284,283	257,624	257,164	270,264
Births	128,981	130,673	129,084	113,784	113,640
Utilization - Outpatient					
Emergency Outpatient Visits	3,227,698	3,149,115	3,128,275	2,854,136	2,731,084
Other Outpatient Visits	9,256,245	8,865,939	8,113,649	7,984,774	7,574,974
Total Outpatient Visits	12,483,943	12,015,054	11,241,924	10,838,910	10,306,058
Outpatient Surgeries	511,906	497,614	459,852	429,526	417,725
Personnel					
Full Time RNs	22,730	21,881	22,259	20,681	21,335
Full Time LPNs	4,063	3,888	3,466	3,854	3,793
Part Time RNs	12,269	12,896	11,977	8,977	8,896
Part Time LPNs	1,189	1,224	1,147	1,147	1,447
Total Full Time	98,246	95,397	92,094	90,711	92,013
Total Part Time	32,518	34,238	32,304	27,457	26,545
Revenue - Inpatient					
Gross Inpatient Revenue	$14,445,750,952	$12,699,629,255	$11,757,965,146	$10,148,108,959	$9,941,881,557
Revenue - Outpatient					
Gross Outpatient Revenue	$9,240,551,617	$7,748,463,309	$7,353,248,681	$5,911,411,142	$5,326,318,708
Revenue and Expenses - Totals					
(Includes Inpatient and Outpatient)					
Total Gross Revenue	$23,686,302,569	$20,448,092,564	$19,111,213,827	$16,059,520,101	$15,268,200,265
Deductions from Revenue	13,112,710,432	10,910,867,874	9,922,910,066	7,822,591,409	7,054,393,279
Net Patient Revenue	10,573,592,137	9,537,224,690	9,188,303,761	8,236,928,692	8,213,806,986
Other Operating Revenue	553,755,731	582,210,731	496,378,760	632,168,142	437,251,429
Other Nonoperating Revenue	29,263,979	247,374,354	242,231,703	227,205,059	252,900,681
Total Net Revenue	11,156,611,847	10,366,809,775	9,926,914,224	9,096,301,893	8,903,959,096
Total Expenses	10,576,054,877	9,839,984,105	9,217,250,307	8,225,718,150	7,934,635,819
HOSPITAL UNIT (Excludes Separate Nursing Home Units)					
Utilization - Inpatient					
Beds	20,655	20,813	20,138	20,540	21,826
Admissions	880,499	898,539	856,482	816,709	815,273
Inpatient Days	4,466,878	4,396,989	4,184,817	4,200,321	4,378,494
Average Length of Stay	5.1	4.9	4.9	5.1	5.4
Personnel					
Total Full Time	95,471	93,155	89,656	88,053	89,896
Total Part Time	31,711	33,610	31,527	26,714	25,932
Revenue and Expenses - Totals					
(Includes Inpatient and Outpatient)					
Total Net Revenue	$11,012,776,470	$10,228,892,959	$9,802,309,486	$8,956,729,154	$8,778,169,228
Total Expenses	10,446,159,150	9,716,646,918	9,104,562,407	8,091,415,980	7,806,605,169
COMMUNITY HEALTH INDICATORS PER 1000 POPULATION					
Total Population (in thousands)	8,560	8,384	8,186	7,788	7,637
Inpatient					
Beds	2.9	2.9	2.9	3.2	3.3
Admissions	103.4	107.8	105.4	105.8	107.6
Inpatient Days	674.6	654.2	669.3	722.3	716.5
Inpatient Surgeries	33.7	33.9	31.5	33.0	35.4
Births	15.1	15.6	15.8	14.6	14.9
Outpatient					
Emergency Outpatient Visits	377.1	375.6	382.1	366.5	357.6
Other Outpatient Visits	1,081.3	1,057.5	991.1	1,025.2	991.9
Total Outpatient Visits	1,458.4	1,433.1	1,373.2	1,391.7	1,349.6
Outpatient Surgeries	59.8	59.4	56.2	55.2	54.7
Expense per Capita (per person)	$1,235.5	$1,173.7	$1,125.9	$1,056.2	$1,039.0

TABLE 6

HAWAII

U.S. Registered Community Hospitals
(Nonfederal, short-term general and other special hospitals)

Overview 1998–2002

	2002	2001	2000	1999	1998
Total U.S. Community Hospitals in Hawaii	25	23	21	22	20
Bed Size Category					
6-24	3	2	2	2	2
25-49	5	4	3	4	3
50-99	3	4	3	3	2
100-199	9	8	8	10	10
200-299	4	4	4	2	2
300-399	0	0	0	0	0
400-499	1	1	1	1	1
500 +	0	0	0	0	0
Location					
Hospitals Urban	13	13	12	12	12
Hospitals Rural	12	10	9	10	8
Control					
State and Local Government	7	8	7	8	6
Not for Profit	18	14	13	13	13
Investor owned	0	1	1	1	1
Physician Models					
Independent Practice Association	3	4	6	5	4
Group Practice without Walls	0	0	0	1	1
Open Physician-Hospital Organization	1	3	4	5	5
Closed Physician-Hospital Organization	1	0	0	0	0
Management Service Organization	0	0	0	1	1
Integrated Salary Model	3	2	2	2	2
Equity Model	0	0	0	1	1
Foundation	1	1	1	1	1
Insurance Products					
Health Maintenance Organization	3	3	3	6	7
Preferred Provider Organization	1	2	2	5	5
Indemnity Fee for Service	0	1	1	1	2
Managed Care Contracts					
Health Maintenance Organization	13	11	11	14	11
Preferred Provider Organization	9	9	7	10	9
Affiliations					
Hospitals in a System	15	13	13	15	10
Hospitals in a Network	1	2	3	2	1
Hospitals in a Group Purchasing Organization	14	16	14	14	7

TABLE 6

HAWAII

U.S. Registered Community Hospitals
(Nonfederal, short-term general and other special hospitals)

Utilization, Personnel, Revenue and Expenses, Community Health Indicators 1998–2002

	2002	2001	2000	1999	1998
TOTAL FACILITY (Includes Hospital and Nursing Home Units)					
Utilization - Inpatient					
Beds..........................	3,191	3,235	3,057	2,913	2,791
Admissions....................	111,498	108,252	99,937	99,191	97,717
Inpatient Days.................	866,160	879,258	847,352	769,824	776,392
Average Length of Stay..........	7.8	8.1	8.5	7.8	7.9
Inpatient Surgeries..............	32,059	31,003	28,912	30,001	31,497
Births.......................	15,845	10,007	9,903	10,148	11,054
Utilization - Outpatient					
Emergency Outpatient Visits.......	311,713	287,017	253,452	239,560	306,804
Other Outpatient Visits..........	1,652,619	2,880,570	2,212,552	2,197,092	2,153,289
Total Outpatient Visits...........	1,964,332	3,167,587	2,466,004	2,436,652	2,460,093
Outpatient Surgeries	52,498	52,624	46,250	45,328	49,842
Personnel					
Full Time RNs	3,328	2,727	3,002	2,738	2,778
Full Time LPNs	410	420	395	423	459
Part Time RNs.................	1,353	1,409	968	1,053	1,198
Part Time LPNs	112	138	93	81	107
Total Full Time.................	13,264	12,621	11,854	11,697	13,116
Total Part Time	3,791	3,953	3,051	2,978	3,521
Revenue - Inpatient					
Gross Inpatient Revenue..........	$2,089,877,140	$1,932,544,979	$1,803,657,551	$1,649,885,281	$1,555,005,916
Revenue - Outpatient					
Gross Outpatient Revenue	$1,175,498,990	$1,063,359,978	$826,991,000	$730,624,505	$668,609,149
Revenue and Expenses - Totals					
(Includes Inpatient and Outpatient)					
Total Gross Revenue.............	$3,265,376,130	$2,995,904,957	$2,630,648,551	$2,380,509,786	$2,223,615,065
Deductions from Revenue.........	1,773,759,884	1,574,104,007	1,382,408,955	1,199,936,747	1,076,694,668
Net Patient Revenue	1,491,616,246	1,421,800,950	1,248,239,596	1,180,573,039	1,146,920,397
Other Operating Revenue	87,285,962	82,464,076	70,164,871	74,945,697	58,805,480
Other Nonoperating Revenue	-1,274,071	30,318,193	33,274,738	28,166,307	29,810,902
Total Net Revenue..............	1,577,628,137	1,534,583,219	1,351,679,205	1,283,685,043	1,235,536,779
Total Expenses.................	1,640,541,613	1,587,146,492	1,360,759,208	1,273,162,963	1,207,907,910
HOSPITAL UNIT (Excludes Separate Nursing Home Units)					
Utilization - Inpatient					
Beds..........................	2,766	2,704	2,511	2,386	2,459
Admissions....................	109,535	106,717	97,822	96,915	95,879
Inpatient Days.................	730,123	704,963	676,735	594,519	664,731
Average Length of Stay...........	6.7	6.6	6.9	6.1	6.9
Personnel					
Total Full Time.................	13,053	12,228	11,517	11,299	12,729
Total Part Time	3,758	3,889	2,992	2,885	3,429
Revenue and Expenses - Totals					
(Includes Inpatient and Outpatient)					
Total Net Revenue..............	$1,555,292,196	$1,513,078,577	$1,331,297,637	$1,255,628,493	$1,215,412,826
Total Expenses.................	1,615,200,267	1,567,775,123	1,342,654,703	1,246,855,789	1,189,371,784
COMMUNITY HEALTH INDICATORS PER 1000 POPULATION					
Total Population (in thousands)	1,245	1,224	1,212	1,185	1,190
Inpatient					
Beds..........................	2.6	2.6	2.5	2.5	2.3
Admissions....................	89.6	88.4	82.5	83.7	82.1
Inpatient Days.................	695.8	718.1	699.4	649.4	652.2
Inpatient Surgeries..............	25.8	25.3	23.9	25.3	26.5
Births.......................	12.7	8.2	8.2	8.6	9.3
Outpatient					
Emergency Outpatient Visits.......	250.4	234.4	209.2	202.1	257.7
Other Outpatient Visits..........	1,327.5	2,352.6	1,826.2	1,853.3	1,808.8
Total Outpatient Visits...........	1,577.9	2,587.1	2,035.4	2,055.4	2,066.5
Outpatient Surgeries	42.2	43.0	38.2	38.2	41.9
Expense per Capita (per person)....	$1,317.8	$1,296.3	$1,123.2	$1,073.9	$1,014.6

States

TABLE 6

IDAHO

U.S. Registered Community Hospitals
(Nonfederal, short-term general and other special hospitals)

Overview 1998–2002

	2002	2001	2000	1999	1998
Total U.S. Community Hospitals in					
Idaho	39	40	42	42	42
Bed Size Category					
6-24	11	9	8	8	8
25-49	8	8	11	10	13
50-99	9	12	12	13	10
100-199	6	6	6	6	6
200-299	3	3	3	4	4
300-399	1	2	2	1	1
400-499	1	0	0	0	0
500 + ...	0	0	0	0	0
Location					
Hospitals Urban......................	6	7	7	7	7
Hospitals Rural	33	33	35	35	35
Control					
State and Local Government	24	27	28	28	26
Not for Profit	13	11	11	11	13
Investor owned	2	2	3	3	3
Physician Models					
Independent Practice Association........	6	6	5	7	5
Group Practice without Walls	1	1	0	2	1
Open Physician-Hospital Organization....	6	6	8	10	12
Closed Physician-Hospital Organization...	5	5	4	2	2
Management Service Organization.......	1	1	1	2	1
Integrated Salary Model	4	7	5	5	7
Equity Model	1	1	0	1	0
Foundation..........................	0	0	0	3	2
Insurance Products					
Health Maintenance Organization........	6	7	6	5	6
Preferred Provider Organization.........	6	8	9	6	6
Indemnity Fee for Service..............	3	4	5	5	4
Managed Care Contracts					
Health Maintenance Organization........	10	12	11	13	17
Preferred Provider Organization.........	17	22	19	19	22
Affiliations					
Hospitals in a System.................	5	6	7	8	7
Hospitals in a Network	13	17	13	14	11
Hospitals in a Group Purchasing					
Organization......................	25	28	29	27	26

States

TABLE **6**

IDAHO

U.S. Registered Community Hospitals
(Nonfederal, short-term general and other special hospitals)

Utilization, Personnel, Revenue and Expenses, Community Health Indicators 1998–2002

	2002	2001	2000	1999	1998
TOTAL FACILITY (Includes Hospital and Nursing Home Units)					
Utilization - Inpatient					
Beds	3,349	3,439	3,485	3,499	3,414
Admissions	123,046	122,510	123,187	119,928	115,248
Inpatient Days	648,640	682,010	669,186	694,361	697,744
Average Length of Stay	5.3	5.6	5.4	5.8	6.1
Inpatient Surgeries	40,816	41,062	38,270	38,624	35,403
Births	19,601	19,672	17,738	17,990	17,258
Utilization - Outpatient					
Emergency Outpatient Visits	445,100	411,533	409,030	414,388	380,805
Other Outpatient Visits	1,942,986	2,228,545	1,748,372	1,767,925	1,795,095
Total Outpatient Visits	2,388,086	2,640,078	2,157,402	2,182,313	2,175,900
Outpatient Surgeries	60,626	57,886	53,171	60,607	66,258
Personnel					
Full Time RNs	3,045	2,411	2,370	2,556	2,337
Full Time LPNs	533	489	502	525	502
Part Time RNs	2,034	1,918	1,759	1,676	1,736
Part Time LPNs	309	275	310	324	330
Total Full Time	13,827	11,650	11,074	11,354	10,698
Total Part Time	6,716	6,681	5,678	5,373	6,036
Revenue - Inpatient					
Gross Inpatient Revenue	$1,689,244,058	$1,311,305,096	$1,243,357,709	$1,132,120,798	$1,028,373,427
Revenue - Outpatient					
Gross Outpatient Revenue	$875,193,822	$841,069,903	$785,301,536	$682,496,769	$625,389,911
Revenue and Expenses - Totals					
(Includes Inpatient and Outpatient)					
Total Gross Revenue	$2,564,437,880	$2,152,374,999	$2,028,659,245	$1,814,617,567	$1,653,763,338
Deductions from Revenue	1,085,024,888	817,619,918	826,933,247	675,699,809	581,633,458
Net Patient Revenue	1,479,412,992	1,334,755,081	1,201,725,998	1,138,917,758	1,072,129,880
Other Operating Revenue	62,644,590	43,219,742	42,583,119	55,873,470	35,587,970
Other Nonoperating Revenue	17,699,166	38,074,932	28,837,697	31,708,471	33,445,442
Total Net Revenue	1,559,756,748	1,416,049,755	1,273,146,814	1,226,499,699	1,141,163,292
Total Expenses	1,488,003,696	1,313,949,886	1,167,101,520	1,116,899,654	1,005,344,536
HOSPITAL UNIT (Excludes Separate Nursing Home Units)					
Utilization - Inpatient					
Beds	2,744	2,828	2,874	2,816	2,785
Admissions	120,656	119,945	120,655	115,670	111,251
Inpatient Days	478,779	504,028	497,049	503,844	512,257
Average Length of Stay	4.0	4.2	4.1	4.4	4.6
Personnel					
Total Full Time	13,513	11,265	10,801	10,839	10,163
Total Part Time	6,443	6,431	5,396	5,097	5,743
Revenue and Expenses - Totals					
(Includes Inpatient and Outpatient)					
Total Net Revenue	$1,529,409,854	$1,390,073,406	$1,249,236,753	$1,191,632,434	$1,104,782,133
Total Expenses	1,465,901,906	1,292,299,636	1,151,521,698	1,093,475,829	978,344,737
COMMUNITY HEALTH INDICATORS PER 1000 POPULATION					
Total Population (in thousands)	1,341	1,321	1,294	1,252	1,231
Inpatient					
Beds	2.5	2.6	2.7	2.8	2.8
Admissions	91.7	92.7	95.2	95.8	93.6
Inpatient Days	483.7	516.3	517.2	554.7	566.8
Inpatient Surgeries	30.4	31.1	29.6	30.9	28.8
Births	14.6	14.9	13.7	14.4	14.0
Outpatient					
Emergency Outpatient Visits	331.9	311.5	316.1	331.1	309.4
Other Outpatient Visits	1,448.8	1,687.0	1,351.2	1,412.4	1,458.3
Total Outpatient Visits	1,780.7	1,998.5	1,667.3	1,743.5	1,767.7
Outpatient Surgeries	45.2	43.8	41.1	48.4	53.8
Expense per Capita (per person)	$1,109.5	$994.7	$902.0	$892.3	$816.7

States

TABLE **6**

ILLINOIS

U.S. Registered Community Hospitals
(Nonfederal, short-term general and other special hospitals)

Overview 1998–2002

	2002	2001	2000	1999	1998
Total U.S. Community Hospitals in					
Illinois	192	192	196	198	203
Bed Size Category					
6-24	6	3	4	3	2
25-49	18	18	18	20	18
50-99	39	36	34	37	42
100-199	63	67	68	66	69
200-299	31	29	33	34	32
300-399	17	21	21	19	18
400-499	6	7	7	6	9
500 + ...	12	11	11	13	13
Location					
Hospitals Urban......................	120	120	124	125	131
Hospitals Rural	72	72	72	73	72
Control					
State and Local Government	29	28	28	30	31
Not for Profit	154	156	159	161	158
Investor owned	9	8	9	7	14
Physician Models					
Independent Practice Association........	36	36	42	42	49
Group Practice without Walls	7	8	9	7	9
Open Physician-Hospital Organization....	50	53	51	51	53
Closed Physician-Hospital Organization...	16	14	19	26	29
Management Service Organization.......	28	37	42	48	50
Integrated Salary Model	52	50	65	65	60
Equity Model	3	2	2	4	3
Foundation.........................	9	9	11	10	15
Insurance Products					
Health Maintenance Organization........	26	27	35	48	57
Preferred Provider Organization.........	28	29	35	44	53
Indemnity Fee for Service..............	7	10	15	11	12
Managed Care Contracts					
Health Maintenance Organization........	121	122	140	143	144
Preferred Provider Organization.........	140	141	153	161	157
Affiliations					
Hospitals in a System.................	95	98	102	103	104
Hospitals in a Network	31	32	32	38	41
Hospitals in a Group Purchasing					
Organization......................	146	150	158	153	143

TABLE 6

ILLINOIS

U.S. Registered Community Hospitals
(Nonfederal, short-term general and other special hospitals)

Utilization, Personnel, Revenue and Expenses, Community Health Indicators 1998–2002

	2002	2001	2000	1999	1998
TOTAL FACILITY (Includes Hospital and Nursing Home Units)					
Utilization - Inpatient					
Beds	36,309	36,834	37,310	37,658	39,218
Admissions	1,615,269	1,559,357	1,530,800	1,508,816	1,466,273
Inpatient Days	8,326,561	8,215,380	8,189,818	8,267,158	8,640,319
Average Length of Stay	5.2	5.3	5.4	5.5	5.9
Inpatient Surgeries	429,366	414,121	404,231	387,355	391,333
Births	172,338	173,967	179,057	176,435	175,567
Utilization - Outpatient					
Emergency Outpatient Visits	4,699,328	4,582,408	4,497,815	4,420,908	4,325,178
Other Outpatient Visits	21,811,988	20,687,505	20,601,748	19,495,093	18,449,726
Total Outpatient Visits	26,511,316	25,269,913	25,099,563	23,916,001	22,774,904
Outpatient Surgeries	745,579	710,346	691,824	654,078	634,897
Personnel					
Full Time RNs	32,720	33,093	33,905	34,481	33,335
Full Time LPNs	2,608	2,781	2,789	3,042	3,280
Part Time RNs	25,875	23,596	21,807	21,044	21,929
Part Time LPNs	1,361	1,116	1,239	1,186	1,332
Total Full Time	156,627	160,545	161,303	157,818	155,054
Total Part Time	80,497	71,502	69,069	65,200	71,091
Revenue - Inpatient					
Gross Inpatient Revenue	$27,722,800,143	$24,926,910,293	$22,597,529,237	$20,652,014,700	$19,762,078,685
Revenue - Outpatient					
Gross Outpatient Revenue	$15,980,470,692	$14,044,549,597	$12,699,517,400	$11,241,559,394	$10,261,730,664
Revenue and Expenses - Totals					
(Includes Inpatient and Outpatient)					
Total Gross Revenue	$43,703,270,835	$38,971,459,890	$35,297,046,637	$31,893,574,094	$30,023,809,349
Deductions from Revenue	25,017,360,640	21,796,610,516	19,210,165,443	17,010,439,012	15,152,657,271
Net Patient Revenue	18,685,910,195	17,174,849,374	16,086,881,194	14,883,135,082	14,871,152,078
Other Operating Revenue	1,174,384,266	1,057,250,792	984,694,243	846,212,294	960,315,367
Other Nonoperating Revenue	56,898,594	384,325,832	937,308,890	975,103,585	804,130,431
Total Net Revenue	19,917,193,055	18,616,425,998	18,008,884,327	16,704,450,961	16,635,597,876
Total Expenses	19,597,944,423	18,304,829,361	17,215,623,885	16,050,659,864	15,467,918,335
HOSPITAL UNIT (Excludes Separate Nursing Home Units)					
Utilization - Inpatient					
Beds	33,876	33,998	33,695	33,806	34,791
Admissions	1,588,707	1,526,030	1,495,873	1,469,587	1,425,365
Inpatient Days	7,652,143	7,417,273	7,180,518	7,202,654	7,335,025
Average Length of Stay	4.8	4.9	4.8	4.9	5.1
Personnel					
Total Full Time	154,973	158,634	158,538	154,891	151,705
Total Part Time	79,653	70,507	67,735	63,943	69,441
Revenue and Expenses - Totals					
(Includes Inpatient and Outpatient)					
Total Net Revenue	$19,771,409,995	$18,410,732,829	$17,824,208,519	$16,449,642,798	$16,317,362,510
Total Expenses	19,476,432,848	18,152,199,024	17,076,598,221	15,858,782,696	15,180,165,418
COMMUNITY HEALTH INDICATORS PER 1000 POPULATION					
Total Population (in thousands)	12,601	12,482	12,419	12,128	12,070
Inpatient					
Beds	2.9	3.0	3.0	3.1	3.2
Admissions	128.2	124.9	123.3	124.4	121.5
Inpatient Days	660.8	658.2	659.4	681.6	715.9
Inpatient Surgeries	34.1	33.2	32.5	31.9	32.4
Births	13.7	13.9	14.4	14.5	14.5
Outpatient					
Emergency Outpatient Visits	372.9	367.1	362.2	364.5	358.3
Other Outpatient Visits	1,731.0	1,657.3	1,658.9	1,607.4	1,528.6
Total Outpatient Visits	2,104.0	2,024.5	2,021.0	1,971.9	1,886.9
Outpatient Surgeries	59.2	56.9	55.7	53.9	52.6
Expense per Capita (per person)	$1,555.3	$1,466.5	$1,386.2	$1,323.4	$1,281.5

TABLE 6

INDIANA

U.S. Registered Community Hospitals
(Nonfederal, short-term general and other special hospitals)

Overview 1998–2002

	2002	2001	2000	1999	1998
Total U.S. Community Hospitals in					
Indiana.............................	112	110	109	111	111
Bed Size Category					
6-24	5	5	4	5	3
25-49	23	21	22	23	22
50-99	33	30	29	30	29
100-199	21	24	24	23	27
200-299	13	13	13	13	13
300-399	6	5	5	5	5
400-499	3	4	3	4	5
500 + ...	8	8	9	8	7
Location					
Hospitals Urban......................	67	64	64	65	65
Hospitals Rural	45	46	45	46	46
Control					
State and Local Government	40	41	41	45	45
Not for Profit	58	57	56	54	55
Investor owned	14	12	12	12	11
Physician Models					
Independent Practice Association........	14	15	15	10	13
Group Practice without Walls	4	4	1	0	2
Open Physician-Hospital Organization....	29	26	32	31	35
Closed Physician-Hospital Organization...	13	14	16	14	14
Management Service Organization.......	16	17	20	19	24
Integrated Salary Model	37	31	32	36	31
Equity Model	0	1	1	1	2
Foundation..........................	3	2	1	4	5
Insurance Products					
Health Maintenance Organization........	17	20	32	34	32
Preferred Provider Organization.........	31	28	42	42	41
Indemnity Fee for Service..............	6	8	11	11	11
Managed Care Contracts					
Health Maintenance Organization........	65	60	73	72	73
Preferred Provider Organization.........	78	71	82	86	89
Affiliations					
Hospitals in a System.................	40	34	41	36	35
Hospitals in a Network	41	36	40	32	37
Hospitals in a Group Purchasing					
Organization......................	87	78	87	84	86

States

TABLE 6

INDIANA

U.S. Registered Community Hospitals
(Nonfederal, short-term general and other special hospitals)

Utilization, Personnel, Revenue and Expenses, Community Health Indicators 1998–2002

	2002	2001	2000	1999	1998
TOTAL FACILITY (Includes Hospital and Nursing Home Units)					
Utilization - Inpatient					
Beds	18,961	19,036	19,160	19,225	19,401
Admissions	715,936	718,369	699,511	683,264	704,396
Inpatient Days	4,077,032	3,944,457	3,943,695	3,998,799	4,076,111
Average Length of Stay...........	5.7	5.5	5.6	5.9	5.8
Inpatient Surgeries..............	199,279	195,206	216,204	189,678	196,317
Births.........................	78,921	80,485	81,052	75,076	76,706
Utilization - Outpatient					
Emergency Outpatient Visits.......	2,437,268	2,385,242	2,187,447	2,120,329	2,154,402
Other Outpatient Visits...........	11,650,167	12,008,043	11,946,547	10,993,509	10,580,210
Total Outpatient Visits	14,087,435	14,393,285	14,133,994	13,113,838	12,734,612
Outpatient Surgeries	416,641	386,704	388,192	408,893	393,135
Personnel					
Full Time RNs	17,176	15,997	17,308	17,831	17,156
Full Time LPNs	2,408	2,486	2,430	2,373	2,222
Part Time RNs	11,544	10,944	11,696	10,222	11,039
Part Time LPNs	1,399	1,344	1,403	1,207	1,286
Total Full Time.................	79,408	77,258	76,219	75,902	76,533
Total Part Time	35,876	35,540	35,901	32,134	33,137
Revenue - Inpatient					
Gross Inpatient Revenue..........	$10,700,904,487	$9,449,404,551	$8,288,484,221	$7,574,440,688	$7,344,203,384
Revenue - Outpatient					
Gross Outpatient Revenue	$7,508,632,761	$6,380,741,910	$5,799,391,724	$5,058,777,890	$4,638,804,328
Revenue and Expenses - Totals					
(Includes Inpatient and Outpatient)					
Total Gross Revenue.............	$18,209,537,248	$15,830,146,461	$14,087,875,945	$12,633,218,578	$11,983,007,712
Deductions from Revenue.........	8,632,745,626	7,243,961,000	6,058,831,246	5,130,679,610	4,768,195,948
Net Patient Revenue	9,576,791,622	8,586,185,461	8,029,044,699	7,502,538,968	7,214,811,764
Other Operating Revenue	433,611,706	501,261,342	496,781,927	439,652,541	416,591,590
Other Nonoperating Revenue	63,204,269	145,445,011	282,308,259	262,145,842	235,353,311
Total Net Revenue..............	10,073,607,597	9,232,891,814	8,808,134,885	8,204,337,351	7,866,756,665
Total Expenses.................	9,272,854,799	8,446,387,337	7,865,789,801	7,490,717,665	7,192,794,077
HOSPITAL UNIT (Excludes Separate Nursing Home Units)					
Utilization - Inpatient					
Beds	17,867	17,157	16,957	16,801	17,110
Admissions	704,094	705,746	684,461	664,977	687,644
Inpatient Days	3,751,265	3,404,916	3,337,863	3,341,593	3,393,449
Average Length of Stay...........	5.3	4.8	4.9	5.0	4.9
Personnel					
Total Full Time.................	78,630	75,807	74,693	74,041	74,493
Total Part Time	35,272	34,952	35,169	31,265	32,362
Revenue and Expenses - Totals					
(Includes Inpatient and Outpatient)					
Total Net Revenue..............	$9,996,393,418	$9,142,546,269	$8,721,330,380	$8,064,204,896	$7,720,270,403
Total Expenses.................	9,204,932,252	8,353,731,881	7,780,952,771	7,368,487,400	7,062,481,912
COMMUNITY HEALTH INDICATORS PER 1000 POPULATION					
Total Population (in thousands)	6,159	6,115	6,080	5,943	5,908
Inpatient					
Beds	3.1	3.1	3.2	3.2	3.3
Admissions	116.2	117.5	115.0	115.0	119.2
Inpatient Days	662.0	645.1	648.6	672.9	690.0
Inpatient Surgeries..............	32.4	31.9	35.6	31.9	33.2
Births.........................	12.8	13.2	13.3	12.6	13.0
Outpatient					
Emergency Outpatient Visits.......	395.7	390.1	359.7	356.8	364.7
Other Outpatient Visits...........	1,891.5	1,963.8	1,964.7	1,849.9	1,790.9
Total Outpatient Visits	2,287.3	2,353.9	2,324.5	2,206.6	2,155.6
Outpatient Surgeries	67.6	63.2	63.8	68.8	66.5
Expense per Capita (per person)....	$1,505.6	$1,381.3	$1,293.6	$1,260.4	$1,217.5

TABLE 6

IOWA

U.S. Registered Community Hospitals
(Nonfederal, short-term general and other special hospitals)

Overview 1998–2002

	2002	2001	2000	1999	1998
Total U.S. Community Hospitals in Iowa..	116	116	115	115	116
Bed Size Category					
6-24	12	12	11	11	12
25-49	45	42	41	40	39
50-99	29	31	29	31	31
100-199	14	15	17	18	18
200-299	7	7	8	6	7
300-399	5	5	5	5	4
400-499	2	2	2	2	3
500 +	2	2	2	2	2
Location					
Hospitals Urban	21	21	21	21	21
Hospitals Rural	95	95	94	94	95
Control					
State and Local Government	59	59	58	59	61
Not for Profit	57	56	57	56	54
Investor owned	0	1	0	0	1
Physician Models					
Independent Practice Association	21	14	15	17	14
Group Practice without Walls	3	4	3	3	4
Open Physician-Hospital Organization	18	21	21	20	20
Closed Physician-Hospital Organization	17	17	19	20	21
Management Service Organization	12	14	13	15	14
Integrated Salary Model	51	44	41	39	35
Equity Model	3	1	1	0	4
Foundation	3	4	6	7	9
Insurance Products					
Health Maintenance Organization	18	17	18	21	20
Preferred Provider Organization	35	34	40	40	39
Indemnity Fee for Service	8	7	6	6	7
Managed Care Contracts					
Health Maintenance Organization	66	69	69	70	64
Preferred Provider Organization	96	98	100	104	97
Affiliations					
Hospitals in a System	52	52	50	49	46
Hospitals in a Network	59	55	52	46	38
Hospitals in a Group Purchasing Organization	105	109	108	104	100

TABLE 6

IOWA

U.S. Registered Community Hospitals
(Nonfederal, short-term general and other special hospitals)

Utilization, Personnel, Revenue and Expenses, Community Health Indicators 1998–2002

	2002	2001	2000	1999	1998
TOTAL FACILITY (Includes Hospital and Nursing Home Units)					
Utilization - Inpatient					
Beds	11,267	11,538	11,811	11,838	12,219
Admissions	370,968	370,885	359,682	359,142	374,245
Inpatient Days	2,447,672	2,491,172	2,493,185	2,498,984	2,528,052
Average Length of Stay...........	6.6	6.7	6.9	7.0	6.8
Inpatient Surgeries..............	106,987	107,252	105,897	105,951	110,705
Births..........................	37,342	37,628	37,692	37,162	37,496
Utilization - Outpatient					
Emergency Outpatient Visits	1,072,319	1,063,304	1,050,606	1,051,682	982,497
Other Outpatient Visits............	8,258,357	8,336,049	8,106,385	7,511,574	6,768,865
Total Outpatient Visits	9,330,676	9,399,353	9,156,991	8,563,256	7,751,362
Outpatient Surgeries	302,995	289,647	289,715	280,264	266,352
Personnel					
Full Time RNs	8,967	8,519	8,855	8,581	9,049
Full Time LPNs	996	904	897	826	940
Part Time RNs..................	7,391	7,027	6,698	6,988	6,848
Part Time LPNs.................	836	818	757	781	887
Total Full Time...............	41,179	40,716	40,602	39,836	39,655
Total Part Time	25,648	25,215	23,512	23,967	23,606
Revenue - Inpatient					
Gross Inpatient Revenue..........	$4,245,474,792	$3,868,944,808	$3,523,992,700	$3,291,048,997	$3,155,651,791
Revenue - Outpatient					
Gross Outpatient Revenue	$3,390,410,867	$2,990,618,965	$2,693,739,475	$2,389,853,804	$2,158,066,967
Revenue and Expenses - Totals					
(Includes Inpatient and Outpatient)					
Total Gross Revenue..............	$7,635,885,659	$6,859,563,773	$6,217,732,175	$5,680,902,801	$5,313,718,758
Deductions from Revenue.........	3,333,435,082	2,824,125,097	2,466,317,174	2,114,838,477	1,958,777,267
Net Patient Revenue	4,302,450,577	4,035,438,676	3,751,415,001	3,566,064,324	3,354,941,491
Other Operating Revenue	328,828,491	319,656,799	308,982,657	265,943,571	257,812,692
Other Nonoperating Revenue	51,699,288	93,484,169	83,255,612	90,128,303	101,543,557
Total Net Revenue..............	4,682,978,356	4,448,579,644	4,143,653,270	3,922,136,198	3,714,297,740
Total Expenses.................	4,483,595,177	4,202,394,287	3,932,103,219	3,669,806,143	3,452,505,145
HOSPITAL UNIT (Excludes Separate Nursing Home Units)					
Utilization - Inpatient					
Beds	9,038	9,251	9,481	9,440	9,677
Admissions	360,065	359,577	347,688	345,654	340,869
Inpatient Days	1,723,431	1,748,201	1,739,816	1,733,617	1,705,889
Average Length of Stay...........	4.8	4.9	5.0	5.0	5.0
Personnel					
Total Full Time...............	40,108	39,690	39,540	38,830	38,421
Total Part Time	24,625	24,220	22,599	23,099	22,445
Revenue and Expenses - Totals					
(Includes Inpatient and Outpatient)					
Total Net Revenue..............	$4,581,452,200	$4,348,039,384	$4,048,875,825	$3,830,086,493	$3,580,062,378
Total Expenses.................	4,406,423,753	4,123,430,546	3,857,836,935	3,590,355,032	3,333,491,525
COMMUNITY HEALTH INDICATORS PER 1000 POPULATION					
Total Population (in thousands)	2,937	2,923	2,926	2,869	2,861
Inpatient					
Beds	3.8	3.9	4.0	4.1	4.3
Admissions	126.3	126.9	122.9	125.2	130.8
Inpatient Days	833.5	852.2	852.0	870.9	883.6
Inpatient Surgeries..............	36.4	36.7	36.2	36.9	38.7
Births..........................	12.7	12.9	12.9	13.0	13.1
Outpatient					
Emergency Outpatient Visits	365.1	363.7	359.0	366.5	343.4
Other Outpatient Visits............	2,812.1	2,851.7	2,770.2	2,617.8	2,365.9
Total Outpatient Visits	3,177.2	3,215.5	3,129.2	2,984.3	2,709.3
Outpatient Surgeries	103.2	99.1	99.0	97.7	93.1
Expense per Capita (per person)....	$1,526.7	$1,437.6	$1,343.7	$1,278.9	$1,206.7

States

TABLE 6

KANSAS

U.S. Registered Community Hospitals
(Nonfederal, short-term general and other special hospitals)

Overview 1998–2002

	2002	2001	2000	1999	1998
Total U.S. Community Hospitals in Kansas..........................	132	133	129	131	129
Bed Size Category					
6-24	15	15	18	17	16
25-49	42	44	39	41	47
50-99	50	46	46	44	36
100-199	14	18	16	17	19
200-299	6	5	5	7	6
300-399	2	2	3	3	2
400-499	2	2	1	0	1
500 + ...	1	1	1	2	2
Location					
Hospitals Urban......................	25	28	25	26	24
Hospitals Rural	107	105	104	105	105
Control					
State and Local Government	61	62	63	63	65
Not for Profit	62	62	60	61	57
Investor owned	9	9	6	7	7
Physician Models					
Independent Practice Association........	16	19	15	12	15
Group Practice without Walls	5	9	7	7	7
Open Physician-Hospital Organization....	18	19	19	21	22
Closed Physician-Hospital Organization...	4	3	4	3	3
Management Service Organization.......	5	5	6	12	15
Integrated Salary Model	45	45	42	43	38
Equity Model	0	0	0	0	1
Foundation.........................	3	2	5	10	9
Insurance Products					
Health Maintenance Organization........	7	9	15	16	18
Preferred Provider Organization.........	22	21	23	27	28
Indemnity Fee for Service..............	6	6	7	6	9
Managed Care Contracts					
Health Maintenance Organization........	41	48	41	45	43
Preferred Provider Organization.........	105	108	106	103	100
Affiliations					
Hospitals in a System.................	56	56	54	55	52
Hospitals in a Network	73	76	79	76	74
Hospitals in a Group Purchasing Organization......................	121	124	119	115	110

TABLE 6

KANSAS

U.S. Registered Community Hospitals
(Nonfederal, short-term general and other special hospitals)

Utilization, Personnel, Revenue and Expenses, Community Health Indicators 1998–2002

	2002	2001	2000	1999	1998
TOTAL FACILITY (Includes Hospital and Nursing Home Units)					
Utilization - Inpatient					
Beds	10,850	11,211	10,821	11,615	10,923
Admissions	328,987	322,067	310,256	326,352	299,701
Inpatient Days	2,165,195	2,175,989	2,081,932	2,232,737	2,148,493
Average Length of Stay	6.6	6.8	6.7	6.8	7.2
Inpatient Surgeries	88,704	86,949	84,051	91,259	81,732
Births	38,591	37,847	37,599	38,971	36,168
Utilization - Outpatient					
Emergency Outpatient Visits	940,408	907,083	889,390	921,066	809,296
Other Outpatient Visits	4,734,607	4,486,945	4,365,883	4,103,314	3,894,843
Total Outpatient Visits	5,675,015	5,394,028	5,255,273	5,024,380	4,704,139
Outpatient Surgeries	155,965	161,789	162,669	176,375	159,197
Personnel					
Full Time RNs	7,600	6,906	7,158	7,601	7,196
Full Time LPNs	1,138	1,079	1,038	1,075	1,025
Part Time RNs	4,088	4,041	4,072	4,415	3,826
Part Time LPNs	558	549	523	590	520
Total Full Time	33,790	32,609	31,548	33,931	34,496
Total Part Time	14,290	14,668	13,944	12,984	11,555
Revenue - Inpatient					
Gross Inpatient Revenue	$4,837,931,215	$4,299,715,760	$3,829,510,816	$3,772,245,204	$3,394,554,236
Revenue - Outpatient					
Gross Outpatient Revenue	$3,020,822,797	$2,632,758,324	$2,374,823,658	$2,198,345,422	$1,926,917,284
Revenue and Expenses - Totals					
(Includes Inpatient and Outpatient)					
Total Gross Revenue	$7,858,754,012	$6,932,474,084	$6,204,334,474	$5,970,590,626	$5,321,471,520
Deductions from Revenue	4,306,839,200	3,693,649,527	3,189,390,696	2,949,255,620	2,551,924,564
Net Patient Revenue	3,551,914,812	3,238,824,557	3,014,943,778	3,021,335,006	2,769,546,956
Other Operating Revenue	150,197,636	162,388,962	147,629,759	144,033,337	128,359,530
Other Nonoperating Revenue	18,174,135	42,943,502	71,565,700	65,565,230	80,111,039
Total Net Revenue	3,720,286,583	3,444,157,021	3,234,139,237	3,230,933,573	2,978,017,525
Total Expenses	3,576,366,207	3,285,567,037	3,065,466,141	3,036,739,861	2,712,003,392
HOSPITAL UNIT (Excludes Separate Nursing Home Units)					
Utilization - Inpatient					
Beds	9,004	9,171	8,658	9,380	8,730
Admissions	322,983	314,556	301,101	316,200	288,353
Inpatient Days	1,630,230	1,576,671	1,489,124	1,615,520	1,506,584
Average Length of Stay	5.0	5.0	4.9	5.1	5.2
Personnel					
Total Full Time	32,669	31,407	30,303	32,649	33,205
Total Part Time	13,618	13,885	13,199	12,225	10,801
Revenue and Expenses - Totals					
(Includes Inpatient and Outpatient)					
Total Net Revenue	$3,656,845,788	$3,372,688,086	$3,169,162,014	$3,160,271,291	$2,901,003,496
Total Expenses	3,520,829,715	3,229,152,871	3,011,711,334	2,981,430,308	2,652,210,976
COMMUNITY HEALTH INDICATORS PER 1000 POPULATION					
Total Population (in thousands)	2,716	2,695	2,688	2,654	2,639
Inpatient					
Beds	4.0	4.2	4.0	4.4	4.1
Admissions	121.1	119.5	115.4	123.0	113.6
Inpatient Days	797.2	807.5	774.4	841.3	814.2
Inpatient Surgeries	32.7	32.3	31.3	34.4	31.0
Births	14.2	14.0	14.0	14.7	13.7
Outpatient					
Emergency Outpatient Visits	346.3	336.6	330.8	347.0	306.7
Other Outpatient Visits	1,743.3	1,665.1	1,624.0	1,546.1	1,476.1
Total Outpatient Visits	2,089.6	2,001.8	1,954.8	1,893.1	1,782.8
Outpatient Surgeries	57.4	60.0	60.5	66.5	60.3
Expense per Capita (per person)	$1,316.8	$1,219.3	$1,140.2	$1,144.2	$1,027.8

States

TABLE 6

KENTUCKY

U.S. Registered Community Hospitals
(Nonfederal, short-term general and other special hospitals)

Overview 1998–2002

	2002	2001	2000	1999	1998
Total U.S. Community Hospitals in Kentucky	104	103	105	105	106
Bed Size Category					
6-24	2	1	3	2	1
25-49	21	20	19	22	19
50-99	33	33	30	29	37
100-199	21	22	27	27	26
200-299	13	14	14	12	9
300-399	6	6	6	9	7
400-499	5	5	4	2	5
500 +	3	2	2	2	2
Location					
Hospitals Urban	32	32	33	33	34
Hospitals Rural	72	71	72	72	72
Control					
State and Local Government	14	14	15	14	13
Not for Profit	73	71	72	73	73
Investor owned	17	18	18	18	20
Physician Models					
Independent Practice Association	8	7	6	8	7
Group Practice without Walls	2	2	3	1	3
Open Physician-Hospital Organization	11	11	12	15	18
Closed Physician-Hospital Organization	1	1	1	6	3
Management Service Organization	3	3	12	14	13
Integrated Salary Model	31	29	24	21	21
Equity Model	0	0	0	1	3
Foundation	9	10	11	10	6
Insurance Products					
Health Maintenance Organization	23	22	17	20	22
Preferred Provider Organization	23	17	8	18	27
Indemnity Fee for Service	1	2	0	3	6
Managed Care Contracts					
Health Maintenance Organization	59	53	48	52	57
Preferred Provider Organization	70	68	54	69	68
Affiliations					
Hospitals in a System	49	52	45	51	47
Hospitals in a Network	15	13	13	15	22
Hospitals in a Group Purchasing Organization	82	76	63	62	57

TABLE 6

KENTUCKY

U.S. Registered Community Hospitals
(Nonfederal, short-term general and other special hospitals)

Utilization, Personnel, Revenue and Expenses, Community Health Indicators 1998–2002

	2002	2001	2000	1999	1998
TOTAL FACILITY (Includes Hospital and Nursing Home Units)					
Utilization - Inpatient					
Beds.........................	15,066	15,001	14,827	14,956	15,240
Admissions....................	601,644	594,899	581,620	569,792	551,325
Inpatient Days	3,393,525	3,315,218	3,333,314	3,296,591	3,173,476
Average Length of Stay...........	5.6	5.6	5.7	5.8	5.8
Inpatient Surgeries..............	180,073	167,283	170,029	164,304	179,309
Births.......................	52,098	52,818	53,547	51,637	51,107
Utilization - Outpatient					
Emergency Outpatient Visits.......	2,109,556	1,985,284	1,953,727	1,990,266	1,761,831
Other Outpatient Visits...........	6,536,556	6,692,104	6,742,993	5,991,574	5,630,880
Total Outpatient Visits	8,646,112	8,677,388	8,696,720	7,981,840	7,392,711
Outpatient Surgeries	363,052	359,153	349,830	333,683	313,438
Personnel					
Full Time RNs	13,224	12,892	13,138	13,532	13,576
Full Time LPNs	2,361	2,427	2,206	2,362	2,496
Part Time RNs	6,354	5,229	5,041	5,217	4,582
Part Time LPNs	714	540	544	648	683
Total Full Time.................	56,104	57,175	55,775	54,147	55,425
Total Part Time	20,611	17,162	17,452	16,457	14,345
Revenue - Inpatient					
Gross Inpatient Revenue..........	$8,677,558,625	$7,787,598,143	$6,926,847,867	$6,349,440,581	$5,934,530,227
Revenue - Outpatient					
Gross Outpatient Revenue	$5,544,182,284	$4,733,719,223	$4,237,568,311	$3,654,809,995	$3,246,317,231
Revenue and Expenses - Totals					
(Includes Inpatient and Outpatient)					
Total Gross Revenue.............	$14,221,740,909	$12,521,317,366	$11,164,416,178	$10,004,250,576	$9,180,847,458
Deductions from Revenue.........	7,943,529,393	6,819,797,436	5,892,730,890	5,113,919,722	4,401,939,860
Net Patient Revenue	6,278,211,516	5,701,519,930	5,271,685,288	4,890,330,854	4,778,907,598
Other Operating Revenue	264,424,862	264,715,481	250,730,317	237,393,468	218,060,479
Other Nonoperating Revenue	55,509,283	61,362,641	91,895,438	108,001,346	132,156,395
Total Net Revenue..............	6,598,145,661	6,027,598,052	5,614,311,043	5,235,725,668	5,129,124,472
Total Expenses.................	6,201,408,483	5,731,885,674	5,262,215,893	4,962,196,037	4,790,309,964
HOSPITAL UNIT (Excludes Separate Nursing Home Units)					
Utilization - Inpatient					
Beds.........................	13,640	13,587	13,295	13,125	13,511
Admissions....................	591,970	584,628	570,135	555,394	539,916
Inpatient Days	2,999,495	2,863,991	2,844,864	2,716,093	2,667,045
Average Length of Stay...........	5.1	4.9	5.0	4.9	4.9
Personnel					
Total Full Time.................	54,958	55,916	54,545	52,598	54,031
Total Part Time	20,115	16,843	17,049	15,919	13,917
Revenue and Expenses - Totals					
(Includes Inpatient and Outpatient)					
Total Net Revenue..............	$6,505,926,611	$5,922,961,820	$5,467,691,050	$5,083,079,627	$5,015,843,495
Total Expenses.................	6,126,969,102	5,659,683,174	5,142,390,665	4,876,938,853	4,713,425,656
COMMUNITY HEALTH INDICATORS PER 1000 POPULATION					
Total Population (in thousands)	4,093	4,066	4,042	3,961	3,934
Inpatient					
Beds.........................	3.7	3.7	3.7	3.8	3.9
Admissions....................	147.0	146.3	143.9	143.9	140.1
Inpatient Days	829.1	815.4	824.7	832.3	806.6
Inpatient Surgeries..............	44.0	41.1	42.1	41.5	45.6
Births.......................	12.7	13.0	13.2	13.0	13.0
Outpatient					
Emergency Outpatient Visits.......	515.4	488.3	483.4	502.5	447.8
Other Outpatient Visits...........	1,597.1	1,646.0	1,668.3	1,512.7	1,431.2
Total Outpatient Visits	2,112.5	2,134.4	2,151.7	2,015.2	1,879.0
Outpatient Surgeries	88.7	88.3	86.6	84.2	79.7
Expense per Capita (per person)....	$1,515.2	$1,409.9	$1,302.0	$1,252.8	$1,217.6

States

TABLE 6

U.S. Registered Community Hospitals
(Nonfederal, short-term general and other special hospitals)

Overview 1998–2002

	2002	2001	2000	1999	1998
Total U.S. Community Hospitals in					
Louisiana..........................	128	125	123	122	126
Bed Size Category					
6-24	10	9	6	5	5
25-49	33	29	29	29	29
50-99	30	30	33	31	32
100-199	28	30	27	32	34
200-299	8	11	11	8	10
300-399	9	6	8	11	8
400-499	5	4	4	4	3
500 + ...	5	6	5	2	5
Location					
Hospitals Urban.....................	77	76	75	74	78
Hospitals Rural	51	49	48	48	48
Control					
State and Local Government	52	55	55	55	57
Not for Profit	35	33	31	30	30
Investor owned	41	37	37	37	39
Physician Models					
Independent Practice Association........	13	17	15	11	12
Group Practice without Walls	5	2	3	1	4
Open Physician-Hospital Organization....	17	17	25	20	19
Closed Physician-Hospital Organization...	8	15	14	13	23
Management Service Organization.......	8	10	15	18	23
Integrated Salary Model	19	16	19	14	18
Equity Model	1	0	0	1	2
Foundation.........................	3	2	2	1	2
Insurance Products					
Health Maintenance Organization........	8	9	12	18	25
Preferred Provider Organization.........	14	15	19	27	37
Indemnity Fee for Service.............	3	2	3	5	7
Managed Care Contracts					
Health Maintenance Organization........	51	54	55	57	66
Preferred Provider Organization.........	62	69	70	72	80
Affiliations					
Hospitals in a System.................	34	39	41	37	44
Hospitals in a Network	18	18	22	17	29
Hospitals in a Group Purchasing					
Organization.......................	64	71	62	60	58

TABLE **6**

LOUISIANA

U.S. Registered Community Hospitals
(Nonfederal, short-term general and other special hospitals)

Utilization, Personnel, Revenue and Expenses, Community Health Indicators 1998–2002

	2002	2001	2000	1999	1998
TOTAL FACILITY (Includes Hospital and Nursing Home Units)					
Utilization - Inpatient					
Beds	17,867	17,975	17,544	16,782	17,820
Admissions	692,011	682,586	654,323	626,801	637,892
Inpatient Days	3,873,634	3,736,536	3,569,621	3,472,409	3,564,901
Average Length of Stay.	5.6	5.5	5.5	5.5	5.6
Inpatient Surgeries.	179,986	172,824	179,651	174,051	173,281
Births.	57,564	63,248	64,904	63,553	63,976
Utilization - Outpatient					
Emergency Outpatient Visits	2,468,832	2,267,490	2,143,846	2,182,109	2,254,789
Other Outpatient Visits.	8,262,795	7,792,891	7,882,211	7,331,885	7,952,356
Total Outpatient Visits	10,731,627	10,060,381	10,026,057	9,513,994	10,207,145
Outpatient Surgeries	287,954	285,927	278,438	272,852	267,370
Personnel					
Full Time RNs	15,320	14,845	15,634	15,460	15,939
Full Time LPNs	3,186	3,202	3,711	3,849	3,787
Part Time RNs	5,973	5,472	5,630	4,586	4,881
Part Time LPNs	921	1,046	1,073	1,018	912
Total Full Time.	69,541	68,540	70,010	68,263	73,149
Total Part Time	19,700	18,200	18,093	16,056	17,568
Revenue - Inpatient					
Gross Inpatient Revenue.	$10,679,535,909	$9,096,048,174	$8,243,500,319	$7,543,819,679	$7,549,027,025
Revenue - Outpatient					
Gross Outpatient Revenue	$5,523,762,540	$4,760,161,472	$4,251,539,053	$3,934,910,084	$3,827,901,719
Revenue and Expenses - Totals					
(Includes Inpatient and Outpatient)					
Total Gross Revenue.	$16,203,298,449	$13,856,209,646	$12,495,039,372	$11,478,729,763	$11,376,928,744
Deductions from Revenue.	9,401,154,343	7,622,952,381	6,598,655,986	5,462,495,406	5,494,978,293
Net Patient Revenue	6,802,144,106	6,233,257,265	5,896,383,386	6,016,234,357	5,881,950,451
Other Operating Revenue	271,896,066	267,094,438	242,589,117	431,151,639	255,734,431
Other Nonoperating Revenue	49,925,463	118,755,497	132,937,013	123,928,310	107,524,057
Total Net Revenue.	7,123,965,635	6,619,107,200	6,271,909,516	6,571,314,306	6,245,208,939
Total Expenses.	6,751,804,011	6,231,829,149	5,944,697,229	5,552,067,184	5,874,665,596
HOSPITAL UNIT (Excludes Separate Nursing Home Units)					
Utilization - Inpatient					
Beds	17,026	16,772	16,724	16,031	17,118
Admissions	687,478	676,446	645,795	617,298	627,610
Inpatient Days	3,657,799	3,433,204	3,333,668	3,256,709	3,361,008
Average Length of Stay.	5.3	5.1	5.2	5.3	5.4
Personnel					
Total Full Time.	68,904	67,852	68,743	67,579	72,324
Total Part Time	19,388	17,972	17,855	15,884	17,368
Revenue and Expenses - Totals					
(Includes Inpatient and Outpatient)					
Total Net Revenue.	$7,079,640,911	$6,575,698,935	$6,196,038,147	$6,306,351,941	$6,173,466,062
Total Expenses.	6,714,901,922	6,196,893,942	5,901,358,320	5,509,175,610	5,814,898,961
COMMUNITY HEALTH INDICATORS PER 1000 POPULATION					
Total Population (in thousands)	4,483	4,465	4,469	4,372	4,363
Inpatient					
Beds	4.0	4.0	3.9	3.8	4.1
Admissions	154.4	152.9	146.4	143.4	146.2
Inpatient Days	864.1	836.8	798.8	794.2	817.1
Inpatient Surgeries.	40.2	38.7	40.2	39.8	39.7
Births.	12.8	14.2	14.5	14.5	14.7
Outpatient					
Emergency Outpatient Visits	550.8	507.8	479.7	499.1	516.8
Other Outpatient Visits.	1,843.3	1,745.2	1,763.8	1,677.0	1,822.8
Total Outpatient Visits	2,394.0	2,252.9	2,243.5	2,176.1	2,339.6
Outpatient Surgeries	64.2	64.0	62.3	62.4	61.3
Expense per Capita (per person). . . .	$1,506.2	$1,395.6	$1,330.2	$1,269.9	$1,346.5

TABLE **6**

MAINE

U.S. Registered Community Hospitals
(Nonfederal, short-term general and other special hospitals)

Overview 1998–2002

	2002	2001	2000	1999	1998
Total U.S. Community Hospitals in Maine.............................	37	37	37	37	38
Bed Size Category					
6-24	3	0	1	2	1
25-49	11	14	13	12	14
50-99	12	11	12	12	13
100-199	8	9	8	8	7
200-299	0	0	0	0	0
300-399	2	2	2	2	2
400-499	0	0	0	0	0
500 + ...	1	1	1	1	1
Location					
Hospitals Urban......................	8	8	8	8	9
Hospitals Rural	29	29	29	29	29
Control					
State and Local Government	2	3	3	3	3
Not for Profit	34	33	33	33	34
Investor owned	1	1	1	1	1
Physician Models					
Independent Practice Association........	4	4	3	3	2
Group Practice without Walls	2	1	1	2	4
Open Physician-Hospital Organization....	15	16	12	13	13
Closed Physician-Hospital Organization...	0	0	2	2	2
Management Service Organization.......	4	4	4	5	5
Integrated Salary Model	14	13	14	16	13
Equity Model	2	2	2	2	2
Foundation.........................	2	2	0	0	0
Insurance Products					
Health Maintenance Organization........	3	2	3	6	7
Preferred Provider Organization.........	4	3	4	7	9
Indemnity Fee for Service..............	2	2	2	2	3
Managed Care Contracts					
Health Maintenance Organization........	24	28	28	27	28
Preferred Provider Organization.........	21	24	25	22	27
Affiliations					
Hospitals in a System..................	21	20	16	18	16
Hospitals in a Network	18	16	15	13	13
Hospitals in a Group Purchasing Organization.......................	34	31	31	30	30

TABLE 6

MAINE

U.S. Registered Community Hospitals
(Nonfederal, short-term general and other special hospitals)

Utilization, Personnel, Revenue and Expenses, Community Health Indicators 1998–2002

	2002	2001	2000	1999	1998
TOTAL FACILITY (Includes Hospital and Nursing Home Units)					
Utilization - Inpatient					
Beds	3,694	3,844	3,700	3,691	3,768
Admissions	145,917	148,612	147,236	146,378	144,363
Inpatient Days	889,005	898,059	867,352	872,635	843,811
Average Length of Stay...........	6.1	6.0	5.9	6.0	5.8
Inpatient Surgeries..............	60,022	45,682	45,114	44,045	41,907
Births.........................	13,072	13,320	13,294	13,284	13,252
Utilization - Outpatient					
Emergency Outpatient Visits.......	709,091	700,510	673,853	579,803	636,973
Other Outpatient Visits...........	3,022,170	2,812,088	2,573,641	2,197,596	2,037,267
Total Outpatient Visits	3,731,261	3,512,598	3,247,494	2,777,399	2,674,240
Outpatient Surgeries	97,665	114,146	108,086	96,653	91,545
Personnel					
Full Time RNs	3,754	3,573	3,628	3,517	3,514
Full Time LPNs	241	270	302	352	364
Part Time RNs..................	3,449	3,005	2,964	2,725	2,652
Part Time LPNs	193	183	212	199	215
Total Full Time.................	17,038	16,599	16,403	15,485	16,028
Total Part Time	10,681	9,641	9,180	7,239	8,293
Revenue - Inpatient					
Gross Inpatient Revenue.........	$2,019,706,879	$1,812,197,212	$1,698,718,945	$1,520,624,429	$1,421,620,856
Revenue - Outpatient					
Gross Outpatient Revenue	$1,567,817,352	$1,304,548,466	$1,154,754,197	$999,290,257	$858,420,867
Revenue and Expenses - Totals					
(Includes Inpatient and Outpatient)					
Total Gross Revenue.............	$3,587,524,231	$3,116,745,678	$2,853,473,142	$2,519,914,686	$2,280,041,723
Deductions from Revenue........	1,488,086,115	1,217,966,635	1,115,439,062	915,152,948	726,791,652
Net Patient Revenue	2,099,438,116	1,898,779,043	1,738,034,080	1,604,761,738	1,553,250,071
Other Operating Revenue	72,149,218	65,237,618	57,843,349	55,504,484	59,938,444
Other Nonoperating Revenue	19,653,975	44,611,020	65,070,578	60,959,561	56,650,639
Total Net Revenue..............	2,191,241,309	2,008,627,681	1,860,948,007	1,721,225,783	1,669,839,154
Total Expenses.................	2,105,062,300	1,895,302,775	1,728,203,811	1,590,697,508	1,529,313,309
HOSPITAL UNIT (Excludes Separate Nursing Home Units)					
Utilization - Inpatient					
Beds	3,151	3,266	3,308	3,146	3,287
Admissions	144,016	146,398	145,274	144,095	142,153
Inpatient Days	714,141	715,018	744,933	702,828	698,519
Average Length of Stay...........	5.0	4.9	5.1	4.9	4.9
Personnel					
Total Full Time.................	16,584	16,166	16,052	15,042	15,485
Total Part Time	10,351	9,376	8,910	6,920	7,946
Revenue and Expenses - Totals					
(Includes Inpatient and Outpatient)					
Total Net Revenue..............	$2,161,952,361	$1,978,598,927	$1,840,086,132	$1,689,929,697	$1,646,474,939
Total Expenses.................	2,081,511,605	1,864,078,445	1,710,294,770	1,569,334,589	1,512,040,904
COMMUNITY HEALTH INDICATORS PER 1000 POPULATION					
Total Population (in thousands)	1,294	1,287	1,275	1,253	1,248
Inpatient					
Beds	2.9	3.0	2.9	2.9	3.0
Admissions	112.7	115.5	115.5	116.8	115.7
Inpatient Days	686.8	698.0	680.3	696.4	676.4
Inpatient Surgeries..............	46.4	35.5	35.4	35.2	33.6
Births.........................	10.1	10.4	10.4	10.6	10.6
Outpatient					
Emergency Outpatient Visits.......	547.8	544.4	528.5	462.7	510.6
Other Outpatient Visits...........	2,334.7	2,185.6	2,018.7	1,753.8	1,633.0
Total Outpatient Visits	2,882.5	2,730.0	2,547.2	2,216.5	2,143.6
Outpatient Surgeries	75.4	88.7	84.8	77.1	73.4
Expense per Capita (per person)....	$1,626.2	$1,473.0	$1,355.5	$1,269.5	$1,225.8

TABLE 6

MARYLAND

U.S. Registered Community Hospitals
(Nonfederal, short-term general and other special hospitals)

Overview 1998–2002

	2002	2001	2000	1999	1998
Total U.S. Community Hospitals in					
Maryland	49	49	49	49	51
Bed Size Category					
6-24	0	0	0	0	0
25-49	4	3	3	3	3
50-99	5	6	5	4	6
100-199	15	15	18	19	19
200-299	11	12	11	9	7
300-399	9	8	6	9	9
400-499	2	2	3	1	3
500 +	3	3	3	4	4
Location					
Hospitals Urban	40	40	40	40	42
Hospitals Rural	9	9	9	9	9
Control					
State and Local Government	0	0	0	0	0
Not for Profit	46	47	47	47	49
Investor owned	3	2	2	2	2
Physician Models					
Independent Practice Association	5	6	7	11	15
Group Practice without Walls	2	1	1	2	3
Open Physician-Hospital Organization	7	7	9	11	14
Closed Physician-Hospital Organization	3	5	4	7	9
Management Service Organization	2	3	5	15	18
Integrated Salary Model	23	23	19	20	19
Equity Model	3	3	4	5	4
Foundation	2	2	2	4	7
Insurance Products					
Health Maintenance Organization	10	16	14	10	11
Preferred Provider Organization	4	8	10	10	14
Indemnity Fee for Service	1	3	3	4	3
Managed Care Contracts					
Health Maintenance Organization	36	38	37	33	32
Preferred Provider Organization	32	34	32	29	34
Affiliations					
Hospitals in a System	34	37	36	32	28
Hospitals in a Network	9	8	6	5	8
Hospitals in a Group Purchasing					
Organization	41	43	41	34	37

States

TABLE 6

MARYLAND

U.S. Registered Community Hospitals
(Nonfederal, short-term general and other special hospitals)

Utilization, Personnel, Revenue and Expenses, Community Health Indicators 1998–2002

	2002	2001	2000	1999	1998
TOTAL FACILITY (Includes Hospital and Nursing Home Units)					
Utilization - Inpatient					
Beds	11,417	11,234	11,192	11,629	12,670
Admissions	634,914	608,165	586,809	576,551	564,913
Inpatient Days	3,049,647	2,981,003	2,993,513	3,023,508	3,144,315
Average Length of Stay.	4.8	4.9	5.1	5.2	5.6
Inpatient Surgeries	186,084	183,287	178,327	175,733	190,587
Births.	63,744	63,843	64,030	62,251	62,307
Utilization - Outpatient					
Emergency Outpatient Visits	1,943,614	1,854,562	1,765,739	1,667,655	1,505,744
Other Outpatient Visits.	4,520,569	4,411,827	4,251,883	4,275,428	3,514,579
Total Outpatient Visits	6,464,183	6,266,389	6,017,622	5,943,083	5,020,323
Outpatient Surgeries	347,715	330,571	335,445	320,799	299,859
Personnel					
Full Time RNs	11,975	11,196	11,629	12,145	12,201
Full Time LPNs	705	593	629	702	795
Part Time RNs	8,418	8,804	8,458	7,152	7,756
Part Time LPNs	357	338	365	515	354
Total Full Time	56,379	54,035	52,045	51,194	50,745
Total Part Time	24,293	25,913	25,896	23,098	24,357
Revenue - Inpatient					
Gross Inpatient Revenue.	$6,314,536,604	$5,524,686,729	$4,869,935,847	$4,872,474,817	$4,945,479,136
Revenue - Outpatient					
Gross Outpatient Revenue	$3,110,642,148	$2,614,614,189	$2,239,872,994	$2,014,087,252	$1,976,311,835
Revenue and Expenses - Totals					
(Includes Inpatient and Outpatient)					
Total Gross Revenue.	$9,425,178,752	$8,139,300,918	$7,109,808,841	$6,886,562,069	$6,921,790,971
Deductions from Revenue	2,597,808,764	1,898,515,253	1,433,510,257	1,603,233,392	1,690,984,916
Net Patient Revenue	6,827,369,988	6,240,785,665	5,676,298,584	5,283,328,677	5,230,806,055
Other Operating Revenue	303,127,043	266,638,563	255,723,354	217,607,190	228,596,574
Other Nonoperating Revenue	25,174,124	43,785,690	91,201,507	82,290,784	103,389,417
Total Net Revenue.	7,155,671,155	6,551,209,918	6,023,223,445	5,583,226,651	5,562,792,046
Total Expenses.	6,971,693,586	6,345,348,924	5,872,418,845	5,457,297,063	5,305,756,896
HOSPITAL UNIT (Excludes Separate Nursing Home Units)					
Utilization - Inpatient					
Beds	10,726	10,575	10,297	10,699	11,350
Admissions	624,477	598,350	574,952	564,358	553,916
Inpatient Days	2,832,577	2,773,678	2,708,689	2,753,302	2,768,381
Average Length of Stay.	4.5	4.6	4.7	4.9	5.0
Personnel					
Total Full Time	55,681	53,463	51,409	50,461	49,810
Total Part Time	23,927	25,579	25,392	22,627	23,861
Revenue and Expenses - Totals					
(Includes Inpatient and Outpatient)					
Total Net Revenue.	$7,070,224,974	$6,462,828,420	$5,938,396,900	$5,486,858,411	$5,441,766,935
Total Expenses.	6,892,430,543	6,281,919,803	5,796,277,170	5,372,382,741	5,198,032,054
COMMUNITY HEALTH INDICATORS PER 1000 POPULATION					
Total Population (in thousands)	5,458	5,375	5,296	5,172	5,130
Inpatient					
Beds	2.1	2.1	2.1	2.2	2.5
Admissions	116.3	113.1	110.8	111.5	110.1
Inpatient Days	558.7	554.6	565.2	584.6	612.9
Inpatient Surgeries	34.1	34.1	33.7	34.0	37.2
Births.	11.7	11.9	12.1	12.0	12.1
Outpatient					
Emergency Outpatient Visits	356.1	345.0	333.4	322.5	293.5
Other Outpatient Visits.	828.2	820.8	802.8	826.7	685.1
Total Outpatient Visits	1,184.3	1,165.8	1,136.2	1,149.2	978.6
Outpatient Surgeries	63.7	61.5	63.3	62.0	58.5
Expense per Capita (per person). . . .	$1,277.3	$1,180.5	$1,108.7	$1,055.2	$1,034.2

States

TABLE 6

MASSACHUSETTS

U.S. Registered Community Hospitals
(Nonfederal, short-term general and other special hospitals)

Overview 1998–2002

	2002	2001	2000	1999	1998
Total U.S. Community Hospitals in Massachusetts	78	80	80	79	82
Bed Size Category					
6-24	4	2	2	3	3
25-49	9	13	13	12	12
50-99	7	6	6	6	9
100-199	27	28	27	29	27
200-299	18	16	16	12	17
300-399	6	8	9	10	6
400-499	1	1	1	1	1
500 +	6	6	6	6	7
Location					
Hospitals Urban	67	69	69	68	71
Hospitals Rural	11	11	11	11	11
Control					
State and Local Government	4	4	4	4	4
Not for Profit	68	70	70	69	72
Investor owned	6	6	6	6	6
Physician Models					
Independent Practice Association	34	31	31	37	31
Group Practice without Walls	8	10	9	9	10
Open Physician-Hospital Organization	17	18	19	21	22
Closed Physician-Hospital Organization	11	10	10	10	11
Management Service Organization	14	17	17	24	19
Integrated Salary Model	30	28	28	24	25
Equity Model	3	1	1	2	2
Foundation	6	5	6	10	10
Insurance Products					
Health Maintenance Organization	9	8	9	8	13
Preferred Provider Organization	6	4	5	6	12
Indemnity Fee for Service	1	1	1	2	4
Managed Care Contracts					
Health Maintenance Organization	62	60	56	62	62
Preferred Provider Organization	58	57	53	57	57
Affiliations					
Hospitals in a System	44	43	40	50	42
Hospitals in a Network	21	22	21	22	18
Hospitals in a Group Purchasing Organization	54	55	50	53	51

TABLE 6

MASSACHUSETTS

U.S. Registered Community Hospitals
(Nonfederal, short-term general and other special hospitals)

Utilization, Personnel, Revenue and Expenses, Community Health Indicators 1998–2002

	2002	2001	2000	1999	1998
TOTAL FACILITY (Includes Hospital and Nursing Home Units)					
Utilization - Inpatient					
Beds	16,033	16,504	16,586	16,309	16,493
Admissions	765,820	766,708	740,286	739,375	738,018
Inpatient Days	4,348,099	4,382,048	4,289,840	4,210,454	4,186,012
Average Length of Stay...........	5.7	5.7	5.8	5.7	5.7
Inpatient Surgeries..............	205,077	212,539	217,649	214,009	219,487
Births.........................	80,034	79,908	81,640	79,484	78,257
Utilization - Outpatient					
Emergency Outpatient Visits	2,882,602	2,717,815	2,715,812	2,726,113	2,473,668
Other Outpatient Visits...........	16,141,885	16,060,322	13,994,541	12,982,756	12,952,045
Total Outpatient Visits	19,024,487	18,778,137	16,710,353	15,708,869	15,425,713
Outpatient Surgeries	486,143	467,917	458,544	440,958	423,601
Personnel					
Full Time RNs	16,799	18,018	16,359	14,936	14,465
Full Time LPNs	1,206	1,236	1,207	854	1,052
Part Time RNs.................	15,846	16,968	18,591	17,782	18,695
Part Time LPNs	961	1,067	1,171	1,111	1,109
Total Full Time.................	99,089	101,474	93,354	87,466	86,242
Total Part Time	51,096	52,916	56,902	56,698	57,013
Revenue - Inpatient					
Gross Inpatient Revenue..........	$12,947,175,259	$12,173,968,661	$11,247,798,711	$9,839,772,237	$9,196,917,700
Revenue - Outpatient					
Gross Outpatient Revenue	$10,988,975,820	$9,610,590,844	$8,231,186,269	$7,625,652,302	$6,711,695,879
Revenue and Expenses - Totals (Includes Inpatient and Outpatient)					
Total Gross Revenue.............	$23,936,151,079	$21,784,559,505	$19,478,984,980	$17,465,424,539	$15,908,613,579
Deductions from Revenue.........	12,756,840,606	11,457,845,346	10,026,437,014	8,646,920,813	7,346,543,961
Net Patient Revenue	11,179,310,473	10,326,714,159	9,452,547,966	8,818,503,726	8,562,069,618
Other Operating Revenue	1,822,811,119	1,636,890,502	1,232,552,918	1,299,771,155	1,364,112,758
Other Nonoperating Revenue	-20,027,456	124,637,693	365,783,979	341,554,169	369,873,327
Total Net Revenue...............	12,982,094,136	12,088,242,354	11,050,884,863	10,459,829,050	10,296,055,703
Total Expenses..................	12,979,804,604	12,055,797,429	11,148,180,478	10,518,160,942	10,315,437,574
HOSPITAL UNIT (Excludes Separate Nursing Home Units)					
Utilization - Inpatient					
Beds	15,301	15,814	15,662	15,515	15,907
Admissions	754,165	757,011	725,509	720,669	726,626
Inpatient Days	4,118,738	4,140,284	3,993,613	3,980,792	4,023,095
Average Length of Stay...........	5.5	5.5	5.5	5.5	5.5
Personnel					
Total Full Time.................	98,795	101,143	92,938	86,618	85,515
Total Part Time	50,699	52,480	56,327	55,971	56,441
Revenue and Expenses - Totals (Includes Inpatient and Outpatient)					
Total Net Revenue...............	$12,931,336,845	$12,032,855,996	$10,993,289,677	$10,367,408,392	$10,176,513,120
Total Expenses..................	12,931,961,619	12,015,811,316	11,098,723,636	10,444,538,511	10,225,709,796
COMMUNITY HEALTH INDICATORS PER 1000 POPULATION					
Total Population (in thousands)	6,428	6,379	6,349	6,175	6,144
Inpatient					
Beds	2.5	2.6	2.6	2.6	2.7
Admissions	119.1	120.2	116.6	119.7	120.1
Inpatient Days	676.5	686.9	675.7	681.8	681.3
Inpatient Surgeries..............	31.9	33.3	34.3	34.7	35.7
Births.........................	12.5	12.5	12.9	12.9	12.7
Outpatient					
Emergency Outpatient Visits	448.5	426.0	427.7	441.5	402.6
Other Outpatient Visits...........	2,511.3	2,517.6	2,204.2	2,102.4	2,107.9
Total Outpatient Visits	2,959.7	2,943.6	2,631.9	2,543.9	2,510.5
Outpatient Surgeries	75.6	73.3	72.2	71.4	68.9
Expense per Capita (per person)....	$2,019.3	$1,889.8	$1,755.9	$1,703.3	$1,678.8

States

TABLE 6

MICHIGAN

U.S. Registered Community Hospitals
(Nonfederal, short-term general and other special hospitals)

Overview 1998–2002

	2002	2001	2000	1999	1998
Total U.S. Community Hospitals in					
Michigan	145	145	146	145	151
Bed Size Category					
6-24	7	7	7	10	11
25-49	24	23	20	17	22
50-99	47	50	51	51	47
100-199	19	17	18	19	20
200-299	16	17	21	18	18
300-399	16	16	13	14	16
400-499	7	7	7	7	8
500 + ...	9	8	9	9	9
Location					
Hospitals Urban......................	86	86	88	87	92
Hospitals Rural	59	59	58	58	59
Control					
State and Local Government	19	20	19	19	21
Not for Profit	122	122	124	122	128
Investor owned	4	3	3	4	2
Physician Models					
Independent Practice Association........	23	22	23	25	32
Group Practice without Walls	12	13	13	7	10
Open Physician-Hospital Organization....	55	58	55	44	46
Closed Physician-Hospital Organization...	17	14	20	23	21
Management Service Organization.......	22	27	26	23	29
Integrated Salary Model	60	59	68	56	59
Equity Model	0	1	1	3	2
Foundation........................	5	4	5	6	8
Insurance Products					
Health Maintenance Organization........	44	45	52	47	50
Preferred Provider Organization........	52	52	66	60	67
Indemnity Fee for Service..............	13	11	18	14	17
Managed Care Contracts					
Health Maintenance Organization........	111	117	114	106	106
Preferred Provider Organization.........	116	125	123	122	121
Affiliations					
Hospitals in a System.................	75	77	79	77	74
Hospitals in a Network	50	50	56	46	45
Hospitals in a Group Purchasing					
Organization......................	124	124	125	119	110

TABLE 6

MICHIGAN

U.S. Registered Community Hospitals
(Nonfederal, short-term general and other special hospitals)

Utilization, Personnel, Revenue and Expenses, Community Health Indicators 1998–2002

	2002	2001	2000	1999	1998
TOTAL FACILITY (Includes Hospital and Nursing Home Units)					
Utilization - Inpatient					
Beds	26,130	25,630	26,074	26,144	27,168
Admissions	1,163,157	1,122,004	1,106,045	1,084,277	1,104,883
Inpatient Days	6,296,654	6,108,896	6,176,230	6,295,931	6,380,260
Average Length of Stay...........	5.4	5.4	5.6	5.8	5.8
Inpatient Surgeries..............	346,641	321,558	334,190	323,881	329,527
Births........................	127,754	126,846	131,092	128,720	127,816
Utilization - Outpatient					
Emergency Outpatient Visits.......	4,029,309	3,753,945	3,703,509	3,528,497	3,462,575
Other Outpatient Visits...........	21,837,056	22,230,144	21,157,782	18,843,667	18,309,759
Total Outpatient Visits	25,866,365	25,984,089	24,861,291	22,372,164	21,772,334
Outpatient Surgeries	739,878	702,275	650,872	661,422	644,153
Personnel					
Full Time RNs	25,067	25,106	25,678	24,608	25,232
Full Time LPNs	2,292	2,768	2,631	2,657	2,996
Part Time RNs..................	19,095	17,888	16,721	17,554	17,752
Part Time LPNs	1,750	2,420	1,764	2,068	2,160
Total Full Time.................	122,075	120,138	122,715	119,054	127,456
Total Part Time	63,009	60,068	54,816	58,407	59,512
Revenue - Inpatient					
Gross Inpatient Revenue..........	$18,067,876,124	$15,269,814,888	$14,753,771,125	$13,703,264,931	$13,735,570,282
Revenue - Outpatient					
Gross Outpatient Revenue	$13,502,108,253	$12,008,967,077	$10,951,098,666	$9,612,610,858	$9,165,570,745
Revenue and Expenses - Totals					
(Includes Inpatient and Outpatient)					
Total Gross Revenue.............	$31,569,984,377	$27,278,781,965	$25,704,869,791	$23,315,875,789	$22,901,141,027
Deductions from Revenue.........	16,694,090,957	13,827,622,183	12,700,091,926	10,906,847,788	10,215,663,891
Net Patient Revenue	14,875,893,420	13,451,159,782	13,004,777,865	12,409,028,001	12,685,477,136
Other Operating Revenue	700,959,929	634,303,135	647,130,579	581,407,288	588,209,470
Other Nonoperating Revenue	19,519,553	122,735,458	687,142,951	515,479,497	471,734,694
Total Net Revenue..............	15,596,372,902	14,208,198,375	14,339,051,395	13,505,914,786	13,745,421,300
Total Expenses.................	15,321,064,736	13,891,061,790	13,456,111,469	12,897,935,106	12,920,233,262
HOSPITAL UNIT (Excludes Separate Nursing Home Units)					
Utilization - Inpatient					
Beds	24,354	23,868	24,012	23,841	24,993
Admissions	1,159,116	1,117,366	1,100,448	1,077,852	1,099,675
Inpatient Days	5,724,932	5,539,802	5,510,749	5,582,723	5,647,658
Average Length of Stay...........	4.9	5.0	5.0	5.2	5.1
Personnel					
Total Full Time.................	120,860	118,969	121,360	117,733	126,146
Total Part Time	62,308	59,286	54,005	57,651	58,775
Revenue and Expenses - Totals					
(Includes Inpatient and Outpatient)					
Total Net Revenue..............	$15,477,617,658	$14,113,345,021	$14,241,432,247	$13,399,295,963	$13,646,478,835
Total Expenses.................	15,232,840,934	13,820,531,836	13,364,180,983	12,804,079,036	12,830,389,161
COMMUNITY HEALTH INDICATORS PER 1000 POPULATION					
Total Population (in thousands)	10,050	9,991	9,938	9,864	9,820
Inpatient					
Beds	2.6	2.6	2.6	2.7	2.8
Admissions	115.7	112.3	111.3	109.9	112.5
Inpatient Days	626.5	611.5	621.4	638.3	649.7
Inpatient Surgeries..............	34.5	32.2	33.6	32.8	33.6
Births........................	12.7	12.7	13.2	13.0	13.0
Outpatient					
Emergency Outpatient Visits.......	400.9	375.7	372.6	357.7	352.6
Other Outpatient Visits...........	2,172.7	2,225.1	2,128.9	1,910.4	1,864.5
Total Outpatient Visits	2,573.7	2,600.8	2,501.5	2,268.1	2,217.1
Outpatient Surgeries	73.6	70.3	65.5	67.1	65.6
Expense per Capita (per person)....	$1,524.4	$1,390.4	$1,353.9	$1,307.6	$1,315.7

TABLE 6

MINNESOTA

U.S. Registered Community Hospitals
(Nonfederal, short-term general and other special hospitals)

Overview 1998–2002

	2002	2001	2000	1999	1998
Total U.S. Community Hospitals in					
Minnesota	133	133	135	134	136
Bed Size Category					
6-24	18	16	16	16	17
25-49	20	23	25	25	26
50-99	38	39	38	40	39
100-199	41	38	39	37	37
200-299	4	6	6	5	6
300-399	3	3	3	6	6
400-499	5	4	4	1	1
500 + ...	4	4	4	4	4
Location					
Hospitals Urban	46	45	45	44	45
Hospitals Rural	87	88	90	90	91
Control					
State and Local Government	44	43	44	42	48
Not for Profit	89	90	91	92	88
Investor owned	0	0	0	0	0
Physician Models					
Independent Practice Association	24	24	21	15	18
Group Practice without Walls	2	2	1	1	4
Open Physician-Hospital Organization	8	9	8	7	12
Closed Physician-Hospital Organization . . .	7	5	4	10	7
Management Service Organization	3	3	3	3	7
Integrated Salary Model	40	37	28	31	31
Equity Model	1	2	2	1	1
Foundation	2	3	1	5	8
Insurance Products					
Health Maintenance Organization	13	19	19	26	24
Preferred Provider Organization	16	18	22	20	25
Indemnity Fee for Service	5	3	5	9	11
Managed Care Contracts					
Health Maintenance Organization	64	70	62	60	64
Preferred Provider Organization	72	78	68	66	63
Affiliations					
Hospitals in a System	50	54	45	49	48
Hospitals in a Network	22	21	17	14	27
Hospitals in a Group Purchasing					
Organization	95	104	94	75	42

States

TABLE 6

MINNESOTA

U.S. Registered Community Hospitals
(Nonfederal, short-term general and other special hospitals)

Utilization, Personnel, Revenue and Expenses, Community Health Indicators 1998–2002

	2002	2001	2000	1999	1998
TOTAL FACILITY (Includes Hospital and Nursing Home Units)					
Utilization - Inpatient					
Beds	16,659	16,508	16,705	16,458	16,486
Admissions	598,852	586,016	570,672	534,692	515,813
Inpatient Days	4,162,994	4,102,576	4,089,075	4,046,050	4,110,360
Average Length of Stay.	7.0	7.0	7.2	7.6	8.0
Inpatient Surgeries.	178,443	173,787	162,709	158,632	157,630
Births.	68,220	67,706	61,900	65,535	65,944
Utilization - Outpatient					
Emergency Outpatient Visits	1,605,237	1,506,825	1,454,970	1,364,802	1,143,117
Other Outpatient Visits.	7,296,661	7,059,035	5,880,642	5,085,822	4,372,094
Total Outpatient Visits	8,901,898	8,565,860	7,335,612	6,450,624	5,515,211
Outpatient Surgeries	279,781	269,459	265,564	267,683	243,258
Personnel					
Full Time RNs	7,750	7,296	7,235	8,404	9,198
Full Time LPNs	1,383	1,463	1,420	1,857	1,922
Part Time RNs	18,637	18,377	16,856	14,906	12,433
Part Time LPNs	2,452	2,612	2,614	2,845	2,356
Total Full Time.	45,546	42,981	40,907	44,027	43,315
Total Part Time	56,063	56,308	52,536	47,798	41,291
Revenue - Inpatient					
Gross Inpatient Revenue.	$10,100,747,850	$8,594,174,827	$7,576,893,093	$6,735,210,305	$5,967,869,859
Revenue - Outpatient					
Gross Outpatient Revenue	$6,116,730,184	$5,096,222,863	$4,321,208,532	$3,755,772,176	$3,119,336,088
Revenue and Expenses - Totals					
(Includes Inpatient and Outpatient)					
Total Gross Revenue.	$16,217,478,034	$13,690,397,690	$11,898,101,625	$10,490,982,481	$9,087,205,947
Deductions from Revenue	8,364,782,672	6,733,859,329	5,560,355,139	4,745,177,001	3,891,787,468
Net Patient Revenue	7,852,695,362	6,956,538,361	6,337,746,486	5,745,805,480	5,195,418,479
Other Operating Revenue	448,432,311	371,921,708	325,155,610	312,210,657	299,354,500
Other Nonoperating Revenue	42,923,367	77,288,116	160,470,734	137,362,929	148,114,241
Total Net Revenue.	8,344,051,040	7,405,748,185	6,823,372,830	6,195,379,066	5,642,887,220
Total Expenses.	7,883,926,731	7,067,072,024	6,411,848,478	5,807,149,050	5,265,388,159
HOSPITAL UNIT (Excludes Separate Nursing Home Units)					
Utilization - Inpatient					
Beds	13,078	12,558	12,669	12,737	11,874
Admissions	594,971	581,569	565,919	528,535	508,463
Inpatient Days	2,918,600	2,715,146	2,714,883	2,789,190	2,540,143
Average Length of Stay.	4.9	4.7	4.8	5.3	5.0
Personnel					
Total Full Time.	43,905	40,988	38,802	42,095	41,327
Total Part Time	53,701	53,557	49,441	45,255	38,314
Revenue and Expenses - Totals					
(Includes Inpatient and Outpatient)					
Total Net Revenue.	$8,180,139,592	$7,227,917,429	$6,659,630,244	$6,039,668,626	$5,453,930,915
Total Expenses.	7,729,649,102	6,891,386,470	6,245,744,327	5,647,638,456	5,088,046,865
COMMUNITY HEALTH INDICATORS PER 1000 POPULATION					
Total Population (in thousands)	5,020	4,972	4,919	4,776	4,726
Inpatient					
Beds	3.3	3.3	3.4	3.4	3.5
Admissions	119.3	117.9	116.0	112.0	109.1
Inpatient Days	829.3	825.1	831.2	847.3	869.7
Inpatient Surgeries.	35.5	35.0	33.1	33.2	33.4
Births.	13.6	13.6	12.6	13.7	14.0
Outpatient					
Emergency Outpatient Visits	319.8	303.0	295.8	285.8	241.9
Other Outpatient Visits.	1,453.6	1,419.7	1,195.4	1,065.0	925.0
Total Outpatient Visits	1,773.4	1,722.7	1,491.1	1,350.8	1,166.9
Outpatient Surgeries	55.7	54.2	54.0	56.1	51.5
Expense per Capita (per person). . . .	$1,570.6	$1,421.3	$1,303.4	$1,216.0	$1,114.0

States

TABLE 6

MISSISSIPPI

U.S. Registered Community Hospitals
(Nonfederal, short-term general and other special hospitals)

Overview 1998–2002

	2002	2001	2000	1999	1998
Total U.S. Community Hospitals in Mississippi	91	96	95	96	96
Bed Size Category					
6-24	2	2	1	1	1
25-49	19	17	18	18	16
50-99	26	29	29	34	36
100-199	29	33	31	27	28
200-299	4	6	8	7	7
300-399	4	2	1	4	3
400-499	2	2	2	0	0
500 + ...	5	5	5	5	5
Location					
Hospitals Urban......................	18	20	19	20	19
Hospitals Rural	73	76	76	76	77
Control					
State and Local Government	42	45	45	46	47
Not for Profit	25	27	26	28	29
Investor owned	24	24	24	22	20
Physician Models					
Independent Practice Association........	11	5	13	11	12
Group Practice without Walls...........	10	4	9	8	5
Open Physician-Hospital Organization....	21	18	22	27	31
Closed Physician-Hospital Organization...	5	5	10	9	6
Management Service Organization.......	10	6	9	8	8
Integrated Salary Model	19	14	16	15	14
Equity Model	0	3	3	3	3
Foundation..........................	11	11	12	13	14
Insurance Products					
Health Maintenance Organization........	12	12	13	13	17
Preferred Provider Organization.........	50	47	48	53	53
Indemnity Fee for Service..............	15	15	15	15	18
Managed Care Contracts					
Health Maintenance Organization........	10	2	0	1	0
Preferred Provider Organization.........	39	38	3	0	0
Affiliations					
Hospitals in a System.................	32	36	33	35	36
Hospitals in a Network	35	32	35	32	32
Hospitals in a Group Purchasing Organization.......................	8	1	—	—	—

States

TABLE 6

MISSISSIPPI

U.S. Registered Community Hospitals
(Nonfederal, short-term general and other special hospitals)

Utilization, Personnel, Revenue and Expenses, Community Health Indicators 1998–2002

	2002	2001	2000	1999	1998
TOTAL FACILITY (Includes Hospital and Nursing Home Units)					
Utilization - Inpatient					
Beds	13,144	13,670	13,598	13,217	13,005
Admissions	416,815	436,100	424,772	415,776	413,907
Inpatient Days	2,745,516	2,990,906	2,929,248	2,916,549	2,949,682
Average Length of Stay...........	6.6	6.9	6.9	7.0	7.1
Inpatient Surgeries.............	121,710	116,292	111,465	120,663	115,790
Births.........................	39,553	42,049	42,199	40,410	39,101
Utilization - Outpatient					
Emergency Outpatient Visits.......	1,556,488	1,501,052	1,478,883	1,429,819	1,425,892
Other Outpatient Visits...........	2,439,892	2,601,447	2,228,914	2,027,658	2,004,076
Total Outpatient Visits	3,996,380	4,102,499	3,707,797	3,457,477	3,429,968
Outpatient Surgeries	152,172	154,317	151,832	145,593	129,570
Personnel					
Full Time RNs	9,091	9,467	9,424	9,594	9,488
Full Time LPNs	1,923	2,025	2,001	2,170	2,478
Part Time RNs..................	3,906	3,636	3,185	2,728	2,701
Part Time LPNs	615	648	583	626	598
Total Full Time..................	40,107	40,936	39,550	40,398	42,165
Total Part Time	11,478	11,627	11,597	10,122	9,973
Revenue - Inpatient					
Gross Inpatient Revenue..........	$5,702,037,800	$5,203,288,483	$4,486,744,256	$4,219,185,699	$3,975,096,989
Revenue - Outpatient					
Gross Outpatient Revenue	$3,320,188,769	$2,891,655,269	$2,471,664,887	$2,196,978,616	$1,932,971,070
Revenue and Expenses - Totals					
(Includes Inpatient and Outpatient)					
Total Gross Revenue.............	$9,022,226,569	$8,094,943,752	$6,958,409,143	$6,416,164,315	$5,908,068,059
Deductions from Revenue.........	4,977,500,289	4,344,923,458	3,645,598,561	3,165,780,811	2,735,462,519
Net Patient Revenue	4,044,726,280	3,750,020,294	3,312,810,582	3,250,383,504	3,172,605,540
Other Operating Revenue	164,171,241	137,215,985	191,115,070	116,160,034	117,184,927
Other Nonoperating Revenue	60,542,992	52,257,480	67,563,680	50,570,163	48,450,755
Total Net Revenue..............	4,269,440,513	3,939,493,759	3,571,489,332	3,417,113,701	3,338,241,222
Total Expenses..................	3,907,203,934	3,614,544,722	3,327,375,432	3,202,825,608	3,138,686,670
HOSPITAL UNIT (Excludes Separate Nursing Home Units)					
Utilization - Inpatient					
Beds	11,579	12,000	11,995	11,633	11,438
Admissions	415,182	434,827	423,739	414,619	412,755
Inpatient Days	2,217,217	2,400,974	2,358,912	2,355,643	2,400,129
Average Length of Stay...........	5.3	5.5	5.6	5.7	5.8
Personnel					
Total Full Time..................	39,009	39,670	38,528	39,375	40,974
Total Part Time	11,212	11,254	11,248	9,815	9,699
Revenue and Expenses - Totals					
(Includes Inpatient and Outpatient)					
Total Net Revenue..............	$4,211,247,202	$3,896,587,199	$3,515,536,637	$3,377,670,317	$3,304,486,181
Total Expenses..................	3,866,957,946	3,583,850,640	3,293,094,874	3,174,354,952	3,113,147,029
COMMUNITY HEALTH INDICATORS PER 1000 POPULATION					
Total Population (in thousands)	2,872	2,858	2,845	2,769	2,751
Inpatient					
Beds	4.6	4.8	4.8	4.8	4.7
Admissions	145.1	152.6	149.3	150.2	150.4
Inpatient Days	956.0	1,046.5	1,029.7	1,053.4	1,072.1
Inpatient Surgeries.............	42.4	40.7	39.2	43.6	42.1
Births.........................	13.8	14.7	14.8	14.6	14.2
Outpatient					
Emergency Outpatient Visits.......	542.0	525.2	519.9	516.4	518.3
Other Outpatient Visits...........	849.6	910.2	783.5	732.4	728.4
Total Outpatient Visits	1,391.6	1,435.4	1,303.4	1,248.8	1,246.7
Outpatient Surgeries	53.0	54.0	53.4	52.6	47.1
Expense per Capita (per person)....	$1,360.6	$1,264.7	$1,169.7	$1,156.8	$1,140.8

TABLE 6

MISSOURI

U.S. Registered Community Hospitals
(Nonfederal, short-term general and other special hospitals)

Overview 1998–2002

	2002	2001	2000	1999	1998
Total U.S. Community Hospitals in Missouri	119	117	119	118	122
Bed Size Category					
6-24	6	4	4	4	3
25-49	31	31	33	29	30
50-99	25	25	24	28	28
100-199	22	22	21	21	25
200-299	17	16	17	13	15
300-399	9	8	9	13	10
400-499	4	5	4	2	3
500 +	5	6	7	8	8
Location					
Hospitals Urban	61	60	61	60	64
Hospitals Rural	58	57	58	58	58
Control					
State and Local Government	36	36	37	35	36
Not for Profit	68	69	71	71	71
Investor owned	15	12	11	12	15
Physician Models					
Independent Practice Association	17	17	22	19	30
Group Practice without Walls	2	4	8	8	9
Open Physician-Hospital Organization	21	26	30	32	35
Closed Physician-Hospital Organization	13	16	17	23	28
Management Service Organization	10	10	9	17	19
Integrated Salary Model	52	50	49	50	44
Equity Model	2	1	3	2	3
Foundation	1	4	3	2	5
Insurance Products					
Health Maintenance Organization	28	31	48	57	56
Preferred Provider Organization	22	22	29	35	48
Indemnity Fee for Service	11	12	11	14	18
Managed Care Contracts					
Health Maintenance Organization	100	99	105	104	107
Preferred Provider Organization	108	106	112	99	108
Affiliations					
Hospitals in a System	68	63	65	63	68
Hospitals in a Network	39	43	44	40	45
Hospitals in a Group Purchasing Organization	107	103	105	100	99

TABLE 6

MISSOURI

U.S. Registered Community Hospitals
(Nonfederal, short-term general and other special hospitals)

Utilization, Personnel, Revenue and Expenses, Community Health Indicators 1998–2002

	2002	2001	2000	1999	1998
TOTAL FACILITY (Includes Hospital and Nursing Home Units)					
Utilization - Inpatient					
Beds	18,891	19,257	20,140	20,253	20,685
Admissions	809,355	800,648	773,261	742,867	741,816
Inpatient Days	4,235,298	4,219,659	4,269,800	4,247,921	4,325,879
Average Length of Stay.	5.2	5.3	5.5	5.7	5.8
Inpatient Surgeries	209,739	210,030	207,476	200,706	205,887
Births.	74,815	75,350	77,333	75,625	76,031
Utilization - Outpatient					
Emergency Outpatient Visits	2,476,194	2,443,744	2,326,906	2,411,820	2,115,060
Other Outpatient Visits.	12,427,894	11,755,063	12,479,871	12,231,541	8,046,012
Total Outpatient Visits	14,904,088	14,198,807	14,806,777	14,643,361	10,161,072
Outpatient Surgeries	393,761	389,098	381,289	362,462	367,983
Personnel					
Full Time RNs	19,236	18,576	18,689	18,685	18,484
Full Time LPNs	3,039	2,881	3,019	2,917	3,432
Part Time RNs	11,417	12,017	11,206	10,562	10,787
Part Time LPNs	1,174	1,171	1,221	1,162	1,380
Total Full Time.	85,983	82,978	82,820	79,501	82,902
Total Part Time	35,177	35,676	34,263	31,230	33,394
Revenue - Inpatient					
Gross Inpatient Revenue.	$13,686,358,547	$12,106,385,281	$11,082,223,366	$9,964,294,835	$9,229,915,545
Revenue - Outpatient					
Gross Outpatient Revenue	$8,390,580,917	$7,685,930,325	$6,685,962,437	$5,791,429,121	$5,196,890,359
Revenue and Expenses - Totals					
(Includes Inpatient and Outpatient)					
Total Gross Revenue.	$22,076,939,464	$19,792,315,606	$17,768,185,803	$15,755,723,956	$14,426,805,904
Deductions from Revenue.	12,532,916,322	10,984,983,535	9,652,801,745	8,213,774,013	7,091,069,076
Net Patient Revenue	9,544,023,142	8,807,332,071	8,115,384,058	7,541,949,943	7,335,736,828
Other Operating Revenue	570,212,535	486,319,667	440,053,995	484,296,906	457,285,200
Other Nonoperating Revenue	89,622,933	154,063,942	196,916,165	197,565,929	291,564,766
Total Net Revenue.	10,203,858,610	9,447,715,680	8,752,354,218	8,223,812,778	8,084,586,794
Total Expenses.	9,747,670,518	9,118,864,692	8,534,174,151	7,953,842,591	7,576,182,640
HOSPITAL UNIT (Excludes Separate Nursing Home Units)					
Utilization - Inpatient					
Beds	17,396	17,642	18,096	18,003	18,049
Admissions	791,849	779,379	746,131	712,942	703,211
Inpatient Days	3,844,365	3,781,344	3,724,585	3,599,897	3,573,987
Average Length of Stay.	4.9	4.9	5.0	5.0	5.1
Personnel					
Total Full Time.	85,531	81,903	81,237	77,895	80,127
Total Part Time	34,767	35,092	33,437	30,530	32,565
Revenue and Expenses - Totals					
(Includes Inpatient and Outpatient)					
Total Net Revenue.	$10,043,647,885	$9,292,053,516	$8,558,718,897	$8,054,357,353	$7,859,783,453
Total Expenses.	9,620,134,560	8,999,337,551	8,392,524,096	7,825,633,137	7,404,638,643
COMMUNITY HEALTH INDICATORS PER 1000 POPULATION					
Total Population (in thousands)	5,673	5,630	5,595	5,468	5,438
Inpatient					
Beds	3.3	3.4	3.6	3.7	3.8
Admissions	142.7	142.2	138.2	135.8	136.4
Inpatient Days	746.6	749.5	763.1	776.8	795.6
Inpatient Surgeries	37.0	37.3	37.1	36.7	37.9
Births.	13.2	13.4	13.8	13.8	14.0
Outpatient					
Emergency Outpatient Visits	436.5	434.1	415.9	441.1	389.0
Other Outpatient Visits.	2,190.9	2,088.0	2,230.5	2,236.8	1,479.7
Total Outpatient Visits	2,627.4	2,522.1	2,646.3	2,677.8	1,868.7
Outpatient Surgeries	69.4	69.1	68.1	66.3	67.7
Expense per Capita (per person). . . .	$1,718.4	$1,619.8	$1,525.3	$1,454.5	$1,393.3

States

TABLE 6

MONTANA

U.S. Registered Community Hospitals
(Nonfederal, short-term general and other special hospitals)

Overview 1998–2002

	2002	2001	2000	1999	1998
Total U.S. Community Hospitals in					
Montana............................	53	53	52	53	53
Bed Size Category					
6-24	8	7	7	7	7
25-49	15	15	14	13	13
50-99	18	17	19	19	20
100-199	9	10	8	9	8
200-299	1	2	2	3	3
300-399	2	1	1	1	1
400-499	0	1	1	1	1
500 + ...	0	0	0	0	0
Location					
Hospitals Urban......................	5	5	3	3	3
Hospitals Rural	48	48	49	50	50
Control					
State and Local Government	10	11	10	12	10
Not for Profit	43	42	42	41	43
Investor owned	0	0	0	0	0
Physician Models					
Independent Practice Association........	6	7	11	5	6
Group Practice without Walls	3	3	3	1	0
Open Physician-Hospital Organization....	7	9	9	9	9
Closed Physician-Hospital Organization...	1	1	1	3	0
Management Service Organization........	6	6	5	2	5
Integrated Salary Model	22	18	16	16	11
Equity Model	1	1	0	0	0
Foundation.........................	2	2	5	1	2
Insurance Products					
Health Maintenance Organization........	4	5	7	7	6
Preferred Provider Organization.........	6	5	6	3	3
Indemnity Fee for Service..............	3	2	2	2	4
Managed Care Contracts					
Health Maintenance Organization........	13	12	14	15	12
Preferred Provider Organization.........	23	24	26	20	20
Affiliations					
Hospitals in a System.................	11	10	10	11	13
Hospitals in a Network	25	23	22	21	16
Hospitals in a Group Purchasing					
Organization......................	47	47	48	42	42

TABLE **6**

MONTANA

U.S. Registered Community Hospitals
(Nonfederal, short-term general and other special hospitals)

Utilization, Personnel, Revenue and Expenses, Community Health Indicators 1998–2002

	2002	2001	2000	1999	1998
TOTAL FACILITY (Includes Hospital and Nursing Home Units)					
Utilization - Inpatient					
Beds..........................	4,263	4,463	4,255	4,668	4,413
Admissions....................	106,758	103,346	99,273	97,875	97,345
Inpatient Days..................	1,071,834	1,058,079	1,045,460	1,161,334	1,090,989
Average Length of Stay...........	10.0	10.2	10.5	11.9	11.2
Inpatient Surgeries.............	32,343	31,774	31,365	30,824	30,475
Births........................	9,963	9,766	9,828	9,826	9,772
Utilization - Outpatient					
Emergency Outpatient Visits.......	276,829	276,175	270,905	263,239	259,462
Other Outpatient Visits...........	2,381,906	2,372,170	2,377,671	2,276,174	2,029,023
Total Outpatient Visits	2,658,735	2,648,345	2,648,576	2,539,413	2,288,485
Outpatient Surgeries	38,792	37,544	38,146	38,123	41,027
Personnel					
Full Time RNs	2,233	2,139	2,262	2,206	2,053
Full Time LPNs	487	493	520	480	538
Part Time RNs.................	1,819	1,695	1,705	1,415	1,643
Part Time LPNs	322	347	375	263	435
Total Full Time.................	11,834	11,464	11,394	11,578	10,846
Total Part Time	6,893	6,492	6,319	5,676	5,982
Revenue - Inpatient					
Gross Inpatient Revenue..........	$1,196,591,796	$1,105,228,828	$999,654,818	$926,618,947	$858,900,634
Revenue - Outpatient					
Gross Outpatient Revenue	$928,260,803	$835,450,580	$737,774,057	$667,505,475	$600,992,951
Revenue and Expenses - Totals					
(Includes Inpatient and Outpatient)					
Total Gross Revenue.............	$2,124,852,599	$1,940,679,408	$1,737,428,875	$1,594,124,422	$1,459,893,585
Deductions from Revenue.........	805,155,142	727,980,516	625,526,349	527,906,272	448,396,455
Net Patient Revenue	1,319,697,457	1,212,698,892	1,111,902,526	1,066,218,150	1,011,497,130
Other Operating Revenue	54,199,364	52,002,157	46,591,161	64,179,153	41,278,334
Other Nonoperating Revenue	11,449,900	29,771,646	37,823,173	29,299,977	57,383,432
Total Net Revenue..............	1,385,346,721	1,294,472,695	1,196,316,860	1,159,697,280	1,110,158,896
Total Expenses.................	1,328,470,349	1,216,570,389	1,145,815,779	1,082,320,886	1,002,984,008
HOSPITAL UNIT (Excludes Separate Nursing Home Units)					
Utilization - Inpatient					
Beds..........................	2,281	2,591	2,301	2,665	2,479
Admissions....................	102,888	99,503	95,295	92,995	92,826
Inpatient Days..................	445,638	466,644	421,283	526,200	460,325
Average Length of Stay...........	4.3	4.7	4.4	5.7	5.0
Personnel					
Total Full Time.................	10,659	10,407	10,273	10,632	9,755
Total Part Time.................	5,944	5,610	5,566	4,994	5,369
Revenue and Expenses - Totals					
(Includes Inpatient and Outpatient)					
Total Net Revenue..............	$1,312,606,078	$1,226,159,560	$1,133,832,079	$1,094,400,649	$1,034,194,455
Total Expenses.................	1,254,156,946	1,149,226,075	1,083,787,392	1,018,250,749	940,693,445
COMMUNITY HEALTH INDICATORS PER 1000 POPULATION					
Total Population (in thousands)	909	904	902	883	880
Inpatient					
Beds..........................	4.7	4.9	4.7	5.3	5.0
Admissions....................	117.4	114.3	110.0	110.9	110.7
Inpatient Days..................	1,178.5	1,169.9	1,158.8	1,315.5	1,240.4
Inpatient Surgeries..............	35.6	35.1	34.8	34.9	34.6
Births........................	11.0	10.8	10.9	11.1	11.1
Outpatient					
Emergency Outpatient Visits.......	304.4	305.4	300.3	298.2	295.0
Other Outpatient Visits...........	2,619.1	2,622.8	2,635.4	2,578.4	2,306.9
Total Outpatient Visits	2,923.4	2,928.2	2,935.7	2,876.6	2,601.9
Outpatient Surgeries	42.7	41.5	42.3	43.2	46.6
Expense per Capita (per person)....	$1,460.7	$1,345.1	$1,270.0	$1,226.0	$1,140.4

States

TABLE 6

NEBRASKA

U.S. Registered Community Hospitals
(Nonfederal, short-term general and other special hospitals)

Overview 1998–2002

	2002	2001	2000	1999	1998
Total U.S. Community Hospitals in					
Nebraska	86	84	85	85	86
Bed Size Category					
6-24	19	18	18	18	21
25-49	30	27	28	27	26
50-99	16	17	19	18	16
100-199	9	10	8	10	11
200-299	6	6	6	6	7
300-399	2	2	2	2	1
400-499	0	0	0	0	0
500 + ...	4	4	4	4	4
Location					
Hospitals Urban	14	14	13	13	13
Hospitals Rural	72	70	72	72	73
Control					
State and Local Government	41	39	41	41	41
Not for Profit	43	43	43	43	43
Investor owned	2	2	1	1	2
Physician Models					
Independent Practice Association	5	6	8	6	6
Group Practice without Walls	2	1	1	1	2
Open Physician-Hospital Organization	14	17	14	16	19
Closed Physician-Hospital Organization . . .	0	0	1	2	1
Management Service Organization	0	0	1	5	5
Integrated Salary Model	22	28	32	34	31
Equity Model	0	0	0	1	1
Foundation	1	1	2	4	4
Insurance Products					
Health Maintenance Organization	4	1	5	5	8
Preferred Provider Organization	17	15	17	21	19
Indemnity Fee for Service	2	2	5	3	3
Managed Care Contracts					
Health Maintenance Organization	21	24	31	28	30
Preferred Provider Organization	46	56	66	64	67
Affiliations					
Hospitals in a System	17	16	22	22	22
Hospitals in a Network	33	40	45	41	42
Hospitals in a Group Purchasing					
Organization	50	63	73	67	69

TABLE 6

NEBRASKA

U.S. Registered Community Hospitals
(Nonfederal, short-term general and other special hospitals)

Utilization, Personnel, Revenue and Expenses, Community Health Indicators 1998–2002

	2002	2001	2000	1999	1998
TOTAL FACILITY (Includes Hospital and Nursing Home Units)					
Utilization - Inpatient					
Beds	8,106	8,324	8,161	8,326	8,133
Admissions	206,208	206,700	209,498	199,471	192,313
Inpatient Days	1,723,683	1,826,566	1,760,490	1,821,925	1,779,579
Average Length of Stay.	8.4	8.8	8.4	9.1	9.3
Inpatient Surgeries.	70,433	68,392	68,738	66,997	71,503
Births.	24,030	24,313	23,479	21,877	22,770
Utilization - Outpatient					
Emergency Outpatient Visits.	511,085	545,607	499,960	491,438	455,953
Other Outpatient Visits.	2,955,952	2,884,235	2,905,439	2,510,386	2,393,171
Total Outpatient Visits	3,467,037	3,429,842	3,405,399	3,001,824	2,849,124
Outpatient Surgeries	132,704	129,154	123,042	114,063	115,114
Personnel					
Full Time RNs	5,548	5,456	5,352	5,185	5,149
Full Time LPNs	997	1,044	1,041	1,059	1,057
Part Time RNs.	4,167	3,695	3,484	3,993	3,703
Part Time LPNs	678	649	692	769	749
Total Full Time.	24,517	24,476	23,898	23,412	23,011
Total Part Time	14,665	14,398	13,454	14,887	13,430
Revenue - Inpatient					
Gross Inpatient Revenue.	$3,420,226,799	$3,052,706,197	$2,675,259,869	$2,371,471,871	$2,195,397,641
Revenue - Outpatient					
Gross Outpatient Revenue	$2,180,716,982	$1,898,195,952	$1,561,380,290	$1,344,021,603	$1,162,909,796
Revenue and Expenses - Totals					
(Includes Inpatient and Outpatient)					
Total Gross Revenue.	$5,600,943,781	$4,950,902,149	$4,236,640,159	$3,715,493,474	$3,358,307,437
Deductions from Revenue.	2,630,090,894	2,221,659,602	1,816,852,259	1,523,396,593	1,293,025,623
Net Patient Revenue	2,970,852,887	2,729,242,547	2,419,787,900	2,192,096,881	2,065,281,814
Other Operating Revenue	146,854,319	131,134,300	122,358,298	111,258,095	97,728,471
Other Nonoperating Revenue	23,940,303	49,150,380	65,215,309	36,446,213	67,326,888
Total Net Revenue.	3,141,647,509	2,909,527,227	2,607,361,507	2,339,801,189	2,230,337,173
Total Expenses.	2,892,566,453	2,645,027,198	2,327,404,184	2,156,055,667	1,988,638,033
HOSPITAL UNIT (Excludes Separate Nursing Home Units)					
Utilization - Inpatient					
Beds	6,414	6,427	6,144	6,216	6,035
Admissions	200,622	201,225	203,541	191,227	186,219
Inpatient Days	1,180,270	1,223,636	1,104,318	1,114,416	1,086,543
Average Length of Stay.	5.9	6.1	5.4	5.8	5.8
Personnel					
Total Full Time.	23,564	23,330	22,725	22,230	22,014
Total Part Time	13,873	13,531	12,561	14,016	12,609
Revenue and Expenses - Totals					
(Includes Inpatient and Outpatient)					
Total Net Revenue.	$3,061,905,470	$2,817,978,178	$2,528,414,477	$2,247,886,654	$2,138,201,381
Total Expenses.	2,805,501,875	2,562,442,544	2,243,914,541	2,078,619,066	1,917,444,766
COMMUNITY HEALTH INDICATORS PER 1000 POPULATION					
Total Population (in thousands)	1,729	1,713	1,711	1,666	1,661
Inpatient					
Beds	4.7	4.9	4.8	5.0	4.9
Admissions	119.3	120.6	122.4	119.7	115.8
Inpatient Days	996.8	1,066.2	1,028.8	1,093.6	1,071.5
Inpatient Surgeries.	40.7	39.9	40.2	40.2	43.1
Births.	13.9	14.2	13.7	13.1	13.7
Outpatient					
Emergency Outpatient Visits.	295.6	318.5	292.2	295.0	274.5
Other Outpatient Visits.	1,709.5	1,683.5	1,697.8	1,506.8	1,441.0
Total Outpatient Visits	2,005.0	2,002.0	1,990.0	1,801.8	1,715.5
Outpatient Surgeries	76.7	75.4	71.9	68.5	69.3
Expense per Capita (per person). . . .	$1,672.8	$1,543.9	$1,360.1	$1,294.1	$1,197.4

States

TABLE 6

NEVADA

U.S. Registered Community Hospitals
(Nonfederal, short-term general and other special hospitals)

Overview 1998–2002

	2002	2001	2000	1999	1998
Total U.S. Community Hospitals in Nevada	26	24	22	22	20
Bed Size Category					
6-24	0	1	1	1	1
25-49	7	5	5	6	5
50-99	5	4	4	3	3
100-199	8	8	6	6	5
200-299	1	2	2	2	2
300-399	2	1	1	1	1
400-499	0	1	1	1	1
500 +	3	2	2	2	2
Location					
Hospitals Urban	17	15	13	14	12
Hospitals Rural	9	9	9	8	8
Control					
State and Local Government	6	7	7	8	7
Not for Profit	9	7	7	6	6
Investor owned	11	10	8	8	7
Physician Models					
Independent Practice Association	5	2	2	4	5
Group Practice without Walls	0	0	0	0	1
Open Physician-Hospital Organization	1	1	1	0	0
Closed Physician-Hospital Organization	0	0	0	0	0
Management Service Organization	1	1	2	3	4
Integrated Salary Model	3	3	2	3	3
Equity Model	0	0	0	0	0
Foundation	0	0	0	1	0
Insurance Products					
Health Maintenance Organization	3	2	3	0	2
Preferred Provider Organization	4	2	3	0	4
Indemnity Fee for Service	2	1	1	0	1
Managed Care Contracts					
Health Maintenance Organization	13	9	8	11	7
Preferred Provider Organization	14	11	9	13	10
Affiliations					
Hospitals in a System	10	11	7	9	9
Hospitals in a Network	4	3	3	4	2
Hospitals in a Group Purchasing Organization	14	14	7	10	7

TABLE 6

NEVADA

U.S. Registered Community Hospitals
(Nonfederal, short-term general and other special hospitals)

Utilization, Personnel, Revenue and Expenses, Community Health Indicators 1998–2002

	2002	2001	2000	1999	1998
TOTAL FACILITY (Includes Hospital and Nursing Home Units)					
Utilization - Inpatient					
Beds	4,495	4,099	3,810	3,706	3,528
Admissions	211,657	207,844	199,455	197,501	171,158
Inpatient Days	1,110,583	1,019,835	984,845	1,000,369	837,270
Average Length of Stay..........	5.2	4.9	4.9	5.1	4.9
Inpatient Surgeries..............	75,406	76,427	72,090	78,969	52,096
Births.........................	29,709	28,040	28,874	30,399	24,799
Utilization - Outpatient					
Emergency Outpatient Visits	626,330	548,798	573,220	527,219	463,706
Other Outpatient Visits............	1,835,894	1,577,315	1,618,898	1,599,270	1,128,937
Total Outpatient Visits	2,462,224	2,126,113	2,192,118	2,126,489	1,592,643
Outpatient Surgeries	87,157	91,748	84,840	111,460	63,138
Personnel					
Full Time RNs	4,605	3,984	4,255	3,992	3,547
Full Time LPNs	422	429	455	581	397
Part Time RNs	1,398	1,523	1,388	1,160	1,252
Part Time LPNs	83	101	72	104	87
Total Full Time................	16,340	15,682	16,173	14,846	13,410
Total Part Time	3,797	4,180	3,783	3,671	3,400
Revenue - Inpatient					
Gross Inpatient Revenue..........	$5,183,035,024	$3,997,307,168	$3,384,346,250	$3,224,856,025	$2,743,705,642
Revenue - Outpatient					
Gross Outpatient Revenue	$1,883,871,488	$1,486,747,093	$1,175,895,927	$1,120,428,723	$858,030,810
Revenue and Expenses - Totals					
(Includes Inpatient and Outpatient)					
Total Gross Revenue.............	$7,066,906,512	$5,484,054,261	$4,560,242,177	$4,345,284,748	$3,601,736,452
Deductions from Revenue.........	4,672,604,272	3,441,708,915	2,795,643,699	2,673,121,276	2,194,873,625
Net Patient Revenue	2,394,302,240	2,042,345,346	1,764,598,478	1,672,163,472	1,406,862,827
Other Operating Revenue	179,018,832	95,047,287	77,338,480	45,314,641	58,226,194
Other Nonoperating Revenue	16,877,884	25,143,034	34,250,055	18,599,731	33,553,971
Total Net Revenue..............	2,590,198,956	2,162,535,667	1,876,187,013	1,736,077,844	1,498,642,992
Total Expenses.................	2,257,000,776	2,087,682,180	1,790,079,467	1,623,910,172	1,392,140,547
HOSPITAL UNIT (Excludes Separate Nursing Home Units)					
Utilization - Inpatient					
Beds	4,416	3,969	3,712	3,600	3,479
Admissions	211,562	207,237	198,904	197,292	170,564
Inpatient Days	1,083,111	977,487	954,823	959,252	822,289
Average Length of Stay..........	5.1	4.7	4.8	4.9	4.8
Personnel					
Total Full Time................	16,270	15,611	16,039	14,788	13,375
Total Part Time	3,779	4,146	3,755	3,657	3,386
Revenue and Expenses - Totals					
(Includes Inpatient and Outpatient)					
Total Net Revenue..............	$2,586,007,972	$2,156,122,530	$1,870,827,186	$1,731,123,484	$1,495,619,656
Total Expenses.................	2,254,904,246	2,083,886,026	1,787,243,271	1,621,429,707	1,390,358,456
COMMUNITY HEALTH INDICATORS PER 1000 POPULATION					
Total Population (in thousands)	2,173	2,106	1,998	1,809	1,744
Inpatient					
Beds	2.1	1.9	1.9	2.0	2.0
Admissions	97.4	98.7	99.8	109.2	98.2
Inpatient Days	511.0	484.2	492.9	552.9	480.1
Inpatient Surgeries..............	34.7	36.3	36.1	43.6	29.9
Births.........................	13.7	13.3	14.4	16.8	14.2
Outpatient					
Emergency Outpatient Visits	288.2	260.6	286.9	291.4	265.9
Other Outpatient Visits............	844.7	748.9	810.2	883.9	647.4
Total Outpatient Visits	1,132.8	1,009.5	1,097.0	1,175.3	913.3
Outpatient Surgeries	40.1	43.6	42.5	61.6	36.2
Expense per Capita (per person)....	$1,038.4	$991.3	$895.8	$897.6	$798.4

States

TABLE 6

NEW HAMPSHIRE

U.S. Registered Community Hospitals
(Nonfederal, short-term general and other special hospitals)

Overview 1998–2002

	2002	2001	2000	1999	1998
Total U.S. Community Hospitals in New Hampshire...........................	28	28	28	28	28
Bed Size Category					
6-24	1	1	1	0	1
25-49	6	6	6	6	6
50-99	11	11	11	12	11
100-199	6	7	7	6	7
200-299	3	2	2	3	2
300-399	1	1	1	1	1
400-499	0	0	0	0	0
500 + ...	0	0	0	0	0
Location					
Hospitals Urban......................	10	10	10	10	10
Hospitals Rural	18	18	18	18	18
Control					
State and Local Government	0	0	0	0	0
Not for Profit	24	24	24	24	24
Investor owned	4	4	4	4	4
Physician Models					
Independent Practice Association........	2	2	2	2	2
Group Practice without Walls	2	2	2	1	0
Open Physician-Hospital Organization....	10	12	14	14	14
Closed Physician-Hospital Organization...	4	4	3	2	3
Management Service Organization.......	4	2	3	3	4
Integrated Salary Model	12	12	11	12	7
Equity Model	0	0	0	0	0
Foundation.........................	1	1	1	3	4
Insurance Products					
Health Maintenance Organization........	2	1	1	2	4
Preferred Provider Organization.........	1	0	0	0	1
Indemnity Fee for Service..............	1	0	0	0	3
Managed Care Contracts					
Health Maintenance Organization........	26	25	26	26	26
Preferred Provider Organization.........	25	23	22	23	24
Affiliations					
Hospitals in a System.................	15	14	14	14	12
Hospitals in a Network	8	8	9	7	6
Hospitals in a Group Purchasing Organization......................	25	25	22	23	22

States

TABLE 6

NEW HAMPSHIRE

U.S. Registered Community Hospitals
(Nonfederal, short-term general and other special hospitals)

Utilization, Personnel, Revenue and Expenses, Community Health Indicators 1998–2002

	2002	2001	2000	1999	1998
TOTAL FACILITY (Includes Hospital and Nursing Home Units)					
Utilization - Inpatient					
Beds	2,879	2,853	2,865	2,974	2,841
Admissions	117,996	116,071	111,227	109,110	108,942
Inpatient Days	646,838	637,239	611,919	599,777	658,884
Average Length of Stay	5.5	5.5	5.5	5.5	6.0
Inpatient Surgeries	33,553	33,702	33,595	32,864	31,291
Births	13,748	13,919	13,715	13,470	13,738
Utilization - Outpatient					
Emergency Outpatient Visits	550,380	537,367	526,103	491,840	476,050
Other Outpatient Visits	2,472,527	2,392,259	2,237,250	1,908,936	1,859,224
Total Outpatient Visits	3,022,907	2,929,626	2,763,353	2,400,776	2,335,274
Outpatient Surgeries	85,056	75,467	68,807	60,607	61,163
Personnel					
Full Time RNs	3,053	3,130	2,825	2,643	2,856
Full Time LPNs	159	175	172	210	166
Part Time RNs	2,720	2,087	2,139	2,261	1,994
Part Time LPNs	135	135	146	180	160
Total Full Time	14,657	14,578	12,923	12,681	12,351
Total Part Time	8,522	7,571	7,905	8,186	7,076
Revenue - Inpatient					
Gross Inpatient Revenue	$1,631,730,543	$1,452,518,894	$1,318,942,481	$1,151,678,573	$1,132,184,877
Revenue - Outpatient					
Gross Outpatient Revenue	$1,730,622,946	$1,422,018,438	$1,189,795,594	$991,577,915	$893,202,730
Revenue and Expenses - Totals					
(Includes Inpatient and Outpatient)					
Total Gross Revenue	$3,362,353,489	$2,874,537,332	$2,508,738,075	$2,143,256,488	$2,025,387,607
Deductions from Revenue	1,525,457,983	1,259,505,490	1,017,348,844	811,801,538	781,467,311
Net Patient Revenue	1,836,895,506	1,615,031,842	1,491,389,231	1,331,454,950	1,243,920,296
Other Operating Revenue	58,980,628	58,806,419	57,582,211	45,891,074	45,890,957
Other Nonoperating Revenue	-13,731,846	-2,412,941	60,358,157	88,389,168	53,492,672
Total Net Revenue	1,882,144,288	1,671,425,320	1,609,329,599	1,465,735,192	1,343,303,925
Total Expenses	1,830,377,475	1,617,994,197	1,466,080,802	1,288,450,986	1,250,170,087
HOSPITAL UNIT (Excludes Separate Nursing Home Units)					
Utilization - Inpatient					
Beds	2,691	2,665	2,677	2,786	2,661
Admissions	117,544	115,645	110,784	108,741	108,707
Inpatient Days	583,999	574,417	548,348	538,451	597,795
Average Length of Stay	5.0	5.0	4.9	5.0	5.5
Personnel					
Total Full Time	14,531	14,458	12,800	12,559	12,257
Total Part Time	8,468	7,510	7,856	8,107	7,006
Revenue and Expenses - Totals					
(Includes Inpatient and Outpatient)					
Total Net Revenue	$1,871,385,906	$1,660,849,124	$1,598,999,933	$1,456,900,913	$1,335,072,570
Total Expenses	1,823,178,785	1,611,350,879	1,459,873,435	1,283,050,412	1,244,489,322
COMMUNITY HEALTH INDICATORS PER 1000 POPULATION					
Total Population (in thousands)	1,275	1,259	1,236	1,201	1,186
Inpatient					
Beds	2.3	2.3	2.3	2.5	2.4
Admissions	92.5	92.2	90.0	90.8	91.9
Inpatient Days	507.3	506.1	495.2	499.3	555.6
Inpatient Surgeries	26.3	26.8	27.2	27.4	26.4
Births	10.8	11.1	11.1	11.2	11.6
Outpatient					
Emergency Outpatient Visits	431.7	426.8	425.7	409.5	401.5
Other Outpatient Visits	1,939.2	1,899.9	1,810.4	1,589.3	1,567.9
Total Outpatient Visits	2,370.8	2,326.6	2,236.1	1,998.8	1,969.3
Outpatient Surgeries	66.7	59.9	55.7	50.5	51.6
Expense per Capita (per person)	$1,435.5	$1,285.0	$1,186.4	$1,072.7	$1,054.3

States

TABLE 6

NEW JERSEY

U.S. Registered Community Hospitals
(Nonfederal, short-term general and other special hospitals)

Overview 1998–2002

	2002	2001	2000	1999	1998
Total U.S. Community Hospitals in New Jersey	81	78	80	81	83
Bed Size Category					
6-24	0	0	0	0	0
25-49	0	0	0	1	0
50-99	5	5	5	4	6
100-199	24	20	23	23	23
200-299	17	20	20	20	20
300-399	16	14	13	14	13
400-499	11	9	11	9	11
500 +	8	10	8	10	10
Location					
Hospitals Urban	81	78	80	81	83
Hospitals Rural	0	0	0	0	0
Control					
State and Local Government	2	2	2	2	3
Not for Profit	76	74	76	77	78
Investor owned	3	2	2	2	2
Physician Models					
Independent Practice Association	36	34	27	27	33
Group Practice without Walls	3	2	4	2	5
Open Physician-Hospital Organization	14	14	15	13	16
Closed Physician-Hospital Organization	5	5	7	7	9
Management Service Organization	23	19	16	21	28
Integrated Salary Model	15	16	15	9	13
Equity Model	2	1	1	2	3
Foundation	0	1	0	1	2
Insurance Products					
Health Maintenance Organization	10	7	14	14	17
Preferred Provider Organization	14	11	15	13	20
Indemnity Fee for Service	3	1	1	5	2
Managed Care Contracts					
Health Maintenance Organization	52	65	58	58	63
Preferred Provider Organization	50	63	57	56	60
Affiliations					
Hospitals in a System	52	51	48	22	37
Hospitals in a Network	32	32	21	6	13
Hospitals in a Group Purchasing Organization	61	61	50	19	35

TABLE 6

NEW JERSEY

U.S. Registered Community Hospitals
(Nonfederal, short-term general and other special hospitals)

Utilization, Personnel, Revenue and Expenses, Community Health Indicators 1998–2002

	2002	2001	2000	1999	1998
TOTAL FACILITY (Includes Hospital and Nursing Home Units)					
Utilization - Inpatient					
Beds	24,094	24,580	25,307	24,570	26,353
Admissions	1,094,781	1,083,798	1,073,619	1,068,664	1,082,668
Inpatient Days	6,190,443	6,165,019	6,340,657	6,150,912	6,790,222
Average Length of Stay...........	5.7	5.7	5.9	5.8	6.3
Inpatient Surgeries..............	303,451	293,850	313,803	307,971	311,540
Births..........................	112,900	109,870	111,057	109,793	104,533
Utilization - Outpatient					
Emergency Outpatient Visits.......	2,940,592	2,936,620	2,853,236	2,882,031	2,675,241
Other Outpatient Visits...........	12,957,409	15,507,940	13,454,037	13,244,138	12,621,673
Total Outpatient Visits	15,898,001	18,444,560	16,307,273	16,126,169	15,296,914
Outpatient Surgeries	416,709	399,564	412,229	414,003	390,589
Personnel					
Full Time RNs	21,384	22,522	23,154	21,826	22,657
Full Time LPNs	1,929	1,931	2,095	2,029	2,272
Part Time RNs.................	12,146	12,624	14,162	14,232	13,616
Part Time LPNs................	770	799	955	1,016	1,139
Total Full Time.................	98,194	98,209	100,557	93,901	99,737
Total Part Time	38,591	42,406	43,732	42,774	41,387
Revenue - Inpatient					
Gross Inpatient Revenue.........	$29,788,891,087	$26,602,275,344	$21,827,720,053	$17,817,044,301	$16,318,478,411
Revenue - Outpatient					
Gross Outpatient Revenue	$10,149,816,977	$8,452,299,275	$7,310,430,959	$5,867,036,075	$5,411,483,046
Revenue and Expenses - Totals					
(Includes Inpatient and Outpatient)					
Total Gross Revenue.............	$39,938,708,064	$35,054,574,619	$29,138,151,012	$23,684,080,376	$21,729,961,457
Deductions from Revenue.........	27,488,534,367	23,885,664,427	18,556,968,225	14,272,643,586	12,181,960,982
Net Patient Revenue	12,450,173,697	11,168,910,192	10,581,182,787	9,411,436,790	9,548,000,475
Other Operating Revenue	667,392,368	644,537,713	730,175,554	594,893,499	648,642,263
Other Nonoperating Revenue	26,399,177	77,244,348	226,655,485	205,235,554	286,808,485
Total Net Revenue..............	13,143,965,242	11,890,692,253	11,538,013,826	10,211,565,843	10,483,451,223
Total Expenses.................	12,841,553,561	11,716,951,020	11,253,553,740	10,079,107,532	10,411,039,349
HOSPITAL UNIT (Excludes Separate Nursing Home Units)					
Utilization - Inpatient					
Beds	23,315	23,716	24,650	23,754	24,756
Admissions	1,091,471	1,080,365	1,070,105	1,065,294	1,077,264
Inpatient Days	5,921,584	5,885,278	6,136,582	5,878,838	6,293,162
Average Length of Stay...........	5.4	5.4	5.7	5.5	5.8
Personnel					
Total Full Time.................	97,573	97,533	99,379	92,941	98,811
Total Part Time	38,411	42,140	43,215	42,320	41,009
Revenue and Expenses - Totals					
(Includes Inpatient and Outpatient)					
Total Net Revenue..............	$13,070,208,862	$11,822,055,392	$11,496,256,093	$10,161,679,983	$10,408,979,933
Total Expenses.................	12,781,447,599	11,659,210,376	11,210,748,330	10,026,590,107	10,344,410,778
COMMUNITY HEALTH INDICATORS PER 1000 POPULATION					
Total Population (in thousands)	8,590	8,484	8,414	8,143	8,096
Inpatient					
Beds	2.8	2.9	3.0	3.0	3.3
Admissions	127.4	127.7	127.6	131.2	133.7
Inpatient Days	720.6	726.6	753.6	755.3	838.8
Inpatient Surgeries..............	35.3	34.6	37.3	37.8	38.5
Births..........................	13.1	12.9	13.2	13.5	12.9
Outpatient					
Emergency Outpatient Visits.......	342.3	346.1	339.1	353.9	330.5
Other Outpatient Visits...........	1,508.4	1,827.8	1,598.9	1,626.4	1,559.1
Total Outpatient Visits	1,850.7	2,173.9	1,938.0	1,980.3	1,889.5
Outpatient Surgeries	48.5	47.1	49.0	50.8	48.2
Expense per Capita (per person)....	$1,494.9	$1,381.0	$1,337.4	$1,237.7	$1,286.0

States

TABLE 6

NEW MEXICO

U.S. Registered Community Hospitals
(Nonfederal, short-term general and other special hospitals)

Overview 1998–2002

	2002	2001	2000	1999	1998
Total U.S. Community Hospitals in New Mexico............................	36	35	35	36	36
Bed Size Category					
6-24	3	2	4	5	4
25-49	11	12	9	8	9
50-99	8	8	9	11	10
100-199	9	8	8	9	8
200-299	4	3	4	2	4
300-399	0	2	1	1	1
400-499	1	0	0	0	0
500 + ...	0	0	0	0	0
Location					
Hospitals Urban......................	14	13	13	13	13
Hospitals Rural	22	22	22	23	23
Control					
State and Local Government	9	10	9	11	12
Not for Profit	19	19	20	20	18
Investor owned	8	6	6	5	6
Physician Models					
Independent Practice Association........	6	5	9	12	11
Group Practice without Walls	0	1	3	4	2
Open Physician-Hospital Organization....	5	4	6	6	9
Closed Physician-Hospital Organization...	2	1	2	4	2
Management Service Organization.......	1	0	1	3	1
Integrated Salary Model	6	9	9	5	4
Equity Model	0	0	0	0	1
Foundation.........................	2	3	2	3	4
Insurance Products					
Health Maintenance Organization........	8	10	8	8	7
Preferred Provider Organization.........	7	6	10	11	10
Indemnity Fee for Service..............	5	4	5	6	4
Managed Care Contracts					
Health Maintenance Organization........	22	20	16	22	19
Preferred Provider Organization.........	20	17	16	18	15
Affiliations					
Hospitals in a System.................	14	16	14	15	16
Hospitals in a Network	4	5	5	9	8
Hospitals in a Group Purchasing Organization......................	24	24	21	21	17

TABLE 6

NEW MEXICO

U.S. Registered Community Hospitals
(Nonfederal, short-term general and other special hospitals)

Utilization, Personnel, Revenue and Expenses, Community Health Indicators 1998–2002

	2002	2001	2000	1999	1998
TOTAL FACILITY (Includes Hospital and Nursing Home Units)					
Utilization - Inpatient					
Beds	3,602	3,584	3,481	3,370	3,489
Admissions	180,041	164,461	173,575	163,700	157,875
Inpatient Days	849,396	758,923	731,708	725,713	707,418
Average Length of Stay	4.7	4.6	4.2	4.4	4.5
Inpatient Surgeries	59,388	45,395	51,466	57,164	54,474
Births	28,178	24,884	24,329	25,526	23,680
Utilization - Outpatient					
Emergency Outpatient Visits	705,643	528,979	532,526	512,645	466,049
Other Outpatient Visits	3,482,019	2,880,249	2,568,108	2,622,325	2,798,522
Total Outpatient Visits	4,187,662	3,409,228	3,100,634	3,134,970	3,264,571
Outpatient Surgeries	103,434	78,047	78,014	86,506	84,918
Personnel					
Full Time RNs	4,300	4,037	3,722	3,467	3,589
Full Time LPNs	626	627	487	508	459
Part Time RNs	2,365	1,330	2,267	2,204	2,860
Part Time LPNs	260	150	225	258	311
Total Full Time	20,133	19,121	15,505	15,616	14,975
Total Part Time	7,114	4,201	6,429	7,608	8,293
Revenue - Inpatient					
Gross Inpatient Revenue	$2,660,033,608	$2,100,619,929	$2,202,879,494	$2,114,743,157	$1,685,266,585
Revenue - Outpatient					
Gross Outpatient Revenue	$1,848,890,309	$1,530,614,098	$1,280,932,571	$1,235,146,668	$1,381,910,309
Revenue and Expenses - Totals					
(Includes Inpatient and Outpatient)					
Total Gross Revenue	$4,508,923,917	$3,631,234,027	$3,483,812,065	$3,349,889,825	$3,067,176,894
Deductions from Revenue	2,451,800,462	1,798,758,901	1,905,810,874	1,454,422,617	1,433,881,000
Net Patient Revenue	2,057,123,455	1,832,475,126	1,578,001,191	1,895,467,208	1,633,295,894
Other Operating Revenue	142,673,861	102,566,160	103,866,572	100,671,605	104,122,520
Other Nonoperating Revenue	30,460,788	32,406,351	30,473,501	33,471,257	34,118,361
Total Net Revenue	2,230,258,104	1,967,447,637	1,712,341,264	2,029,610,070	1,771,536,775
Total Expenses	2,129,702,267	1,868,614,170	1,695,651,227	1,847,553,034	1,599,265,050
HOSPITAL UNIT (Excludes Separate Nursing Home Units)					
Utilization - Inpatient					
Beds	3,592	3,498	3,426	3,279	3,411
Admissions	179,996	163,080	172,543	161,933	156,490
Inpatient Days	849,127	739,270	715,831	699,736	685,831
Average Length of Stay	4.7	4.5	4.1	4.3	4.4
Personnel					
Total Full Time	20,133	19,094	15,434	15,526	14,954
Total Part Time	7,114	4,196	6,401	7,573	8,292
Revenue and Expenses - Totals					
(Includes Inpatient and Outpatient)					
Total Net Revenue	$2,230,225,516	$1,961,248,667	$1,709,281,550	$2,023,848,425	$1,760,937,195
Total Expenses	2,129,675,083	1,865,267,433	1,693,109,995	1,845,065,340	1,593,743,179
COMMUNITY HEALTH INDICATORS PER 1000 POPULATION					
Total Population (in thousands)	1,855	1,829	1,819	1,740	1,734
Inpatient					
Beds	1.9	2.0	1.9	1.9	2.0
Admissions	97.1	89.9	95.4	94.1	91.1
Inpatient Days	457.9	414.9	402.2	417.1	408.1
Inpatient Surgeries	32.0	24.8	28.3	32.9	31.4
Births	15.2	13.6	13.4	14.7	13.7
Outpatient					
Emergency Outpatient Visits	380.4	289.2	292.8	294.6	268.8
Other Outpatient Visits	1,877.0	1,574.6	1,411.8	1,507.2	1,614.3
Total Outpatient Visits	2,257.4	1,863.8	1,704.5	1,801.9	1,883.2
Outpatient Surgeries	55.8	42.7	42.9	49.7	49.0
Expense per Capita (per person)	$1,148.1	$1,021.6	$932.2	$1,061.9	$922.5

States

TABLE **6**

NEW YORK

U.S. Registered Community Hospitals
(Nonfederal, short-term general and other special hospitals)

Overview 1998–2002

	2002	2001	2000	1999	1998
Total U.S. Community Hospitals in New York	211	212	215	218	222
Bed Size Category					
6-24	4	4	4	2	3
25-49	8	8	8	12	12
50-99	23	23	25	21	21
100-199	53	51	50	50	53
200-299	46	49	53	54	50
300-399	25	24	23	27	30
400-499	18	21	20	19	19
500 +	34	32	32	33	34
Location					
Hospitals Urban	173	176	180	182	186
Hospitals Rural	38	36	35	36	36
Control					
State and Local Government	26	25	24	25	24
Not for Profit	181	181	183	185	189
Investor owned	4	6	8	8	9
Physician Models					
Independent Practice Association	45	44	70	70	74
Group Practice without Walls	8	6	10	5	6
Open Physician-Hospital Organization	22	28	36	34	41
Closed Physician-Hospital Organization	11	10	11	13	14
Management Service Organization	13	21	32	36	32
Integrated Salary Model	46	30	44	31	35
Equity Model	3	2	2	3	5
Foundation	4	3	5	7	8
Insurance Products					
Health Maintenance Organization	47	38	51	51	61
Preferred Provider Organization	26	30	42	38	48
Indemnity Fee for Service	6	10	10	5	6
Managed Care Contracts					
Health Maintenance Organization	116	115	140	140	141
Preferred Provider Organization	107	108	128	117	111
Affiliations					
Hospitals in a System	74	81	92	90	84
Hospitals in a Network	67	71	77	87	86
Hospitals in a Group Purchasing Organization	128	138	133	133	121

TABLE **6**

NEW YORK

U.S. Registered Community Hospitals
(Nonfederal, short-term general and other special hospitals)

Utilization, Personnel, Revenue and Expenses, Community Health Indicators 1998–2002

	2002	2001	2000	1999	1998
TOTAL FACILITY (Includes Hospital and Nursing Home Units)					
Utilization - Inpatient					
Beds	65,570	67,296	66,434	68,924	68,511
Admissions	2,463,447	2,410,906	2,416,112	2,406,327	2,364,608
Inpatient Days	18,394,472	19,021,960	19,074,063	19,349,127	19,176,323
Average Length of Stay	7.5	7.9	7.9	8.0	8.1
Inpatient Surgeries	698,796	692,769	722,083	710,183	725,774
Births	251,311	249,035	254,165	256,910	249,782
Utilization - Outpatient					
Emergency Outpatient Visits	7,474,440	7,452,574	7,275,122	7,141,070	6,785,222
Other Outpatient Visits	39,286,094	38,193,199	39,096,732	38,601,503	36,888,203
Total Outpatient Visits	46,760,534	45,645,773	46,371,854	45,742,573	43,673,425
Outpatient Surgeries	1,379,645	1,254,924	1,263,783	1,176,107	1,224,017
Personnel					
Full Time RNs	62,771	63,798	63,283	62,747	61,620
Full Time LPNs	7,361	7,538	7,424	7,318	7,282
Part Time RNs	21,022	18,869	20,945	19,568	19,064
Part Time LPNs	2,240	2,094	2,208	2,188	2,102
Total Full Time	307,318	308,267	301,182	305,163	298,813
Total Part Time	69,818	65,664	70,536	66,143	62,730
Revenue - Inpatient					
Gross Inpatient Revenue	$47,822,780,230	$42,992,186,646	$37,492,283,644	$34,644,592,681	$33,644,430,383
Revenue - Outpatient					
Gross Outpatient Revenue	$22,679,522,539	$19,539,156,438	$16,875,958,120	$15,564,285,898	$14,046,961,332
Revenue and Expenses - Totals					
(Includes Inpatient and Outpatient)					
Total Gross Revenue	$70,502,302,769	$62,531,343,084	$54,368,241,764	$50,208,878,579	$47,691,391,715
Deductions from Revenue	37,481,624,861	31,905,296,191	25,694,206,309	22,649,391,683	21,019,392,047
Net Patient Revenue	33,020,677,908	30,626,046,893	28,674,035,455	27,559,486,896	26,671,999,668
Other Operating Revenue	3,204,465,501	3,163,011,300	2,641,649,037	2,645,639,145	2,248,627,300
Other Nonoperating Revenue	338,322,872	482,220,705	500,659,020	587,485,474	663,053,669
Total Net Revenue	36,563,466,281	34,271,278,898	31,816,343,512	30,792,611,515	29,583,680,637
Total Expenses	36,549,754,047	34,352,757,050	31,963,065,624	31,023,119,426	29,269,407,269
HOSPITAL UNIT (Excludes Separate Nursing Home Units)					
Utilization - Inpatient					
Beds	57,534	60,609	58,655	61,313	61,617
Admissions	2,448,584	2,398,757	2,404,711	2,395,003	2,355,270
Inpatient Days	15,627,829	16,630,275	16,229,578	16,680,325	16,782,177
Average Length of Stay	6.4	6.9	6.7	7.0	7.1
Personnel					
Total Full Time	301,508	302,961	294,588	300,691	294,622
Total Part Time	67,801	63,968	68,570	64,730	61,220
Revenue and Expenses - Totals					
(Includes Inpatient and Outpatient)					
Total Net Revenue	$35,990,827,886	$33,722,096,947	$31,324,367,381	$30,300,120,420	$29,118,978,713
Total Expenses	35,915,200,955	33,937,745,908	31,557,256,923	30,613,692,890	28,898,772,886
COMMUNITY HEALTH INDICATORS PER 1000 POPULATION					
Total Population (in thousands)	19,158	19,011	18,976	18,197	18,159
Inpatient					
Beds	3.4	3.5	3.5	3.8	3.8
Admissions	128.6	126.8	127.3	132.2	130.2
Inpatient Days	960.2	1,000.6	1,005.1	1,063.3	1,056.0
Inpatient Surgeries	36.5	36.4	38.1	39.0	40.0
Births	13.1	13.1	13.4	14.1	13.8
Outpatient					
Emergency Outpatient Visits	390.2	392.0	383.4	392.4	373.7
Other Outpatient Visits	2,050.7	2,009.0	2,060.3	2,121.4	2,031.4
Total Outpatient Visits	2,440.8	2,401.0	2,443.7	2,513.8	2,405.0
Outpatient Surgeries	72.0	66.0	66.6	64.6	67.4
Expense per Capita (per person)	$1,907.9	$1,807.0	$1,684.4	$1,704.9	$1,611.8

States

TABLE 6

NORTH CAROLINA

U.S. Registered Community Hospitals
(Nonfederal, short-term general and other special hospitals)

Overview 1998–2002

	2002	2001	2000	1999	1998
Total U.S. Community Hospitals in North Carolina	113	111	113	114	116
Bed Size Category					
6-24	4	2	2	2	3
25-49	10	11	12	12	11
50-99	27	23	22	22	24
100-199	37	38	41	43	42
200-299	13	14	14	14	16
300-399	8	8	9	9	7
400-499	1	3	1	0	1
500 +	13	12	12	12	12
Location					
Hospitals Urban	51	50	51	52	54
Hospitals Rural	62	61	62	62	62
Control					
State and Local Government	30	32	32	33	33
Not for Profit	75	70	71	72	72
Investor owned	8	9	10	9	11
Physician Models					
Independent Practice Association	10	10	14	24	19
Group Practice without Walls	4	3	2	1	3
Open Physician-Hospital Organization	25	24	25	31	24
Closed Physician-Hospital Organization	4	5	3	7	17
Management Service Organization	16	14	17	16	21
Integrated Salary Model	35	31	27	31	30
Equity Model	1	0	1	1	4
Foundation	7	6	5	9	13
Insurance Products					
Health Maintenance Organization	10	11	21	31	31
Preferred Provider Organization	22	19	28	39	40
Indemnity Fee for Service	5	4	5	10	8
Managed Care Contracts					
Health Maintenance Organization	66	67	71	73	76
Preferred Provider Organization	81	82	83	88	90
Affiliations					
Hospitals in a System	47	45	46	47	47
Hospitals in a Network	41	42	42	55	63
Hospitals in a Group Purchasing Organization	86	86	86	96	88

TABLE 6

NORTH CAROLINA

U.S. Registered Community Hospitals
(Nonfederal, short-term general and other special hospitals)

Utilization, Personnel, Revenue and Expenses, Community Health Indicators 1998–2002

	2002	2001	2000	1999	1998
TOTAL FACILITY (Includes Hospital and Nursing Home Units)					
Utilization - Inpatient					
Beds..........................	23,583	23,755	23,081	23,391	23,297
Admissions.....................	966,722	973,451	970,742	930,747	907,911
Inpatient Days	5,929,916	5,959,143	5,859,282	5,726,618	5,813,321
Average Length of Stay...........	6.1	6.1	6.0	6.2	6.4
Inpatient Surgeries...............	291,914	289,260	278,532	279,057	267,831
Births..........................	108,967	110,585	112,885	107,946	104,193
Utilization - Outpatient					
Emergency Outpatient Visits.......	3,322,226	3,230,198	2,983,548	2,844,680	2,885,802
Other Outpatient Visits...........	10,500,582	10,200,478	9,395,105	8,695,722	8,181,231
Total Outpatient Visits	13,822,808	13,430,676	12,378,653	11,540,402	11,067,033
Outpatient Surgeries	519,494	460,545	435,210	442,859	398,481
Personnel					
Full Time RNs	26,990	25,892	25,047	25,390	24,800
Full Time LPNs	2,221	2,381	2,393	2,441	2,515
Part Time RNs..................	11,510	10,855	10,575	9,506	8,517
Part Time LPNs	738	711	829	778	828
Total Full Time..................	107,239	105,994	104,926	102,981	102,539
Total Part Time	32,029	30,745	31,480	29,055	27,862
Revenue - Inpatient					
Gross Inpatient Revenue..........	$13,579,832,889	$12,324,492,251	$11,353,688,447	$10,061,207,112	$9,313,486,463
Revenue - Outpatient					
Gross Outpatient Revenue	$8,591,785,373	$7,225,934,040	$6,225,077,316	$5,345,769,802	$4,754,725,497
Revenue and Expenses - Totals					
(Includes Inpatient and Outpatient)					
Total Gross Revenue..............	$22,171,618,262	$19,550,426,291	$17,578,765,763	$15,406,976,914	$14,068,211,960
Deductions from Revenue..........	10,719,115,151	8,934,901,143	7,748,738,093	6,466,123,700	5,495,522,936
Net Patient Revenue	11,452,503,111	10,615,525,148	9,830,027,670	8,940,853,214	8,572,689,024
Other Operating Revenue	645,286,961	651,522,219	604,076,521	516,615,284	411,891,798
Other Nonoperating Revenue	81,728,986	181,114,779	376,862,714	311,116,988	362,764,227
Total Net Revenue...............	12,179,519,058	11,448,162,146	10,810,966,905	9,768,585,486	9,347,345,049
Total Expenses..................	11,563,648,159	10,625,022,294	10,028,178,236	8,980,841,368	8,364,935,329
HOSPITAL UNIT (Excludes Separate Nursing Home Units)					
Utilization - Inpatient					
Beds..........................	20,627	21,040	20,047	20,130	20,119
Admissions.....................	957,259	964,357	961,312	919,616	897,079
Inpatient Days	4,968,309	5,064,097	4,881,713	4,623,084	4,756,240
Average Length of Stay...........	5.2	5.3	5.1	5.0	5.3
Personnel					
Total Full Time..................	105,030	103,658	102,369	100,023	100,191
Total Part Time	31,000	29,819	30,453	28,139	27,031
Revenue and Expenses - Totals					
(Includes Inpatient and Outpatient)					
Total Net Revenue...............	$12,041,087,073	$11,322,622,945	$10,665,778,056	$9,617,095,929	$9,189,418,129
Total Expenses..................	11,418,905,299	10,504,024,494	9,896,919,542	8,840,059,827	8,223,397,759
COMMUNITY HEALTH INDICATORS PER 1000 POPULATION					
Total Population (in thousands)	8,320	8,186	8,049	7,651	7,546
Inpatient					
Beds..........................	2.8	2.9	2.9	3.1	3.1
Admissions.....................	116.2	118.9	120.6	121.7	120.3
Inpatient Days	712.7	727.9	727.9	748.5	770.4
Inpatient Surgeries...............	35.1	35.3	34.6	36.5	35.5
Births..........................	13.1	13.5	14.0	14.1	13.8
Outpatient					
Emergency Outpatient Visits.......	399.3	394.6	370.7	371.8	382.4
Other Outpatient Visits...........	1,262.1	1,246.0	1,167.2	1,136.6	1,084.2
Total Outpatient Visits	1,661.4	1,640.6	1,537.9	1,508.4	1,466.6
Outpatient Surgeries	62.4	56.3	54.1	57.9	52.8
Expense per Capita (per person)....	$1,389.8	$1,297.9	$1,245.8	$1,173.8	$1,108.6

States

TABLE 6

NORTH DAKOTA

U.S. Registered Community Hospitals
(Nonfederal, short-term general and other special hospitals)

Overview 1998–2002

	2002	2001	2000	1999	1998
Total U.S. Community Hospitals in North Dakota	42	40	42	41	43
Bed Size Category					
6-24	7	7	7	6	6
25-49	11	11	10	11	12
50-99	16	14	15	13	14
100-199	2	1	3	4	4
200-299	4	5	5	5	5
300-399	0	1	1	1	1
400-499	1	0	1	1	1
500 +	1	1	0	0	0
Location					
Hospitals Urban	7	7	6	6	6
Hospitals Rural	35	33	36	35	37
Control					
State and Local Government	0	0	0	0	0
Not for Profit	41	39	40	39	41
Investor owned	1	1	2	2	2
Physician Models					
Independent Practice Association	4	4	5	7	7
Group Practice without Walls	1	0	1	1	2
Open Physician-Hospital Organization	2	1	1	2	2
Closed Physician-Hospital Organization	2	3	1	1	1
Management Service Organization	0	0	1	1	1
Integrated Salary Model	13	13	15	10	12
Equity Model	1	0	0	1	1
Foundation	2	1	0	1	2
Insurance Products					
Health Maintenance Organization	0	0	1	1	1
Preferred Provider Organization	4	3	4	5	6
Indemnity Fee for Service	1	1	2	1	1
Managed Care Contracts					
Health Maintenance Organization	5	7	8	9	9
Preferred Provider Organization	19	21	21	19	16
Affiliations					
Hospitals in a System	13	13	15	14	18
Hospitals in a Network	9	10	8	7	9
Hospitals in a Group Purchasing Organization	27	28	28	28	28

States

TABLE 6

NORTH DAKOTA

U.S. Registered Community Hospitals
(Nonfederal, short-term general and other special hospitals)

Utilization, Personnel, Revenue and Expenses, Community Health Indicators 1998–2002

	2002	2001	2000	1999	1998
TOTAL FACILITY (Includes Hospital and Nursing Home Units)					
Utilization - Inpatient					
Beds	3,880	3,717	3,865	3,884	3,978
Admissions	94,630	91,530	89,219	86,931	85,176
Inpatient Days	845,194	787,722	841,256	852,457	873,623
Average Length of Stay...........	8.9	8.6	9.4	9.8	10.3
Inpatient Surgeries..............	27,650	23,814	25,052	29,603	29,012
Births...........................	9,337	8,691	8,282	8,366	8,523
Utilization - Outpatient					
Emergency Outpatient Visits.......	295,074	259,673	248,562	249,955	221,797
Other Outpatient Visits...........	1,621,700	1,599,065	1,446,407	1,381,484	1,200,140
Total Outpatient Visits	1,916,774	1,858,738	1,694,969	1,631,439	1,421,937
Outpatient Surgeries	48,213	45,718	43,764	42,656	46,070
Personnel					
Full Time RNs	1,884	1,734	2,075	1,634	1,931
Full Time LPNs	531	524	458	438	405
Part Time RNs..................	2,453	2,409	1,910	2,191	2,523
Part Time LPNs	583	524	376	560	542
Total Full Time..................	11,676	11,343	10,921	9,834	9,946
Total Part Time	9,379	8,618	7,529	7,749	8,620
Revenue - Inpatient					
Gross Inpatient Revenue..........	$1,302,289,738	$1,068,649,264	$1,003,041,889	$919,295,692	$947,292,506
Revenue - Outpatient					
Gross Outpatient Revenue	$1,134,691,244	$879,815,286	$766,845,547	$759,586,932	$752,533,518
Revenue and Expenses - Totals **(Includes Inpatient and Outpatient)**					
Total Gross Revenue..............	$2,436,980,982	$1,948,464,550	$1,769,887,436	$1,678,882,624	$1,699,826,024
Deductions from Revenue.........	1,094,215,330	798,865,633	705,636,353	648,667,094	667,836,387
Net Patient Revenue	1,342,765,652	1,149,598,917	1,064,251,083	1,030,215,530	1,031,989,637
Other Operating Revenue	63,807,911	65,081,910	66,992,430	66,044,016	60,404,086
Other Nonoperating Revenue	8,085,712	20,055,117	32,833,000	20,696,900	35,634,346
Total Net Revenue..............	1,414,659,275	1,234,735,944	1,164,076,513	1,116,956,446	1,128,028,069
Total Expenses..................	1,351,763,031	1,220,687,431	1,111,495,262	1,063,751,582	1,052,697,761
HOSPITAL UNIT (Excludes Separate Nursing Home Units)					
Utilization - Inpatient					
Beds	2,883	2,762	3,099	2,935	3,069
Admissions	92,446	90,169	87,453	84,780	83,464
Inpatient Days	515,332	479,300	606,974	536,949	566,947
Average Length of Stay...........	5.6	5.3	6.9	6.3	6.8
Personnel					
Total Full Time..................	11,066	10,726	10,496	9,077	9,315
Total Part Time	8,878	8,119	7,126	7,134	7,921
Revenue and Expenses - Totals **(Includes Inpatient and Outpatient)**					
Total Net Revenue..............	$1,365,837,644	$1,196,091,770	$1,136,148,987	$1,075,514,346	$1,090,055,879
Total Expenses..................	1,314,789,098	1,188,642,681	1,088,906,965	1,032,134,787	1,022,248,824
COMMUNITY HEALTH INDICATORS PER 1000 POPULATION					
Total Population (in thousands)	634	634	642	634	638
Inpatient					
Beds	6.1	5.9	6.0	6.1	6.2
Admissions	149.2	144.3	138.9	137.2	133.5
Inpatient Days	1,332.9	1,241.6	1,310.0	1,345.3	1,369.7
Inpatient Surgeries..............	43.6	37.5	39.0	46.7	45.5
Births...........................	14.7	13.7	12.9	13.2	13.4
Outpatient					
Emergency Outpatient Visits.......	465.3	409.3	387.0	394.5	347.7
Other Outpatient Visits...........	2,557.4	2,520.4	2,252.3	2,180.1	1,881.7
Total Outpatient Visits	3,022.8	2,929.7	2,639.3	2,574.6	2,229.4
Outpatient Surgeries	76.0	72.1	68.1	67.3	72.2
Expense per Capita (per person)....	$2,131.7	$1,924.0	$1,730.8	$1,678.7	$1,650.5

TABLE 6

OHIO

U.S. Registered Community Hospitals
(Nonfederal, short-term general and other special hospitals)

Overview 1998–2002

	2002	2001	2000	1999	1998
Total U.S. Community Hospitals in Ohio	168	166	163	167	172
Bed Size Category					
6-24	2	2	2	3	3
25-49	27	22	21	21	20
50-99	27	33	31	33	33
100-199	50	50	50	52	50
200-299	27	26	24	23	32
300-399	16	14	15	14	14
400-499	9	9	9	10	10
500 +	10	10	11	11	10
Location					
Hospitals Urban	116	114	111	114	120
Hospitals Rural	52	52	52	53	52
Control					
State and Local Government	23	23	22	23	23
Not for Profit	141	139	137	139	139
Investor owned	4	4	4	5	10
Physician Models					
Independent Practice Association	17	23	15	19	16
Group Practice without Walls	11	12	10	11	10
Open Physician-Hospital Organization	47	46	51	63	66
Closed Physician-Hospital Organization	18	26	19	20	22
Management Service Organization	33	33	39	44	44
Integrated Salary Model	44	53	44	52	47
Equity Model	7	9	7	7	8
Foundation	14	21	18	21	26
Insurance Products					
Health Maintenance Organization	27	32	38	45	44
Preferred Provider Organization	32	36	37	44	46
Indemnity Fee for Service	12	12	11	12	13
Managed Care Contracts					
Health Maintenance Organization	104	110	110	112	123
Preferred Provider Organization	112	115	116	118	126
Affiliations					
Hospitals in a System	75	84	75	79	78
Hospitals in a Network	60	68	52	54	56
Hospitals in a Group Purchasing Organization	126	134	130	133	124

TABLE **6**

OHIO

U.S. Registered Community Hospitals
(Nonfederal, short-term general and other special hospitals)

Utilization, Personnel, Revenue and Expenses, Community Health Indicators 1998–2002

	2002	2001	2000	1999	1998
TOTAL FACILITY (Includes Hospital and Nursing Home Units)					
Utilization - Inpatient					
Beds	33,706	33,310	33,849	34,164	35,187
Admissions	1,475,630	1,439,252	1,404,467	1,358,662	1,355,186
Inpatient Days	7,657,394	7,483,873	7,556,261	7,362,468	7,289,259
Average Length of Stay	5.2	5.2	5.4	5.4	5.4
Inpatient Surgeries	431,329	417,023	400,999	390,732	409,404
Births	150,298	151,371	149,565	147,506	151,247
Utilization - Outpatient					
Emergency Outpatient Visits	5,125,829	5,124,561	5,133,276	4,906,178	5,003,406
Other Outpatient Visits	23,229,558	23,252,713	21,724,028	19,980,036	19,794,816
Total Outpatient Visits	28,355,387	28,377,274	26,857,304	24,886,214	24,798,222
Outpatient Surgeries	810,253	793,989	798,907	765,459	790,645
Personnel					
Full Time RNs	35,036	34,676	33,921	34,424	35,530
Full Time LPNs	4,011	3,961	3,644	4,039	4,019
Part Time RNs	22,467	22,713	22,568	19,371	18,419
Part Time LPNs	2,211	2,123	2,028	2,140	2,031
Total Full Time	161,392	159,239	151,382	151,875	154,471
Total Part Time	66,399	66,944	66,769	60,642	56,449
Revenue - Inpatient					
Gross Inpatient Revenue	$23,112,708,865	$20,613,914,515	$17,881,757,694	$15,806,982,496	$15,196,210,325
Revenue - Outpatient					
Gross Outpatient Revenue	$16,391,385,950	$14,224,448,482	$11,888,253,297	$10,278,820,338	$9,119,353,937
Revenue and Expenses - Totals					
(Includes Inpatient and Outpatient)					
Total Gross Revenue	$39,504,094,815	$34,838,362,997	$29,770,010,991	$26,085,802,834	$24,315,564,262
Deductions from Revenue	20,841,549,318	17,753,807,229	14,553,540,678	11,859,000,198	10,533,346,817
Net Patient Revenue	18,662,545,497	17,084,555,768	15,216,470,313	14,226,802,636	13,782,217,445
Other Operating Revenue	1,069,165,656	1,084,169,641	727,705,267	834,560,047	781,078,239
Other Nonoperating Revenue	60,979,408	132,770,316	558,247,388	446,576,015	506,628,141
Total Net Revenue	19,792,690,561	18,301,495,725	16,502,422,968	15,507,938,698	15,069,923,825
Total Expenses	19,132,292,794	17,866,114,856	15,550,349,910	14,881,546,876	14,354,350,789
HOSPITAL UNIT (Excludes Separate Nursing Home Units)					
Utilization - Inpatient					
Beds	31,729	31,471	31,413	31,118	33,036
Admissions	1,458,479	1,421,435	1,381,778	1,328,866	1,329,828
Inpatient Days	7,051,923	6,925,175	6,775,436	6,471,288	6,632,608
Average Length of Stay	4.8	4.9	4.9	4.9	5.0
Personnel					
Total Full Time	159,965	157,884	149,237	149,246	152,222
Total Part Time	65,646	66,306	65,817	59,403	55,358
Revenue and Expenses - Totals					
(Includes Inpatient and Outpatient)					
Total Net Revenue	$19,619,443,053	$18,146,551,602	$16,331,999,691	$15,247,381,253	$14,860,887,528
Total Expenses	18,970,939,986	17,752,957,340	15,427,132,070	14,660,321,444	14,197,589,490
COMMUNITY HEALTH INDICATORS PER 1000 POPULATION					
Total Population (in thousands)	11,421	11,374	11,353	11,257	11,238
Inpatient					
Beds	3.0	2.9	3.0	3.0	3.1
Admissions	129.2	126.5	123.7	120.7	120.6
Inpatient Days	670.5	658.0	665.6	654.1	648.6
Inpatient Surgeries	37.8	36.7	35.3	34.7	36.4
Births	13.2	13.3	13.2	13.1	13.5
Outpatient					
Emergency Outpatient Visits	448.8	450.6	452.1	435.8	445.2
Other Outpatient Visits	2,033.9	2,044.5	1,913.5	1,775.0	1,761.5
Total Outpatient Visits	2,482.7	2,495.0	2,365.6	2,210.8	2,206.7
Outpatient Surgeries	70.9	69.8	70.4	68.0	70.4
Expense per Capita (per person)	$1,675.1	$1,570.8	$1,369.7	$1,322.0	$1,277.3

TABLE 6

OKLAHOMA

U.S. Registered Community Hospitals
(Nonfederal, short-term general and other special hospitals)

Overview 1998–2002

	2002	2001	2000	1999	1998
Total U.S. Community Hospitals in Oklahoma	105	108	108	109	109
Bed Size Category					
6-24	15	15	14	15	16
25-49	36	38	41	40	40
50-99	24	22	22	21	21
100-199	15	18	15	17	16
200-299	6	7	8	8	7
300-399	3	2	2	3	3
400-499	2	3	3	1	2
500 +	4	3	3	4	4
Location					
Hospitals Urban	38	40	40	41	41
Hospitals Rural	67	68	68	68	68
Control					
State and Local Government	44	45	45	50	49
Not for Profit	46	48	49	44	41
Investor owned	15	15	14	15	19
Physician Models					
Independent Practice Association	14	12	16	16	16
Group Practice without Walls	3	1	3	3	4
Open Physician-Hospital Organization	15	14	22	23	24
Closed Physician-Hospital Organization	8	10	6	8	14
Management Service Organization	11	11	15	11	17
Integrated Salary Model	22	16	16	19	18
Equity Model	0	1	2	1	2
Foundation	0	4	4	2	3
Insurance Products					
Health Maintenance Organization	11	18	26	28	28
Preferred Provider Organization	17	18	32	32	34
Indemnity Fee for Service	6	5	6	6	10
Managed Care Contracts					
Health Maintenance Organization	37	40	42	55	48
Preferred Provider Organization	54	61	65	82	68
Affiliations					
Hospitals in a System	31	33	39	42	42
Hospitals in a Network	17	18	22	29	30
Hospitals in a Group Purchasing Organization	66	67	63	—	—

States

TABLE **6**

OKLAHOMA

U.S. Registered Community Hospitals
(Nonfederal, short-term general and other special hospitals)

Utilization, Personnel, Revenue and Expenses, Community Health Indicators 1998–2002

	2002	2001	2000	1999	1998
TOTAL FACILITY (Includes Hospital and Nursing Home Units)					
Utilization - Inpatient					
Beds	11,122	11,207	11,112	11,075	11,022
Admissions	445,952	434,831	428,927	411,025	391,243
Inpatient Days	2,371,009	2,360,979	2,280,050	2,273,850	2,169,379
Average Length of Stay	5.3	5.4	5.3	5.5	5.5
Inpatient Surgeries	109,770	120,417	117,785	123,765	107,628
Births	43,564	43,053	43,461	44,295	38,639
Utilization - Outpatient					
Emergency Outpatient Visits	1,292,652	1,226,716	1,134,337	1,172,259	1,101,327
Other Outpatient Visits	3,510,111	3,343,188	3,567,619	3,452,578	3,285,675
Total Outpatient Visits	4,802,763	4,569,904	4,701,956	4,624,837	4,387,002
Outpatient Surgeries	173,030	173,752	182,488	186,624	165,150
Personnel					
Full Time RNs	8,738	8,403	8,194	8,054	8,184
Full Time LPNs	2,302	2,422	2,087	2,312	2,253
Part Time RNs	3,469	3,708	3,453	3,041	2,801
Part Time LPNs	698	758	618	701	574
Total Full Time	41,470	43,342	41,964	39,901	40,712
Total Part Time	13,105	12,815	11,583	11,864	11,276
Revenue - Inpatient					
Gross Inpatient Revenue	$6,358,250,635	$5,478,614,594	$5,218,973,104	$4,678,294,998	$4,207,669,067
Revenue - Outpatient					
Gross Outpatient Revenue	$3,123,729,308	$2,830,596,281	$2,560,162,792	$2,337,006,164	$2,103,831,457
Revenue and Expenses - Totals **(Includes Inpatient and Outpatient)**					
Total Gross Revenue	$9,481,979,943	$8,309,210,875	$7,779,135,896	$7,015,301,162	$6,311,500,524
Deductions from Revenue	5,455,901,182	4,548,324,907	4,263,955,656	3,677,580,563	3,167,902,504
Net Patient Revenue	4,026,078,761	3,760,885,968	3,515,180,240	3,337,720,599	3,143,598,020
Other Operating Revenue	253,147,564	234,843,029	268,105,178	238,136,668	190,021,268
Other Nonoperating Revenue	26,110,536	39,695,513	28,871,537	64,910,590	33,155,610
Total Net Revenue	4,305,336,861	4,035,424,510	3,812,156,955	3,640,767,857	3,366,774,898
Total Expenses	3,986,180,785	3,722,315,467	3,689,668,282	3,433,636,312	3,217,517,307
HOSPITAL UNIT (Excludes Separate Nursing Home Units)					
Utilization - Inpatient					
Beds	10,877	10,857	10,788	10,577	10,615
Admissions	443,327	431,093	423,287	406,459	385,731
Inpatient Days	2,295,445	2,248,489	2,179,541	2,123,082	2,051,482
Average Length of Stay	5.2	5.2	5.1	5.2	5.3
Personnel					
Total Full Time	41,248	42,873	41,541	39,636	40,498
Total Part Time	13,022	12,693	11,436	11,809	11,239
Revenue and Expenses - Totals **(Includes Inpatient and Outpatient)**					
Total Net Revenue	$4,290,663,306	$4,008,168,171	$3,774,861,696	$3,624,098,673	$3,336,083,870
Total Expenses	3,977,214,712	3,697,330,894	3,669,710,412	3,421,100,441	3,195,565,729
COMMUNITY HEALTH INDICATORS PER 1000 POPULATION					
Total Population (in thousands)	3,494	3,460	3,451	3,358	3,339
Inpatient					
Beds	3.2	3.2	3.2	3.3	3.3
Admissions	127.6	125.7	124.3	122.4	117.2
Inpatient Days	678.6	682.3	660.8	677.1	649.6
Inpatient Surgeries	31.4	34.8	34.1	36.9	32.2
Births	12.5	12.4	12.6	13.2	11.6
Outpatient					
Emergency Outpatient Visits	370.0	354.5	328.7	349.1	329.8
Other Outpatient Visits	1,004.7	966.2	1,033.9	1,028.2	983.9
Total Outpatient Visits	1,374.7	1,320.7	1,362.6	1,377.2	1,313.7
Outpatient Surgeries	49.5	50.2	52.9	55.6	49.5
Expense per Capita (per person)	$1,141.0	$1,075.8	$1,069.3	$1,022.5	$963.5

States

TABLE 6

OREGON

U.S. Registered Community Hospitals
(Nonfederal, short-term general and other special hospitals)

Overview 1998–2002

	2002	2001	2000	1999	1998
Total U.S. Community Hospitals in Oregon..........................	60	60	59	59	60
Bed Size Category					
6-24	5	5	5	5	4
25-49	18	19	21	21	20
50-99	17	17	13	11	12
100-199	11	10	10	12	14
200-299	3	3	4	4	4
300-399	3	3	3	4	5
400-499	3	3	3	2	1
500 + ...	0	0	0	0	0
Location					
Hospitals Urban......................	29	28	27	27	27
Hospitals Rural	31	32	32	32	33
Control					
State and Local Government	12	12	15	15	15
Not for Profit	44	44	41	41	41
Investor owned	4	4	3	3	4
Physician Models					
Independent Practice Association........	26	26	22	19	22
Group Practice without Walls	3	3	0	1	1
Open Physician-Hospital Organization....	4	7	3	7	6
Closed Physician-Hospital Organization...	4	5	3	4	4
Management Service Organization.......	7	8	7	6	5
Integrated Salary Model	21	24	23	21	14
Equity Model	0	0	0	0	0
Foundation	2	2	1	1	0
Insurance Products					
Health Maintenance Organization........	14	13	12	17	17
Preferred Provider Organization.........	15	12	12	13	9
Indemnity Fee for Service.............	2	2	1	1	1
Managed Care Contracts					
Health Maintenance Organization........	41	44	40	41	41
Preferred Provider Organization.........	47	49	43	42	40
Affiliations					
Hospitals in a System.................	32	35	28	29	27
Hospitals in a Network	19	21	16	17	21
Hospitals in a Group Purchasing Organization......................	53	56	48	49	46

TABLE 6

OREGON

U.S. Registered Community Hospitals
(Nonfederal, short-term general and other special hospitals)

Utilization, Personnel, Revenue and Expenses, Community Health Indicators 1998–2002

	2002	2001	2000	1999	1998
TOTAL FACILITY (Includes Hospital and Nursing Home Units)					
Utilization - Inpatient					
Beds	6,798	6,660	6,631	6,643	6,809
Admissions	345,193	334,862	329,932	317,808	313,350
Inpatient Days	1,511,420	1,449,556	1,435,545	1,409,906	1,401,720
Average Length of Stay	4.4	4.3	4.4	4.4	4.5
Inpatient Surgeries	113,669	108,024	105,967	103,162	104,239
Births	45,409	45,279	46,065	45,328	44,610
Utilization - Outpatient					
Emergency Outpatient Visits	1,117,313	1,098,201	1,008,428	921,414	958,415
Other Outpatient Visits	7,058,865	6,559,929	6,264,342	5,736,216	4,830,333
Total Outpatient Visits	8,176,178	7,658,130	7,272,770	6,657,630	5,788,748
Outpatient Surgeries	191,717	172,400	167,938	163,147	164,553
Personnel					
Full Time RNs	7,114	7,975	8,054	6,426	6,692
Full Time LPNs	547	420	448	409	524
Part Time RNs	7,454	6,588	6,224	6,315	5,983
Part Time LPNs	568	314	285	349	348
Total Full Time	32,765	32,473	31,121	26,971	29,348
Total Part Time	22,952	18,793	17,828	17,324	17,885
Revenue - Inpatient					
Gross Inpatient Revenue	$4,563,875,879	$3,859,967,211	$3,485,892,570	$3,113,689,297	$2,933,384,377
Revenue - Outpatient					
Gross Outpatient Revenue	$3,183,571,829	$2,728,455,375	$2,350,061,380	$2,048,806,236	$1,829,620,648
Revenue and Expenses - Totals					
(Includes Inpatient and Outpatient)					
Total Gross Revenue	$7,747,447,708	$6,588,422,586	$5,835,953,950	$5,162,495,533	$4,763,005,025
Deductions from Revenue	3,206,030,580	2,617,704,367	2,306,496,669	1,947,905,128	1,730,229,358
Net Patient Revenue	4,541,417,128	3,970,718,219	3,529,457,281	3,214,590,405	3,032,775,667
Other Operating Revenue	220,287,872	225,753,818	233,238,786	201,378,271	181,708,607
Other Nonoperating Revenue	6,824,416	63,051,233	69,416,016	75,147,493	102,764,290
Total Net Revenue	4,768,529,416	4,259,523,270	3,832,112,083	3,491,116,169	3,317,248,564
Total Expenses	4,468,834,030	3,951,387,339	3,600,487,783	3,286,343,045	3,095,154,279
HOSPITAL UNIT (Excludes Separate Nursing Home Units)					
Utilization - Inpatient					
Beds	6,452	6,184	6,111	6,027	6,288
Admissions	344,564	331,985	326,453	313,845	309,453
Inpatient Days	1,406,690	1,325,563	1,294,908	1,251,063	1,269,063
Average Length of Stay	4.1	4.0	4.0	4.0	4.1
Personnel					
Total Full Time	32,601	32,229	30,783	26,646	29,039
Total Part Time	22,777	18,651	17,669	17,145	17,733
Revenue and Expenses - Totals					
(Includes Inpatient and Outpatient)					
Total Net Revenue	$4,756,252,635	$4,234,725,706	$3,810,739,241	$3,469,658,693	$3,295,734,830
Total Expenses	4,455,142,703	3,927,287,050	3,582,438,850	3,271,980,437	3,075,675,635
COMMUNITY HEALTH INDICATORS PER 1000 POPULATION					
Total Population (in thousands)	3,522	3,473	3,421	3,316	3,282
Inpatient					
Beds	1.9	1.9	1.9	2.0	2.1
Admissions	98.0	96.4	96.4	95.8	95.5
Inpatient Days	429.2	417.4	419.6	425.2	427.1
Inpatient Surgeries	32.3	31.1	31.0	31.1	31.8
Births	12.9	13.0	13.5	13.7	13.6
Outpatient					
Emergency Outpatient Visits	317.3	316.2	294.7	277.9	292.0
Other Outpatient Visits	2,004.5	1,888.9	1,830.9	1,729.8	1,471.7
Total Outpatient Visits	2,321.8	2,205.1	2,125.7	2,007.6	1,763.8
Outpatient Surgeries	54.4	49.6	49.1	49.2	50.1
Expense per Capita (per person)	$1,269.0	$1,137.8	$1,052.3	$991.0	$943.1

States

TABLE 6

PENNSYLVANIA

U.S. Registered Community Hospitals
(Nonfederal, short-term general and other special hospitals)

Overview 1998–2002

	2002	2001	2000	1999	1998
Total U.S. Community Hospitals in Pennsylvania	201	205	207	210	212
Bed Size Category					
6-24	4	3	4	5	4
25-49	13	14	12	12	11
50-99	36	33	34	34	33
100-199	71	74	79	78	82
200-299	40	42	39	42	40
300-399	14	14	11	11	12
400-499	11	12	15	13	14
500 +	12	13	13	15	16
Location					
Hospitals Urban	158	161	163	165	167
Hospitals Rural	43	44	44	45	45
Control					
State and Local Government	2	2	2	1	1
Not for Profit	184	189	194	199	203
Investor owned	15	14	11	10	8
Physician Models					
Independent Practice Association	18	20	23	29	29
Group Practice without Walls	10	12	12	13	11
Open Physician-Hospital Organization	40	39	53	54	63
Closed Physician-Hospital Organization	10	10	15	24	25
Management Service Organization	28	32	41	39	40
Integrated Salary Model	57	53	53	53	52
Equity Model	4	3	11	8	3
Foundation	7	5	9	9	18
Insurance Products					
Health Maintenance Organization	25	25	32	36	47
Preferred Provider Organization	39	38	41	46	55
Indemnity Fee for Service	8	6	4	5	13
Managed Care Contracts					
Health Maintenance Organization	149	150	153	153	150
Preferred Provider Organization	143	144	147	148	145
Affiliations					
Hospitals in a System	109	104	108	108	103
Hospitals in a Network	53	45	57	53	61
Hospitals in a Group Purchasing Organization	161	151	151	137	131

TABLE 6

PENNSYLVANIA

U.S. Registered Community Hospitals
(Nonfederal, short-term general and other special hospitals)

Utilization, Personnel, Revenue and Expenses, Community Health Indicators 1998–2002

	2002	2001	2000	1999	1998
TOTAL FACILITY (Includes Hospital and Nursing Home Units)					
Utilization - Inpatient					
Beds	40,534	42,131	42,303	42,999	44,739
Admissions	1,798,243	1,808,531	1,796,081	1,755,029	1,752,298
Inpatient Days	10,340,276	10,395,360	10,558,152	10,652,791	10,927,224
Average Length of Stay	5.8	5.7	5.9	6.1	6.2
Inpatient Surgeries	537,857	544,254	534,894	555,367	578,008
Births	139,489	143,463	139,408	139,888	142,896
Utilization - Outpatient					
Emergency Outpatient Visits	5,059,150	4,873,595	4,727,149	4,615,588	4,620,945
Other Outpatient Visits	27,349,887	27,189,829	27,122,027	24,653,538	25,959,042
Total Outpatient Visits	32,409,037	32,063,424	31,849,176	29,269,126	30,579,987
Outpatient Surgeries	983,477	1,034,191	997,911	969,895	983,299
Personnel					
Full Time RNs	40,679	39,444	39,290	39,819	39,327
Full Time LPNs	4,910	4,962	4,807	5,287	5,306
Part Time RNs	24,880	23,733	22,678	22,707	23,391
Part Time LPNs	2,557	2,515	2,541	2,735	2,929
Total Full Time	185,944	181,276	178,775	179,851	180,604
Total Part Time	74,311	71,386	68,530	70,841	74,102
Revenue - Inpatient					
Gross Inpatient Revenue	$36,887,336,442	$33,160,635,367	$29,235,892,623	$27,097,518,634	$25,636,639,265
Revenue - Outpatient					
Gross Outpatient Revenue	$20,349,623,193	$17,751,314,945	$15,605,206,965	$13,919,316,631	$12,554,243,341
Revenue and Expenses - Totals					
(Includes Inpatient and Outpatient)					
Total Gross Revenue	$57,236,959,635	$50,911,950,312	$44,841,099,588	$41,016,835,265	$38,190,882,606
Deductions from Revenue	36,862,617,072	31,902,707,556	27,167,023,083	24,081,858,092	21,495,641,201
Net Patient Revenue	20,374,342,563	19,009,242,756	17,674,076,505	16,934,977,173	16,695,241,405
Other Operating Revenue	1,073,805,639	1,050,625,699	1,001,303,780	918,424,356	871,307,419
Other Nonoperating Revenue	109,263,545	320,138,109	473,372,882	436,390,618	604,119,011
Total Net Revenue	21,557,411,747	20,380,006,564	19,148,753,167	18,289,792,147	18,170,667,835
Total Expenses	20,669,545,292	19,668,618,568	18,449,395,399	17,762,016,623	17,561,776,794
HOSPITAL UNIT (Excludes Separate Nursing Home Units)					
Utilization - Inpatient					
Beds	37,613	38,652	38,642	38,320	40,334
Admissions	1,765,118	1,772,168	1,753,702	1,704,806	1,707,740
Inpatient Days	9,427,742	9,322,503	9,424,533	9,224,935	9,514,173
Average Length of Stay	5.3	5.3	5.4	5.4	5.6
Personnel					
Total Full Time	183,198	178,633	175,754	176,561	177,072
Total Part Time	72,709	69,755	66,833	69,104	72,322
Revenue and Expenses - Totals					
(Includes Inpatient and Outpatient)					
Total Net Revenue	$21,296,239,697	$20,087,923,397	$18,857,929,952	$17,920,002,342	$17,747,827,775
Total Expenses	20,474,291,752	19,453,873,721	18,267,250,601	17,508,949,084	17,276,532,062
COMMUNITY HEALTH INDICATORS PER 1000 POPULATION					
Total Population (in thousands)	12,335	12,287	12,281	11,994	12,002
Inpatient					
Beds	3.3	3.4	3.4	3.6	3.7
Admissions	145.8	147.2	146.2	146.3	146.0
Inpatient Days	838.3	846.0	859.7	888.2	910.4
Inpatient Surgeries	43.6	44.3	43.6	46.3	48.2
Births	11.3	11.7	11.4	11.7	11.9
Outpatient					
Emergency Outpatient Visits	410.1	396.6	384.9	384.8	385.0
Other Outpatient Visits	2,217.2	2,212.9	2,208.4	2,055.5	2,162.8
Total Outpatient Visits	2,627.4	2,609.5	2,593.4	2,440.3	2,547.8
Outpatient Surgeries	79.7	84.2	81.3	80.9	81.9
Expense per Capita (per person)	$1,675.7	$1,600.7	$1,502.3	$1,480.9	$1,463.2

States

TABLE **6**

RHODE ISLAND

U.S. Registered Community Hospitals
(Nonfederal, short-term general and other special hospitals)

Overview 1998–2002

	2002	2001	2000	1999	1998
Total U.S. Community Hospitals in Rhode Island.	11	11	11	11	12
Bed Size Category					
6-24	0	0	0	0	0
25-49	0	0	0	0	0
50-99	1	1	1	1	1
100-199	5	5	5	6	8
200-299	3	3	3	2	1
300-399	1	1	1	1	1
400-499	0	0	0	0	0
500 + ...	1	1	1	1	1
Location					
Hospitals Urban.	10	10	10	10	11
Hospitals Rural	1	1	1	1	1
Control					
State and Local Government	0	0	0	0	0
Not for Profit	11	11	11	11	12
Investor owned	0	0	0	0	0
Physician Models					
Independent Practice Association.	7	7	3	3	5
Group Practice without Walls	1	1	0	0	0
Open Physician-Hospital Organization. . . .	6	6	7	8	8
Closed Physician-Hospital Organization. . .	2	3	2	1	1
Management Service Organization.	2	3	2	3	3
Integrated Salary Model	4	5	4	5	5
Equity Model	1	1	1	0	0
Foundation.	3	4	4	4	4
Insurance Products					
Health Maintenance Organization.	2	2	0	0	0
Preferred Provider Organization	2	2	0	0	2
Indemnity Fee for Service.	1	1	0	0	0
Managed Care Contracts					
Health Maintenance Organization.	10	11	11	11	12
Preferred Provider Organization	8	9	10	10	10
Affiliations					
Hospitals in a System.	6	7	7	6	6
Hospitals in a Network	1	1	3	2	2
Hospitals in a Group Purchasing Organization.	10	11	11	9	10

States

TABLE 6

RHODE ISLAND

U.S. Registered Community Hospitals
(Nonfederal, short-term general and other special hospitals)

Utilization, Personnel, Revenue and Expenses, Community Health Indicators 1998–2002

	2002	2001	2000	1999	1998
TOTAL FACILITY (Includes Hospital and Nursing Home Units)					
Utilization - Inpatient					
Beds	2,428	2,449	2,400	2,400	2,581
Admissions	122,741	120,901	119,070	117,163	117,320
Inpatient Days	649,451	638,571	625,939	623,306	659,966
Average Length of Stay	5.3	5.3	5.3	5.3	5.6
Inpatient Surgeries	36,943	35,543	35,483	35,116	35,232
Births	13,328	13,375	13,064	13,320	13,398
Utilization - Outpatient					
Emergency Outpatient Visits	468,530	451,325	440,098	421,667	407,366
Other Outpatient Visits	1,743,459	1,699,915	1,640,847	1,489,890	1,762,581
Total Outpatient Visits	2,211,989	2,151,240	2,080,945	1,911,557	2,169,947
Outpatient Surgeries	105,833	99,423	94,146	86,783	80,546
Personnel					
Full Time RNs	1,583	1,539	1,630	1,545	1,588
Full Time LPNs	183	184	183	161	192
Part Time RNs	2,720	3,056	3,087	3,145	2,748
Part Time LPNs	200	221	206	197	220
Total Full Time	11,440	10,793	10,894	10,491	11,224
Total Part Time	8,071	8,620	8,409	8,558	8,733
Revenue - Inpatient					
Gross Inpatient Revenue	$1,954,502,575	$1,738,042,664	$1,512,132,670	$1,415,053,397	$1,393,271,369
Revenue - Outpatient					
Gross Outpatient Revenue	$1,625,894,089	$1,342,251,100	$1,154,392,267	$1,041,727,122	$933,791,131
Revenue and Expenses - Totals					
(Includes Inpatient and Outpatient)					
Total Gross Revenue	$3,580,396,664	$3,080,293,764	$2,666,524,937	$2,456,780,519	$2,327,062,500
Deductions from Revenue	1,965,189,964	1,626,498,267	1,338,811,208	1,230,336,909	1,098,641,571
Net Patient Revenue	1,615,206,700	1,453,795,497	1,327,713,729	1,226,443,610	1,228,420,929
Other Operating Revenue	113,085,707	97,199,257	101,392,569	84,757,555	86,452,618
Other Nonoperating Revenue	45,373,163	18,363,394	48,479,673	28,358,285	30,473,011
Total Net Revenue	1,773,665,570	1,569,358,148	1,477,585,971	1,339,559,450	1,345,346,558
Total Expenses	1,791,383,545	1,592,333,629	1,488,194,792	1,362,140,752	1,278,223,306
HOSPITAL UNIT (Excludes Separate Nursing Home Units)					
Utilization - Inpatient					
Beds	2,373	2,405	2,337	2,361	2,542
Admissions	121,485	119,649	117,446	116,370	116,611
Inpatient Days	633,715	622,075	604,416	612,307	648,796
Average Length of Stay	5.2	5.2	5.1	5.3	5.6
Personnel					
Total Full Time	11,421	10,718	10,811	10,485	11,210
Total Part Time	8,010	8,538	8,315	8,520	8,692
Revenue and Expenses - Totals					
(Includes Inpatient and Outpatient)					
Total Net Revenue	$1,761,520,237	$1,557,626,889	$1,465,522,013	$1,333,633,808	$1,337,590,292
Total Expenses	1,780,279,260	1,582,522,184	1,479,990,940	1,356,396,823	1,271,503,480
COMMUNITY HEALTH INDICATORS PER 1000 POPULATION					
Total Population (in thousands)	1,070	1,059	1,048	991	988
Inpatient					
Beds	2.3	2.3	2.3	2.4	2.6
Admissions	114.7	114.2	113.6	118.2	118.8
Inpatient Days	607.1	603.0	597.1	629.1	668.2
Inpatient Surgeries	34.5	33.6	33.8	35.4	35.7
Births	12.5	12.6	12.5	13.4	13.6
Outpatient					
Emergency Outpatient Visits	438.0	426.2	419.8	425.6	412.4
Other Outpatient Visits	1,629.8	1,605.3	1,565.2	1,503.7	1,784.5
Total Outpatient Visits	2,067.8	2,031.5	1,985.0	1,929.3	2,197.0
Outpatient Surgeries	98.9	93.9	89.8	87.6	81.5
Expense per Capita (per person)	$1,674.6	$1,503.7	$1,419.6	$1,374.8	$1,294.1

TABLE 6

SOUTH CAROLINA

U.S. Registered Community Hospitals
(Nonfederal, short-term general and other special hospitals)

Overview 1998–2002

	2002	2001	2000	1999	1998
Total U.S. Community Hospitals in South Carolina	62	62	63	64	65
Bed Size Category					
6-24	2	1	1	1	1
25-49	10	9	11	9	12
50-99	14	13	12	13	12
100-199	14	16	15	18	18
200-299	13	14	14	12	12
300-399	4	4	4	6	5
400-499	2	2	3	2	2
500 +	3	3	3	3	3
Location					
Hospitals Urban	35	35	35	36	37
Hospitals Rural	27	27	28	28	28
Control					
State and Local Government	21	22	23	24	24
Not for Profit	23	20	20	20	20
Investor owned	18	20	20	20	21
Physician Models					
Independent Practice Association	3	6	6	4	4
Group Practice without Walls	0	0	0	0	1
Open Physician-Hospital Organization	11	13	13	11	21
Closed Physician-Hospital Organization	1	1	4	7	2
Management Service Organization	8	9	9	4	7
Integrated Salary Model	8	6	9	8	5
Equity Model	5	1	7	6	5
Foundation	0	1	1	1	0
Insurance Products					
Health Maintenance Organization	4	4	8	10	11
Preferred Provider Organization	10	11	11	14	20
Indemnity Fee for Service	1	1	1	1	3
Managed Care Contracts					
Health Maintenance Organization	37	34	38	41	40
Preferred Provider Organization	42	38	41	46	46
Affiliations					
Hospitals in a System	34	35	34	34	33
Hospitals in a Network	22	20	22	23	29
Hospitals in a Group Purchasing Organization	0	0	0	—	—

States

TABLE 6

SOUTH CAROLINA

U.S. Registered Community Hospitals
(Nonfederal, short-term general and other special hospitals)

Utilization, Personnel, Revenue and Expenses, Community Health Indicators 1998–2002

	2002	2001	2000	1999	1998
TOTAL FACILITY (Includes Hospital and Nursing Home Units)					
Utilization - Inpatient					
Beds	11,107	11,282	11,520	11,629	11,518
Admissions	513,136	505,294	495,410	478,936	457,347
Inpatient Days	2,914,964	2,940,707	2,916,386	2,816,481	2,763,146
Average Length of Stay	5.7	5.8	5.9	5.9	6.0
Inpatient Surgeries	179,098	173,046	173,645	150,556	140,781
Births	48,864	50,304	51,355	48,875	47,634
Utilization - Outpatient					
Emergency Outpatient Visits	1,799,127	1,840,819	1,831,462	1,675,252	1,531,231
Other Outpatient Visits	5,467,718	5,788,476	5,947,571	4,684,820	4,327,410
Total Outpatient Visits	7,266,845	7,629,295	7,779,033	6,360,072	5,858,641
Outpatient Surgeries	278,897	262,308	253,389	220,015	218,676
Personnel					
Full Time RNs	12,161	11,674	10,921	11,437	11,276
Full Time LPNs	1,545	1,689	1,623	1,687	1,662
Part Time RNs	5,116	5,366	4,911	5,061	3,927
Part Time LPNs	648	622	585	599	613
Total Full Time	48,661	48,615	45,230	46,006	45,568
Total Part Time	15,356	15,342	14,772	13,878	12,808
Revenue - Inpatient					
Gross Inpatient Revenue	$9,137,079,254	$7,754,863,580	$6,462,086,026	$6,267,433,167	$5,599,831,497
Revenue - Outpatient					
Gross Outpatient Revenue	$4,772,097,600	$4,036,284,822	$3,446,830,663	$3,111,764,599	$2,700,429,264
Revenue and Expenses - Totals					
(Includes Inpatient and Outpatient)					
Total Gross Revenue	$13,909,176,854	$11,791,148,402	$9,908,916,689	$9,379,197,766	$8,300,260,761
Deductions from Revenue	7,966,264,098	6,352,960,698	4,892,874,213	4,637,273,635	3,895,425,584
Net Patient Revenue	5,942,912,756	5,438,187,704	5,016,042,476	4,741,924,131	4,404,835,177
Other Operating Revenue	221,416,734	214,469,378	198,031,960	206,800,122	225,359,463
Other Nonoperating Revenue	48,721,284	60,313,151	85,852,895	55,842,812	98,172,230
Total Net Revenue	6,213,050,774	5,712,970,233	5,299,927,331	5,004,567,065	4,728,366,870
Total Expenses	5,829,536,908	5,211,814,991	5,017,991,441	4,714,616,676	4,348,407,394
HOSPITAL UNIT (Excludes Separate Nursing Home Units)					
Utilization - Inpatient					
Beds	10,182	10,229	10,411	10,676	10,640
Admissions	506,957	499,396	488,626	472,693	451,827
Inpatient Days	2,603,383	2,600,069	2,570,557	2,512,213	2,487,633
Average Length of Stay	5.1	5.2	5.3	5.3	5.5
Personnel					
Total Full Time	47,852	47,744	44,175	45,228	44,814
Total Part Time	15,120	15,057	14,394	13,615	12,538
Revenue and Expenses - Totals					
(Includes Inpatient and Outpatient)					
Total Net Revenue	$6,100,277,342	$5,647,774,666	$4,478,643,578	$4,912,849,352	$4,655,195,598
Total Expenses	5,764,072,107	5,160,720,870	4,960,782,656	4,658,570,962	4,301,557,086
COMMUNITY HEALTH INDICATORS PER 1000 POPULATION					
Total Population (in thousands)	4,107	4,063	4,012	3,886	3,840
Inpatient					
Beds	2.7	2.8	2.9	3.0	3.0
Admissions	124.9	124.4	123.5	123.3	119.1
Inpatient Days	709.7	723.8	726.9	724.8	719.6
Inpatient Surgeries	43.6	42.6	43.3	38.7	36.7
Births	11.9	12.4	12.8	12.6	12.4
Outpatient					
Emergency Outpatient Visits	438.0	453.1	456.5	431.1	398.8
Other Outpatient Visits	1,331.3	1,424.7	1,482.4	1,205.6	1,127.1
Total Outpatient Visits	1,769.3	1,877.7	1,938.9	1,636.8	1,525.9
Outpatient Surgeries	67.9	64.6	63.2	56.6	57.0
Expense per Capita (per person)	$1,419.4	$1,282.7	$1,250.7	$1,213.3	$1,132.5

States

TABLE **6**

SOUTH DAKOTA

U.S. Registered Community Hospitals
(Nonfederal, short-term general and other special hospitals)

Overview 1998–2002

	2002	2001	2000	1999	1998
Total U.S. Community Hospitals in South Dakota.............................	51	50	48	48	49
Bed Size Category					
6-24	12	13	13	13	13
25-49	13	10	10	10	8
50-99	12	13	11	11	16
100-199	9	8	9	9	7
200-299	2	3	1	2	2
300-399	1	1	2	1	1
400-499	1	1	1	1	0
500 + ...	1	1	1	1	2
Location					
Hospitals Urban......................	6	6	5	5	5
Hospitals Rural	45	44	43	43	44
Control					
State and Local Government	6	6	7	8	7
Not for Profit	44	43	41	40	42
Investor owned	1	1	0	0	0
Physician Models					
Independent Practice Association........	9	11	9	7	5
Group Practice without Walls	3	2	3	2	4
Open Physician-Hospital Organization....	5	4	6	5	3
Closed Physician-Hospital Organization...	2	2	4	3	3
Management Service Organization........	3	3	4	4	7
Integrated Salary Model	17	13	14	12	13
Equity Model	1	1	1	0	0
Foundation...........................	1	1	0	2	2
Insurance Products					
Health Maintenance Organization........	14	13	13	13	13
Preferred Provider Organization	21	17	17	14	11
Indemnity Fee for Service..............	6	6	5	6	7
Managed Care Contracts					
Health Maintenance Organization........	24	21	21	22	22
Preferred Provider Organization	39	34	35	36	32
Affiliations					
Hospitals in a System.................	33	33	32	28	26
Hospitals in a Network	22	17	17	15	20
Hospitals in a Group Purchasing Organization.......................	46	46	43	38	35

TABLE 6

SOUTH DAKOTA

U.S. Registered Community Hospitals
(Nonfederal, short-term general and other special hospitals)

Utilization, Personnel, Revenue and Expenses, Community Health Indicators 1998–2002

	2002	2001	2000	1999	1998
TOTAL FACILITY (Includes Hospital and Nursing Home Units)					
Utilization - Inpatient					
Beds	4,624	4,465	4,339	4,344	4,401
Admissions	100,141	103,907	98,508	97,316	96,055
Inpatient Days	1,001,800	1,046,760	1,035,027	1,052,039	1,032,566
Average Length of Stay	10.0	10.1	10.5	10.8	10.7
Inpatient Surgeries	38,478	32,462	32,993	32,627	32,976
Births	9,537	10,261	10,006	9,363	9,445
Utilization - Outpatient					
Emergency Outpatient Visits	208,068	211,200	196,054	192,035	183,556
Other Outpatient Visits	1,296,030	1,616,898	1,522,147	1,361,718	1,324,908
Total Outpatient Visits	1,504,098	1,828,098	1,718,201	1,553,753	1,508,464
Outpatient Surgeries	156,648	44,596	43,642	46,065	43,081
Personnel					
Full Time RNs	3,070	2,719	2,486	2,147	2,029
Full Time LPNs	307	267	226	186	209
Part Time RNs	1,390	1,508	1,822	2,058	1,915
Part Time LPNs	122	142	201	197	196
Total Full Time	12,760	12,093	10,774	9,989	9,510
Total Part Time	6,209	6,074	7,124	7,034	6,658
Revenue - Inpatient					
Gross Inpatient Revenue	$1,261,059,667	$1,134,749,973	$1,000,043,131	$925,396,063	$863,704,037
Revenue - Outpatient					
Gross Outpatient Revenue	$695,088,937	$613,055,802	$550,896,116	$457,270,200	$415,256,677
Revenue and Expenses - Totals					
(Includes Inpatient and Outpatient)					
Total Gross Revenue	$1,956,148,604	$1,747,805,775	$1,550,939,247	$1,382,666,263	$1,278,960,714
Deductions from Revenue	772,856,470	647,480,234	527,471,606	434,728,043	377,142,751
Net Patient Revenue	1,183,292,134	1,100,325,541	1,023,467,641	947,938,220	901,817,963
Other Operating Revenue	86,084,094	77,627,200	60,933,637	57,779,801	51,660,847
Other Nonoperating Revenue	4,988,767	11,008,624	43,912,340	28,755,729	29,569,700
Total Net Revenue	1,274,364,995	1,188,961,365	1,128,313,618	1,034,473,750	983,048,510
Total Expenses	1,195,193,697	1,106,276,599	1,058,129,155	942,471,403	923,990,512
HOSPITAL UNIT (Excludes Separate Nursing Home Units)					
Utilization - Inpatient					
Beds	2,937	2,763	2,619	2,659	2,802
Admissions	98,694	102,468	97,152	96,048	94,853
Inpatient Days	519,705	503,878	475,240	485,592	495,477
Average Length of Stay	5.3	4.9	4.9	5.1	5.2
Personnel					
Total Full Time	11,801	11,146	9,803	9,299	8,789
Total Part Time	5,369	5,249	6,324	6,271	5,865
Revenue and Expenses - Totals					
(Includes Inpatient and Outpatient)					
Total Net Revenue	$1,210,167,076	$1,129,594,457	$1,075,161,508	$979,061,301	$932,548,108
Total Expenses	1,142,543,091	1,048,181,427	1,010,362,656	895,701,751	878,640,302
COMMUNITY HEALTH INDICATORS PER 1000 POPULATION					
Total Population (in thousands)	761	757	755	733	731
Inpatient					
Beds	6.1	5.9	5.7	5.9	6.0
Admissions	131.6	137.3	130.5	132.7	131.4
Inpatient Days	1,316.3	1,383.5	1,371.2	1,435.0	1,412.9
Inpatient Surgeries	50.6	42.9	43.7	44.5	45.1
Births	12.5	13.6	13.3	12.8	12.9
Outpatient					
Emergency Outpatient Visits	273.4	279.1	259.7	261.9	251.2
Other Outpatient Visits	1,702.9	2,137.1	2,016.5	1,857.4	1,813.0
Total Outpatient Visits	1,976.3	2,416.2	2,276.2	2,119.3	2,064.2
Outpatient Surgeries	205.8	58.9	57.8	62.8	59.0
Expense per Capita (per person)	$1,570.4	$1,462.2	$1,401.8	$1,285.5	$1,264.4

States

TABLE 6

TENNESSEE

U.S. Registered Community Hospitals
(Nonfederal, short-term general and other special hospitals)

Overview 1998–2002

	2002	2001	2000	1999	1998
Total U.S. Community Hospitals in Tennessee..........................	125	123	121	121	122
Bed Size Category					
6-24	5	1	0	0	2
25-49	28	26	25	20	23
50-99	29	30	33	39	35
100-199	33	36	34	33	33
200-299	11	11	10	11	13
300-399	6	6	7	5	4
400-499	4	5	3	3	3
500 + ...	9	8	9	10	9
Location					
Hospitals Urban......................	61	60	58	58	59
Hospitals Rural	64	63	63	63	63
Control					
State and Local Government	26	26	27	27	30
Not for Profit	64	61	57	56	58
Investor owned	35	36	37	38	34
Physician Models					
Independent Practice Association........	27	21	19	22	21
Group Practice without Walls	2	1	0	1	4
Open Physician-Hospital Organization....	24	25	15	19	24
Closed Physician-Hospital Organization...	9	5	4	3	6
Management Service Organization.......	32	31	23	24	27
Integrated Salary Model	22	18	11	12	10
Equity Model	2	0	0	2	3
Foundation.........................	2	3	4	4	1
Insurance Products					
Health Maintenance Organization........	19	17	16	21	19
Preferred Provider Organization.........	44	35	27	36	34
Indemnity Fee for Service.............	13	11	10	10	8
Managed Care Contracts					
Health Maintenance Organization........	82	80	62	65	63
Preferred Provider Organization.........	93	92	70	71	73
Affiliations					
Hospitals in a System.................	63	73	52	53	51
Hospitals in a Network	41	44	24	30	26
Hospitals in a Group Purchasing Organization......................	83	90	69	69	57

TABLE 6

TENNESSEE

U.S. Registered Community Hospitals
(Nonfederal, short-term general and other special hospitals)

Utilization, Personnel, Revenue and Expenses, Community Health Indicators 1998–2002

	2002	2001	2000	1999	1998
TOTAL FACILITY (Includes Hospital and Nursing Home Units)					
Utilization - Inpatient					
Beds	20,446	20,600	20,561	20,627	20,682
Admissions	797,318	751,495	737,313	751,523	744,913
Inpatient Days	4,473,786	4,122,419	4,225,812	4,296,679	4,292,500
Average Length of Stay..........	5.6	5.5	5.7	5.7	5.8
Inpatient Surgeries..............	227,882	238,914	241,938	236,298	228,702
Births.........................	77,090	76,722	71,854	76,194	74,433
Utilization - Outpatient					
Emergency Outpatient Visits	2,815,655	2,710,481	2,601,659	2,589,171	2,443,232
Other Outpatient Visits............	7,136,086	6,826,446	7,673,605	6,890,695	6,787,328
Total Outpatient Visits	9,951,741	9,536,927	10,275,264	9,479,866	9,230,560
Outpatient Surgeries	391,725	406,248	399,184	378,646	372,857
Personnel					
Full Time RNs	18,073	16,806	18,265	19,220	18,900
Full Time LPNs	3,895	3,799	3,273	3,388	3,581
Part Time RNs.................	7,661	6,683	6,880	5,037	4,430
Part Time LPNs	1,154	1,070	916	723	854
Total Full Time.................	78,261	79,904	78,784	80,276	81,263
Total Part Time	23,695	18,899	20,550	15,446	15,274
Revenue - Inpatient					
Gross Inpatient Revenue..........	$11,947,904,647	$11,374,599,693	$10,080,668,101	$9,327,573,723	$8,743,361,839
Revenue - Outpatient					
Gross Outpatient Revenue	$7,268,386,224	$6,608,725,588	$5,810,556,366	$5,004,878,950	$4,463,657,836
Revenue and Expenses - Totals **(Includes Inpatient and Outpatient)**					
Total Gross Revenue.............	$19,216,290,871	$17,983,325,281	$15,891,224,467	$14,332,452,673	$13,207,019,675
Deductions from Revenue.........	10,705,040,668	10,088,328,741	8,531,972,395	7,456,932,016	6,508,958,847
Net Patient Revenue	8,511,250,203	7,894,996,540	7,359,252,072	6,875,520,657	6,698,060,828
Other Operating Revenue	340,382,627	395,634,694	361,920,349	419,276,199	383,930,905
Other Nonoperating Revenue	63,525,859	310,696,758	328,615,366	163,624,734	134,814,577
Total Net Revenue..............	8,915,158,689	8,601,327,992	8,049,787,787	7,458,421,590	7,216,806,310
Total Expenses.................	8,386,650,030	8,143,131,226	7,554,623,035	7,233,873,814	6,530,695,662
HOSPITAL UNIT (Excludes Separate Nursing Home Units)					
Utilization - Inpatient					
Beds	18,928	19,170	19,273	19,104	19,310
Admissions	784,003	739,360	726,271	738,689	734,223
Inpatient Days	3,902,204	3,621,415	3,801,360	3,827,904	3,862,873
Average Length of Stay..........	5.0	4.9	5.2	5.2	5.3
Personnel					
Total Full Time.................	76,883	78,783	77,416	78,259	79,829
Total Part Time	23,351	18,561	20,230	15,095	15,065
Revenue and Expenses - Totals **(Includes Inpatient and Outpatient)**					
Total Net Revenue..............	$8,781,164,810	$8,500,355,125	$7,950,369,293	$7,321,010,015	$7,116,667,493
Total Expenses.................	8,276,736,830	8,058,017,723	7,475,659,236	7,128,551,841	6,446,647,305
COMMUNITY HEALTH INDICATORS PER 1000 POPULATION					
Total Population (in thousands)	5,797	5,740	5,689	5,484	5,433
Inpatient					
Beds	3.5	3.6	3.6	3.8	3.8
Admissions	137.5	130.9	129.6	137.1	137.1
Inpatient Days	771.7	718.2	742.8	783.6	790.1
Inpatient Surgeries..............	39.3	41.6	42.5	43.1	42.1
Births.........................	13.3	13.4	12.6	13.9	13.7
Outpatient					
Emergency Outpatient Visits	485.7	472.2	457.3	472.2	449.7
Other Outpatient Visits............	1,230.9	1,189.3	1,348.8	1,256.6	1,249.4
Total Outpatient Visits	1,716.6	1,661.5	1,806.1	1,728.8	1,699.1
Outpatient Surgeries	67.6	70.8	70.2	69.1	68.6
Expense per Capita (per person)....	$1,446.7	$1,418.7	$1,327.9	$1,319.2	$1,202.1

TABLE 6

TEXAS

U.S. Registered Community Hospitals
(Nonfederal, short-term general and other special hospitals)

Overview 1998–2002

	2002	2001	2000	1999	1998
Total U.S. Community Hospitals in Texas............................	416	411	403	408	400
Bed Size Category					
6-24	51	48	48	54	47
25-49	110	111	108	101	104
50-99	78	75	68	70	69
100-199	87	88	86	91	88
200-299	39	34	41	40	40
300-399	27	31	28	26	22
400-499	9	8	7	9	14
500 + ...	15	16	17	17	16
Location					
Hospitals Urban......................	255	250	241	245	238
Hospitals Rural	161	161	162	163	162
Control					
State and Local Government	129	128	130	131	133
Not for Profit	155	146	142	143	138
Investor owned	132	137	131	134	129
Physician Models					
Independent Practice Association........	79	76	82	103	107
Group Practice without Walls	14	18	20	18	23
Open Physician-Hospital Organization....	91	96	104	109	124
Closed Physician-Hospital Organization...	20	21	23	30	31
Management Service Organization.......	53	53	79	98	105
Integrated Salary Model	62	58	55	64	68
Equity Model	7	8	15	22	30
Foundation..........................	30	34	41	50	59
Insurance Products					
Health Maintenance Organization........	59	60	73	100	101
Preferred Provider Organization.........	85	76	95	118	126
Indemnity Fee for Service.............	23	22	27	39	44
Managed Care Contracts					
Health Maintenance Organization........	311	311	309	330	316
Preferred Provider Organization.........	352	351	350	370	350
Affiliations					
Hospitals in a System.................	242	233	226	228	217
Hospitals in a Network	94	93	102	121	136
Hospitals in a Group Purchasing Organization......................	344	335	326	306	280

TABLE 6

TEXAS

U.S. Registered Community Hospitals
(Nonfederal, short-term general and other special hospitals)

Utilization, Personnel, Revenue and Expenses, Community Health Indicators 1998–2002

	2002	2001	2000	1999	1998
TOTAL FACILITY (Includes Hospital and Nursing Home Units)					
Utilization - Inpatient					
Beds	56,833	56,354	55,877	56,824	56,573
Admissions	2,533,821	2,461,016	2,366,652	2,302,892	2,227,166
Inpatient Days	13,187,000	12,650,063	12,122,361	12,015,612	11,732,621
Average Length of Stay.	5.2	5.1	5.1	5.2	5.3
Inpatient Surgeries.	752,465	725,998	716,990	695,394	709,815
Births.	371,677	366,373	357,906	339,105	332,825
Utilization - Outpatient					
Emergency Outpatient Visits.	8,243,642	7,806,334	7,375,580	7,071,236	6,722,059
Other Outpatient Visits.	25,258,993	23,647,614	22,017,896	21,187,640	20,616,924
Total Outpatient Visits	33,502,635	31,453,948	29,393,476	28,258,876	27,338,983
Outpatient Surgeries	1,093,705	1,049,923	1,043,853	1,033,349	986,411
Personnel					
Full Time RNs	58,370	55,139	52,889	53,028	51,559
Full Time LPNs	12,137	11,908	11,420	12,738	12,681
Part Time RNs	18,458	18,430	17,165	16,782	17,951
Part Time LPNs	3,396	3,484	3,197	3,199	3,610
Total Full Time.	243,520	235,495	227,471	231,401	225,409
Total Part Time	58,389	57,901	53,904	53,137	57,372
Revenue - Inpatient					
Gross Inpatient Revenue.	$48,954,346,337	$42,086,234,028	$36,110,028,792	$32,577,994,295	$29,472,655,033
Revenue - Outpatient					
Gross Outpatient Revenue	$24,518,438,912	$20,856,680,055	$17,722,021,020	$15,630,753,126	$13,914,506,461
Revenue and Expenses - Totals					
(Includes Inpatient and Outpatient)					
Total Gross Revenue.	$73,472,785,249	$62,942,914,083	$53,832,049,812	$48,168,747,421	$43,387,161,494
Deductions from Revenue.	45,004,634,205	37,784,174,261	31,935,698,552	27,344,870,806	23,349,445,508
Net Patient Revenue	28,468,151,044	25,158,739,822	21,896,351,260	20,823,876,615	20,037,715,986
Other Operating Revenue	2,760,139,848	2,466,963,729	2,311,583,837	2,071,860,033	2,000,853,453
Other Nonoperating Revenue	162,526,064	397,849,826	476,653,999	457,181,324	418,580,724
Total Net Revenue.	31,390,816,956	28,023,553,377	24,684,589,096	23,352,917,972	22,457,150,163
Total Expenses.	28,457,791,824	25,906,399,927	23,494,693,306	21,811,587,994	20,578,760,550
HOSPITAL UNIT (Excludes Separate Nursing Home Units)					
Utilization - Inpatient					
Beds	55,040	54,430	53,335	53,570	53,128
Admissions	2,508,127	2,427,696	2,323,817	2,246,168	2,165,772
Inpatient Days	12,719,345	12,142,510	11,498,881	11,180,783	10,839,457
Average Length of Stay.	5.1	5.0	4.9	5.0	5.0
Personnel					
Total Full Time.	241,964	233,563	225,255	228,566	221,876
Total Part Time	57,963	57,471	53,479	52,351	56,306
Revenue and Expenses - Totals					
(Includes Inpatient and Outpatient)					
Total Net Revenue.	$31,211,712,467	$27,788,903,511	$24,508,683,378	$23,037,586,558	$22,079,657,603
Total Expenses.	28,313,376,914	25,757,452,142	23,374,693,756	21,595,696,612	20,334,411,518
COMMUNITY HEALTH INDICATORS PER 1000 POPULATION					
Total Population (in thousands)	21,780	21,325	20,852	20,044	19,712
Inpatient					
Beds	2.6	2.6	2.7	2.8	2.9
Admissions	116.3	115.4	113.5	114.9	113.0
Inpatient Days	605.5	593.2	581.4	599.5	595.2
Inpatient Surgeries.	34.5	34.0	34.4	34.7	36.0
Births.	17.1	17.2	17.2	16.9	16.9
Outpatient					
Emergency Outpatient Visits.	378.5	366.1	353.7	352.8	341.0
Other Outpatient Visits.	1,159.7	1,108.9	1,055.9	1,057.0	1,045.9
Total Outpatient Visits	1,538.2	1,475.0	1,409.6	1,409.8	1,386.9
Outpatient Surgeries	50.2	49.2	50.1	51.6	50.0
Expense per Capita (per person). . . .	$1,306.6	$1,214.8	$1,126.7	$1,088.2	$1,044.0

States

TABLE 6

UTAH

U.S. Registered Community Hospitals
(Nonfederal, short-term general and other special hospitals)

Overview 1998–2002

	2002	2001	2000	1999	1998
Total U.S. Community Hospitals in Utah..	42	42	42	42	41
Bed Size Category					
6-24	6	8	7	7	7
25-49	13	11	14	12	12
50-99	8	8	5	7	7
100-199	9	9	10	11	10
200-299	3	3	3	2	2
300-399	2	1	2	2	2
400-499	1	2	1	1	1
500 +	0	0	0	0	0
Location					
Hospitals Urban	21	21	20	20	19
Hospitals Rural	21	21	22	22	22
Control					
State and Local Government	6	7	7	9	9
Not for Profit	22	22	22	20	20
Investor owned	14	13	13	13	12
Physician Models					
Independent Practice Association	8	11	16	15	16
Group Practice without Walls	2	1	1	1	3
Open Physician-Hospital Organization	4	4	5	3	4
Closed Physician-Hospital Organization	0	0	0	1	0
Management Service Organization	2	2	4	5	8
Integrated Salary Model	13	17	18	16	18
Equity Model	0	0	0	0	0
Foundation	0	0	0	1	3
Insurance Products					
Health Maintenance Organization	15	18	19	15	22
Preferred Provider Organization	15	20	20	16	25
Indemnity Fee for Service	8	12	11	6	15
Managed Care Contracts					
Health Maintenance Organization	17	21	25	24	24
Preferred Provider Organization	20	23	28	26	27
Affiliations					
Hospitals in a System	21	28	32	26	30
Hospitals in a Network	10	11	14	8	8
Hospitals in a Group Purchasing Organization	26	33	32	24	30

States

TABLE 6

UTAH

U.S. Registered Community Hospitals
(Nonfederal, short-term general and other special hospitals)

Utilization, Personnel, Revenue and Expenses, Community Health Indicators 1998–2002

	2002	2001	2000	1999	1998
TOTAL FACILITY (Includes Hospital and Nursing Home Units)					
Utilization - Inpatient					
Beds	4,403	4,437	4,330	4,170	4,010
Admissions	206,344	203,037	194,047	189,430	192,357
Inpatient Days	876,524	902,313	886,846	871,864	885,746
Average Length of Stay	4.2	4.4	4.6	4.6	4.6
Inpatient Surgeries	72,489	59,425	58,729	56,992	60,493
Births	48,792	47,319	47,389	45,831	44,259
Utilization - Outpatient					
Emergency Outpatient Visits	797,951	699,934	697,703	687,822	625,879
Other Outpatient Visits	4,016,360	3,718,415	3,771,285	3,677,904	3,598,412
Total Outpatient Visits	4,814,311	4,418,349	4,468,988	4,365,726	4,224,291
Outpatient Surgeries	156,769	122,692	125,430	120,031	128,033
Personnel					
Full Time RNs	4,939	4,442	4,143	4,405	5,078
Full Time LPNs	627	566	413	493	856
Part Time RNs	3,145	2,749	3,426	3,134	2,604
Part Time LPNs	405	387	359	326	330
Total Full Time	21,063	20,005	18,807	18,880	19,692
Total Part Time	10,564	10,822	11,987	9,852	8,223
Revenue - Inpatient					
Gross Inpatient Revenue	$3,062,158,326	$2,559,345,455	$2,168,015,062	$2,124,901,031	$1,888,753,714
Revenue - Outpatient					
Gross Outpatient Revenue	$1,897,673,822	$1,582,419,304	$1,347,153,458	$1,328,671,681	$1,104,236,886
Revenue and Expenses - Totals (Includes Inpatient and Outpatient)					
Total Gross Revenue	$4,959,832,148	$4,141,764,759	$3,515,168,520	$3,453,572,712	$2,992,990,600
Deductions from Revenue	2,384,893,655	1,865,061,006	1,391,174,618	1,439,113,434	1,144,878,464
Net Patient Revenue	2,574,938,493	2,276,703,753	2,123,993,902	2,014,459,278	1,848,112,136
Other Operating Revenue	139,121,419	158,563,665	115,758,563	105,790,033	119,057,672
Other Nonoperating Revenue	23,585,217	21,198,879	12,177,408	16,489,703	5,226,424
Total Net Revenue	2,737,645,129	2,456,466,297	2,251,929,873	2,136,739,014	1,972,396,232
Total Expenses	2,505,242,473	2,242,551,322	2,069,630,397	1,927,577,263	1,826,222,339
HOSPITAL UNIT (Excludes Separate Nursing Home Units)					
Utilization - Inpatient					
Beds	4,257	4,283	4,187	3,967	3,737
Admissions	204,612	200,838	191,941	187,940	189,316
Inpatient Days	831,512	857,332	844,301	825,693	807,010
Average Length of Stay	4.1	4.3	4.4	4.4	4.3
Personnel					
Total Full Time	21,007	19,858	18,739	18,803	19,433
Total Part Time	10,462	10,689	11,891	9,772	7,958
Revenue and Expenses - Totals (Includes Inpatient and Outpatient)					
Total Net Revenue	$2,728,571,258	$2,435,680,792	$2,239,569,389	$2,124,836,350	$1,957,383,056
Total Expenses	2,500,424,658	2,230,611,574	2,064,796,222	1,921,753,908	1,818,502,949
COMMUNITY HEALTH INDICATORS PER 1000 POPULATION					
Total Population (in thousands)	2,316	2,270	2,233	2,130	2,101
Inpatient					
Beds	1.9	2.0	1.9	2.0	1.9
Admissions	89.1	89.5	86.9	88.9	91.6
Inpatient Days	378.4	397.5	397.1	409.4	421.7
Inpatient Surgeries	31.3	26.2	26.3	26.8	28.8
Births	21.1	20.8	21.2	21.5	21.1
Outpatient					
Emergency Outpatient Visits	344.5	308.4	312.4	322.9	298.0
Other Outpatient Visits	1,734.0	1,638.2	1,688.8	1,726.8	1,713.1
Total Outpatient Visits	2,078.5	1,946.6	2,001.2	2,049.8	2,011.0
Outpatient Surgeries	67.7	54.1	56.2	56.4	61.0
Expense per Capita (per person)	$1,081.6	$988.0	$926.8	$905.0	$869.4

TABLE 6

VERMONT

U.S. Registered Community Hospitals
(Nonfederal, short-term general and other special hospitals)

Overview 1998–2002

	2002	2001	2000	1999	1998
Total U.S. Community Hospitals in Vermont	14	14	14	14	14
Bed Size Category					
6-24	0	0	0	0	0
25-49	6	5	5	5	4
50-99	5	5	4	5	6
100-199	1	2	3	2	2
200-299	1	1	1	1	1
300-399	0	0	0	0	0
400-499	0	0	0	0	1
500 +	1	1	1	1	0
Location					
Hospitals Urban	2	2	2	2	2
Hospitals Rural	12	12	12	12	12
Control					
State and Local Government	0	0	0	0	0
Not for Profit	14	14	14	14	14
Investor owned	0	0	0	0	0
Physician Models					
Independent Practice Association	1	1	1	1	1
Group Practice without Walls	2	2	0	1	1
Open Physician-Hospital Organization	5	6	5	5	5
Closed Physician-Hospital Organization	1	1	2	2	2
Management Service Organization	3	3	2	3	2
Integrated Salary Model	7	8	5	6	6
Equity Model	0	0	0	0	0
Foundation	1	1	0	0	0
Insurance Products					
Health Maintenance Organization	5	6	6	6	7
Preferred Provider Organization	4	3	2	2	2
Indemnity Fee for Service	0	1	2	1	1
Managed Care Contracts					
Health Maintenance Organization	9	11	8	11	11
Preferred Provider Organization	7	9	8	10	7
Affiliations					
Hospitals in a System	6	7	5	3	3
Hospitals in a Network	2	3	3	4	4
Hospitals in a Group Purchasing Organization	11	13	9	7	7

TABLE 6

VERMONT

U.S. Registered Community Hospitals
(Nonfederal, short-term general and other special hospitals)

Utilization, Personnel, Revenue and Expenses, Community Health Indicators 1998–2002

	2002	2001	2000	1999	1998
TOTAL FACILITY (Includes Hospital and Nursing Home Units)					
Utilization - Inpatient					
Beds	1,576	1,694	1,674	1,669	1,671
Admissions	52,236	54,701	52,413	50,820	50,076
Inpatient Days	348,528	403,993	407,915	394,752	393,539
Average Length of Stay	6.7	7.4	7.8	7.8	7.9
Inpatient Surgeries	14,971	14,507	14,677	15,890	15,763
Births	6,003	5,982	6,086	6,521	6,366
Utilization - Outpatient					
Emergency Outpatient Visits	230,643	237,773	236,337	220,500	213,367
Other Outpatient Visits	1,239,885	1,053,731	1,006,715	1,193,334	938,260
Total Outpatient Visits	1,470,528	1,291,504	1,243,052	1,413,834	1,151,627
Outpatient Surgeries	39,468	37,983	34,739	33,443	32,198
Personnel					
Full Time RNs	1,040	939	977	948	868
Full Time LPNs	216	202	167	170	183
Part Time RNs	1,770	1,201	1,651	1,505	1,491
Part Time LPNs	240	216	265	222	233
Total Full Time	7,981	7,317	5,977	5,911	5,594
Total Part Time	5,589	4,134	5,307	4,958	4,351
Revenue - Inpatient					
Gross Inpatient Revenue	$632,612,094	$594,629,834	$574,346,167	$518,323,168	$554,981,205
Revenue - Outpatient					
Gross Outpatient Revenue	$683,857,958	$583,052,967	$496,200,352	$435,098,015	$399,689,481
Revenue and Expenses - Totals					
(Includes Inpatient and Outpatient)					
Total Gross Revenue	$1,316,470,052	$1,177,682,801	$1,070,546,519	$953,421,183	$954,670,686
Deductions from Revenue	514,087,762	406,248,096	373,526,131	321,690,952	404,255,939
Net Patient Revenue	802,382,290	771,434,705	697,020,388	631,730,231	550,414,747
Other Operating Revenue	17,504,386	16,049,961	15,403,343	15,793,813	24,695,865
Other Nonoperating Revenue	260,503	-17,559,247	27,208,270	15,736,174	13,200,342
Total Net Revenue	820,147,179	769,925,419	739,632,001	663,260,218	588,310,954
Total Expenses	812,757,084	771,202,476	696,036,667	646,945,630	572,807,035
HOSPITAL UNIT (Excludes Separate Nursing Home Units)					
Utilization - Inpatient					
Beds	1,325	1,318	1,425	1,302	1,263
Admissions	51,785	54,016	52,048	50,270	49,593
Inpatient Days	263,456	275,686	320,624	270,279	251,889
Average Length of Stay	5.1	5.1	6.2	5.4	5.1
Personnel					
Total Full Time	7,778	7,062	5,844	5,712	5,358
Total Part Time	5,469	3,936	5,192	4,753	4,112
Revenue and Expenses - Totals					
(Includes Inpatient and Outpatient)					
Total Net Revenue	$807,750,162	$749,316,386	$727,972,770	$645,310,922	$569,552,051
Total Expenses	798,095,694	751,409,578	685,479,802	629,980,592	554,130,892
COMMUNITY HEALTH INDICATORS PER 1000 POPULATION					
Total Population (in thousands)	617	613	609	594	591
Inpatient					
Beds	2.6	2.8	2.7	2.8	2.8
Admissions	84.7	89.2	86.1	85.6	84.8
Inpatient Days	565.2	658.9	670.0	664.9	666.4
Inpatient Surgeries	24.3	23.7	24.1	26.8	26.7
Births	9.7	9.8	10.0	11.0	10.8
Outpatient					
Emergency Outpatient Visits	374.1	387.8	388.2	371.4	361.3
Other Outpatient Visits	2,010.9	1,718.7	1,653.5	2,009.9	1,588.7
Total Outpatient Visits	2,384.9	2,106.5	2,041.7	2,381.2	1,950.0
Outpatient Surgeries	64.0	62.0	57.1	56.3	54.5
Expense per Capita (per person)	$1,318.1	$1,257.9	$1,143.2	$1,089.6	$969.9

States

TABLE **6**

VIRGINIA

U.S. Registered Community Hospitals
(Nonfederal, short-term general and other special hospitals)

Overview 1998–2002

	2002	2001	2000	1999	1998
Total U.S. Community Hospitals in					
Virginia	86	87	88	89	93
Bed Size Category					
6-24	1	2	4	2	2
25-49	11	10	7	7	8
50-99	18	18	17	20	18
100-199	25	25	29	28	33
200-299	15	17	15	16	15
300-399	5	5	7	8	8
400-499	3	3	3	2	2
500 + ...	8	7	6	6	7
Location					
Hospitals Urban.....................	51	52	53	54	58
Hospitals Rural	35	35	35	35	35
Control					
State and Local Government	5	5	5	5	5
Not for Profit	67	67	66	68	70
Investor owned	14	15	17	16	18
Physician Models					
Independent Practice Association........	8	6	11	11	14
Group Practice without Walls	1	1	6	10	8
Open Physician-Hospital Organization....	20	22	24	30	30
Closed Physician-Hospital Organization...	3	2	4	8	12
Management Service Organization.......	6	9	11	21	21
Integrated Salary Model	28	23	28	32	26
Equity Model	2	1	3	6	6
Foundation........................	5	3	4	4	5
Insurance Products					
Health Maintenance Organization........	26	23	25	31	28
Preferred Provider Organization........	33	30	37	41	42
Indemnity Fee for Service..............	9	7	13	17	19
Managed Care Contracts					
Health Maintenance Organization........	56	51	55	55	60
Preferred Provider Organization.........	64	57	64	64	72
Affiliations					
Hospitals in a System.................	49	45	48	51	51
Hospitals in a Network	28	28	32	29	38
Hospitals in a Group Purchasing					
Organization.....................	66	60	65	62	60

TABLE 6

VIRGINIA

U.S. Registered Community Hospitals
(Nonfederal, short-term general and other special hospitals)

Utilization, Personnel, Revenue and Expenses, Community Health Indicators 1998–2002

	2002	2001	2000	1999	1998
TOTAL FACILITY (Includes Hospital and Nursing Home Units)					
Utilization - Inpatient					
Beds	17,241	16,775	16,869	17,295	17,890
Admissions	746,686	743,992	726,772	723,803	716,976
Inpatient Days	4,278,445	4,239,227	4,161,981	4,133,834	4,090,018
Average Length of Stay	5.7	5.7	5.7	5.7	5.7
Inpatient Surgeries	236,774	235,109	221,837	215,568	219,878
Births	90,401	90,043	88,419	87,384	85,573
Utilization - Outpatient					
Emergency Outpatient Visits	2,606,320	2,482,380	2,476,006	2,291,867	2,255,094
Other Outpatient Visits	8,183,177	7,266,153	7,067,468	6,439,017	6,068,901
Total Outpatient Visits	10,789,497	9,748,533	9,543,474	8,730,884	8,323,995
Outpatient Surgeries	503,094	468,427	424,570	399,995	373,869
Personnel					
Full Time RNs	18,038	17,572	17,875	17,243	17,657
Full Time LPNs	2,764	2,690	2,704	2,778	2,872
Part Time RNs	8,110	7,902	7,432	6,990	6,952
Part Time LPNs	844	865	861	1,090	1,006
Total Full Time	72,397	72,228	71,430	68,276	68,914
Total Part Time	23,323	24,196	23,153	22,200	21,451
Revenue - Inpatient					
Gross Inpatient Revenue	$12,167,189,859	$10,850,288,232	$9,441,736,067	$8,879,124,657	$8,168,485,435
Revenue - Outpatient					
Gross Outpatient Revenue	$7,232,253,089	$6,253,409,826	$5,348,095,706	$4,761,310,776	$4,098,142,024
Revenue and Expenses - Totals (Includes Inpatient and Outpatient)					
Total Gross Revenue	$19,399,442,948	$17,103,698,058	$14,789,831,773	$13,640,435,433	$12,266,627,459
Deductions from Revenue	10,621,457,968	8,992,877,116	7,349,786,545	6,565,622,328	5,636,877,770
Net Patient Revenue	8,777,984,980	8,110,820,942	7,440,045,228	7,074,813,105	6,629,749,689
Other Operating Revenue	241,242,013	302,761,541	273,304,634	261,032,965	197,884,519
Other Nonoperating Revenue	-14,532,952	131,168,071	126,490,381	226,795,432	117,590,421
Total Net Revenue	9,004,694,041	8,544,750,554	7,839,840,243	7,562,641,502	6,945,224,629
Total Expenses	8,779,480,958	7,961,019,921	7,109,751,133	6,637,854,513	6,294,405,851
HOSPITAL UNIT (Excludes Separate Nursing Home Units)					
Utilization - Inpatient					
Beds	15,938	15,866	15,709	15,872	16,430
Admissions	743,372	740,997	723,853	720,497	712,640
Inpatient Days	3,875,511	3,927,254	3,769,912	3,653,766	3,595,253
Average Length of Stay	5.2	5.3	5.2	5.1	5.0
Personnel					
Total Full Time	71,403	71,289	70,525	67,346	67,693
Total Part Time	23,004	23,845	22,889	21,770	21,131
Revenue and Expenses - Totals (Includes Inpatient and Outpatient)					
Total Net Revenue	$8,947,350,583	$8,501,564,931	$7,795,125,327	$7,500,435,588	$6,874,805,160
Total Expenses	8,727,817,754	7,921,569,817	7,069,123,980	6,592,027,665	6,233,864,195
COMMUNITY HEALTH INDICATORS PER 1000 POPULATION					
Total Population (in thousands)	7,294	7,188	7,079	6,873	6,789
Inpatient					
Beds	2.4	2.3	2.4	2.5	2.6
Admissions	102.4	103.5	102.7	105.3	105.6
Inpatient Days	586.6	589.8	588.0	601.5	602.4
Inpatient Surgeries	32.5	32.7	31.3	31.4	32.4
Births	12.4	12.5	12.5	12.7	12.6
Outpatient					
Emergency Outpatient Visits	357.3	345.4	349.8	333.5	332.2
Other Outpatient Visits	1,122.0	1,010.9	998.4	936.9	893.9
Total Outpatient Visits	1,479.3	1,356.3	1,348.2	1,270.3	1,226.1
Outpatient Surgeries	69.0	65.2	60.0	58.2	55.1
Expense per Capita (per person)	$1,203.7	$1,107.6	$1,004.4	$965.8	$927.1

States

TABLE 6

WASHINGTON

U.S. Registered Community Hospitals
(Nonfederal, short-term general and other special hospitals)

Overview 1998–2002

	2002	2001	2000	1999	1998
Total U.S. Community Hospitals in Washington..........................	86	84	84	86	86
Bed Size Category					
6-24	9	5	6	8	6
25-49	20	22	22	22	25
50-99	18	18	17	17	17
100-199	16	17	16	18	19
200-299	14	12	15	13	10
300-399	6	7	6	6	7
400-499	1	1	0	0	0
500 + ...	2	2	2	2	2
Location					
Hospitals Urban......................	45	44	44	46	46
Hospitals Rural	41	40	40	40	40
Control					
State and Local Government	40	39	38	40	41
Not for Profit	42	41	42	43	42
Investor owned	4	4	4	3	3
Physician Models					
Independent Practice Association........	3	9	9	11	10
Group Practice without Walls	3	5	2	2	2
Open Physician-Hospital Organization....	11	10	13	14	10
Closed Physician-Hospital Organization...	1	3	3	6	5
Management Service Organization.......	6	7	7	9	9
Integrated Salary Model	36	22	22	20	17
Equity Model	0	1	2	2	1
Foundation.........................	0	2	3	3	3
Insurance Products					
Health Maintenance Organization........	9	6	7	13	11
Preferred Provider Organization.........	12	9	11	17	16
Indemnity Fee for Service..............	3	3	4	6	6
Managed Care Contracts					
Health Maintenance Organization........	41	35	37	43	35
Preferred Provider Organization.........	54	39	43	48	38
Affiliations					
Hospitals in a System.................	27	27	24	24	21
Hospitals in a Network	16	19	15	17	11
Hospitals in a Group Purchasing Organization......................	62	53	49	52	47

States

TABLE 6

WASHINGTON

U.S. Registered Community Hospitals
(Nonfederal, short-term general and other special hospitals)

Utilization, Personnel, Revenue and Expenses, Community Health Indicators 1998–2002

	2002	2001	2000	1999	1998
TOTAL FACILITY (Includes Hospital and Nursing Home Units)					
Utilization - Inpatient					
Beds	11,338	11,382	11,136	11,092	10,739
Admissions	518,562	522,624	504,836	490,659	474,394
Inpatient Days	2,486,925	2,501,066	2,432,089	2,375,711	2,295,333
Average Length of Stay	4.8	4.8	4.8	4.8	4.8
Inpatient Surgeries	162,809	163,263	163,298	164,275	144,499
Births	72,586	74,134	73,816	72,814	72,506
Utilization - Outpatient					
Emergency Outpatient Visits	1,936,458	2,063,313	1,932,238	1,887,881	1,602,826
Other Outpatient Visits	7,811,926	7,369,191	7,656,940	8,072,113	7,118,236
Total Outpatient Visits	9,748,384	9,432,504	9,589,178	9,959,994	8,721,062
Outpatient Surgeries	280,786	312,357	261,219	247,937	239,312
Personnel					
Full Time RNs	10,214	10,991	10,083	8,427	9,154
Full Time LPNs	1,060	1,098	1,175	932	1,026
Part Time RNs	11,477	9,567	11,165	11,467	9,579
Part Time LPNs	866	595	1,155	1,176	992
Total Full Time	53,490	54,672	50,106	45,373	42,071
Total Part Time	32,880	27,551	33,201	33,715	28,849
Revenue - Inpatient					
Gross Inpatient Revenue	$8,210,414,712	$7,463,136,201	$6,558,652,349	$5,936,579,978	$5,037,900,244
Revenue - Outpatient					
Gross Outpatient Revenue	$6,583,605,589	$5,100,762,752	$4,446,084,034	$3,979,924,518	$3,089,214,485
Revenue and Expenses - Totals					
(Includes Inpatient and Outpatient)					
Total Gross Revenue	$14,794,020,301	$12,563,898,953	$11,004,736,383	$9,916,504,496	$8,127,114,729
Deductions from Revenue	7,178,544,115	5,870,547,412	4,776,586,811	3,981,377,196	3,055,762,073
Net Patient Revenue	7,615,476,186	6,693,351,541	6,228,149,572	5,935,127,300	5,071,352,656
Other Operating Revenue	473,047,880	438,253,314	344,678,358	329,844,922	289,826,305
Other Nonoperating Revenue	45,762,585	81,540,504	160,620,397	127,455,356	117,922,748
Total Net Revenue	8,134,286,651	7,213,145,359	6,733,448,327	6,392,427,578	5,479,101,709
Total Expenses	7,830,121,368	6,971,690,572	6,384,423,283	6,091,763,363	5,240,148,977
HOSPITAL UNIT (Excludes Separate Nursing Home Units)					
Utilization - Inpatient					
Beds	10,494	10,696	10,326	10,217	10,148
Admissions	513,922	516,955	501,157	484,728	470,529
Inpatient Days	2,219,549	2,292,820	2,211,500	2,125,679	2,107,302
Average Length of Stay	4.3	4.4	4.4	4.4	4.5
Personnel					
Total Full Time	52,927	54,120	49,627	44,769	41,514
Total Part Time	32,525	27,177	32,905	33,403	28,527
Revenue and Expenses - Totals					
(Includes Inpatient and Outpatient)					
Total Net Revenue	$8,082,984,927	$7,171,721,867	$6,697,390,270	$6,346,757,006	$5,449,820,746
Total Expenses	7,788,632,966	6,932,850,141	6,352,247,750	6,054,313,545	5,215,161,786
COMMUNITY HEALTH INDICATORS PER 1000 POPULATION					
Total Population (in thousands)	6,069	5,988	5,894	5,756	5,688
Inpatient					
Beds	1.9	1.9	1.9	1.9	1.9
Admissions	85.4	87.3	85.7	85.2	83.4
Inpatient Days	409.8	417.7	412.6	412.7	403.6
Inpatient Surgeries	26.8	27.3	27.7	28.5	25.4
Births	12.0	12.4	12.5	12.6	12.7
Outpatient					
Emergency Outpatient Visits	319.1	344.6	327.8	328.0	281.8
Other Outpatient Visits	1,287.2	1,230.7	1,299.1	1,402.3	1,251.5
Total Outpatient Visits	1,606.3	1,575.2	1,626.9	1,730.3	1,533.3
Outpatient Surgeries	46.3	52.2	44.3	43.1	42.1
Expense per Capita (per person)	$1,290.2	$1,164.3	$1,083.2	$1,058.3	$921.3

States

TABLE 6

WEST VIRGINIA

U.S. Registered Community Hospitals
(Nonfederal, short-term general and other special hospitals)

Overview 1998–2002

	2002	2001	2000	1999	1998
Total U.S. Community Hospitals in West Virginia	57	57	57	58	58
Bed Size Category					
6-24	4	3	3	3	3
25-49	11	13	13	13	13
50-99	17	16	16	16	16
100-199	12	10	10	10	10
200-299	8	10	10	10	11
300-399	3	3	2	3	2
400-499	1	1	2	2	2
500 +	1	1	1	1	1
Location					
Hospitals Urban	18	18	18	18	18
Hospitals Rural	39	39	39	40	40
Control					
State and Local Government	10	10	10	10	10
Not for Profit	33	33	33	34	33
Investor owned	14	14	14	14	15
Physician Models					
Independent Practice Association	3	3	3	0	2
Group Practice without Walls	1	2	2	3	6
Open Physician-Hospital Organization	16	17	17	19	20
Closed Physician-Hospital Organization	1	1	3	1	1
Management Service Organization	4	4	7	10	13
Integrated Salary Model	21	20	17	14	11
Equity Model	1	1	1	1	1
Foundation	0	0	0	1	3
Insurance Products					
Health Maintenance Organization	6	4	8	7	8
Preferred Provider Organization	9	8	12	12	15
Indemnity Fee for Service	5	4	6	4	5
Managed Care Contracts					
Health Maintenance Organization	34	35	37	38	35
Preferred Provider Organization	48	45	47	46	42
Affiliations					
Hospitals in a System	25	29	30	28	24
Hospitals in a Network	30	28	28	26	21
Hospitals in a Group Purchasing Organization	52	52	48	45	42

States

TABLE 6

WEST VIRGINIA

U.S. Registered Community Hospitals
(Nonfederal, short-term general and other special hospitals)

Utilization, Personnel, Revenue and Expenses, Community Health Indicators 1998–2002

	2002	2001	2000	1999	1998
TOTAL FACILITY (Includes Hospital and Nursing Home Units)					
Utilization - Inpatient					
Beds	7,821	7,906	7,966	8,109	8,117
Admissions	295,011	297,079	288,095	289,427	280,729
Inpatient Days	1,775,869	1,806,411	1,772,580	1,792,038	1,778,264
Average Length of Stay	6.0	6.1	6.2	6.2	6.3
Inpatient Surgeries	79,711	82,783	81,969	100,693	77,859
Births	20,659	20,775	20,917	20,785	21,030
Utilization - Outpatient					
Emergency Outpatient Visits	1,100,258	1,057,155	1,007,028	1,002,071	1,020,060
Other Outpatient Visits	4,585,150	4,705,105	4,188,510	4,093,375	3,987,301
Total Outpatient Visits	5,685,408	5,762,260	5,195,538	5,095,446	5,007,361
Outpatient Surgeries	201,288	203,775	185,222	196,421	189,507
Personnel					
Full Time RNs	6,836	7,005	7,013	6,869	7,049
Full Time LPNs	1,599	1,656	1,639	1,599	1,603
Part Time RNs	3,191	3,019	2,435	2,426	2,327
Part Time LPNs	532	452	512	468	514
Total Full Time	29,733	29,730	29,191	29,397	29,089
Total Part Time	9,691	9,679	8,528	8,212	8,421
Revenue - Inpatient					
Gross Inpatient Revenue	$3,247,995,766	$3,059,121,057	$2,738,379,228	$2,558,226,357	$2,414,070,698
Revenue - Outpatient					
Gross Outpatient Revenue	$2,395,425,269	$2,108,241,241	$1,896,927,001	$1,702,148,428	$1,624,810,990
Revenue and Expenses - Totals					
(Includes Inpatient and Outpatient)					
Total Gross Revenue	$5,643,421,035	$5,167,362,298	$4,635,306,229	$4,260,374,785	$4,038,881,688
Deductions from Revenue	2,606,272,014	2,318,812,349	2,018,286,724	1,717,929,145	1,534,687,947
Net Patient Revenue	3,037,149,021	2,848,549,949	2,617,019,505	2,542,445,640	2,504,193,741
Other Operating Revenue	87,401,673	94,610,622	83,958,168	67,331,452	54,616,020
Other Nonoperating Revenue	16,381,152	42,442,849	62,118,544	73,508,215	72,933,826
Total Net Revenue	3,140,931,846	2,985,603,420	2,763,096,217	2,683,285,307	2,631,743,587
Total Expenses	3,068,384,987	2,867,459,406	2,672,667,972	2,569,940,576	2,476,492,231
HOSPITAL UNIT (Excludes Separate Nursing Home Units)					
Utilization - Inpatient					
Beds	6,756	6,835	6,904	7,063	7,022
Admissions	286,752	288,941	279,560	280,887	270,905
Inpatient Days	1,435,794	1,475,652	1,442,082	1,463,906	1,428,662
Average Length of Stay	5.0	5.1	5.2	5.2	5.3
Personnel					
Total Full Time	28,849	28,817	28,286	28,402	28,173
Total Part Time	9,386	9,398	8,251	7,907	8,130
Revenue and Expenses - Totals					
(Includes Inpatient and Outpatient)					
Total Net Revenue	$3,073,370,762	$2,917,661,986	$2,707,349,521	$2,628,108,392	$2,562,192,400
Total Expenses	3,005,319,455	2,818,658,157	2,625,906,089	2,521,864,295	2,419,075,794
COMMUNITY HEALTH INDICATORS PER 1000 POPULATION					
Total Population (in thousands)	1,802	1,802	1,808	1,807	1,812
Inpatient					
Beds	4.3	4.4	4.4	4.5	4.5
Admissions	163.7	164.9	159.3	160.2	155.0
Inpatient Days	985.6	1,002.5	980.2	991.8	981.6
Inpatient Surgeries	44.2	45.9	45.3	55.7	43.0
Births	11.5	11.5	11.6	11.5	11.6
Outpatient					
Emergency Outpatient Visits	610.6	586.7	556.9	554.6	563.0
Other Outpatient Visits	2,544.7	2,611.2	2,316.2	2,265.4	2,200.9
Total Outpatient Visits	3,155.3	3,197.9	2,873.1	2,819.9	2,763.9
Outpatient Surgeries	111.7	113.1	102.4	108.7	104.6
Expense per Capita (per person)	$1,702.9	$1,591.3	$1,478.0	$1,422.3	$1,367.0

States

TABLE **6**

WISCONSIN

U.S. Registered Community Hospitals
(Nonfederal, short-term general and other special hospitals)

Overview 1998–2002

	2002	2001	2000	1999	1998
Total U.S. Community Hospitals in					
Wisconsin..........................	120	121	118	123	123
Bed Size Category					
6-24	8	5	5	6	6
25-49	29	30	27	26	24
50-99	27	29	26	29	30
100-199	36	35	40	40	39
200-299	14	15	13	15	15
300-399	4	2	2	2	4
400-499	1	3	3	3	2
500 + ...	1	2	2	2	3
Location					
Hospitals Urban......................	55	56	56	57	57
Hospitals Rural	65	65	62	66	66
Control					
State and Local Government	2	2	2	2	2
Not for Profit	117	118	115	120	120
Investor owned	1	1	1	1	1
Physician Models					
Independent Practice Association........	12	12	16	14	15
Group Practice without Walls	9	10	8	11	6
Open Physician-Hospital Organization....	8	12	17	14	14
Closed Physician-Hospital Organization...	8	6	8	5	3
Management Service Organization.......	7	6	9	7	6
Integrated Salary Model	42	36	35	38	36
Equity Model	2	3	7	3	3
Foundation.........................	2	2	6	2	1
Insurance Products					
Health Maintenance Organization........	28	30	22	25	29
Preferred Provider Organization.........	21	20	27	35	31
Indemnity Fee for Service.............	5	5	7	10	10
Managed Care Contracts					
Health Maintenance Organization........	102	106	93	112	111
Preferred Provider Organization.........	108	113	101	115	111
Affiliations					
Hospitals in a System.................	68	69	58	66	62
Hospitals in a Network	41	39	38	41	40
Hospitals in a Group Purchasing					
Organization......................	109	107	93	61	—

TABLE 6

WISCONSIN

U.S. Registered Community Hospitals
(Nonfederal, short-term general and other special hospitals)

Utilization, Personnel, Revenue and Expenses, Community Health Indicators 1998–2002

	2002	2001	2000	1999	1998
TOTAL FACILITY (Includes Hospital and Nursing Home Units)					
Utilization - Inpatient					
Beds..........................	14,610	15,597	15,329	15,870	16,693
Admissions.....................	579,830	579,089	558,357	553,337	553,810
Inpatient Days	3,396,381	3,455,633	3,331,095	3,394,502	3,442,860
Average Length of Stay...........	5.9	6.0	6.0	6.1	6.2
Inpatient Surgeries...............	181,674	184,704	181,028	179,457	180,783
Births..........................	65,588	67,772	66,406	65,961	65,751
Utilization - Outpatient					
Emergency Outpatient Visits	1,833,344	1,866,201	1,785,771	1,723,490	1,608,391
Other Outpatient Visits...........	9,778,893	9,163,082	9,068,481	8,787,589	8,025,131
Total Outpatient Visits	11,612,237	11,029,283	10,854,252	10,511,079	9,633,522
Outpatient Surgeries	388,879	358,874	346,742	329,008	309,459
Personnel					
Full Time RNs	10,225	9,873	9,982	10,002	10,297
Full Time LPNs	794	751	689	712	919
Part Time RNs.................	12,915	13,772	13,399	12,989	13,169
Part Time LPNs	1,125	1,114	1,139	1,163	1,307
Total Full Time...............	53,737	51,379	49,099	50,249	49,216
Total Part Time	42,826	43,352	41,266	42,222	40,726
Revenue - Inpatient					
Gross Inpatient Revenue..........	$7,802,749,118	$6,991,429,425	$6,098,946,220	$5,948,871,964	$5,786,700,159
Revenue - Outpatient					
Gross Outpatient Revenue	$6,112,204,146	$5,291,918,670	$4,468,653,347	$4,013,180,391	$3,539,897,672
Revenue and Expenses - Totals					
(Includes Inpatient and Outpatient)					
Total Gross Revenue.............	$13,914,953,264	$12,283,348,095	$10,567,599,567	$9,962,052,355	$9,326,597,831
Deductions from Revenue........	5,950,993,178	5,054,991,610	3,975,769,894	3,784,662,896	3,476,564,635
Net Patient Revenue	7,963,960,086	7,228,356,485	6,591,829,673	6,177,389,459	5,850,033,196
Other Operating Revenue	437,318,773	330,549,912	318,938,842	308,659,328	310,750,930
Other Nonoperating Revenue	92,711,281	132,446,055	153,176,880	139,860,357	166,270,056
Total Net Revenue.............	8,493,990,140	7,691,352,452	7,063,945,395	6,625,909,144	6,327,054,182
Total Expenses.................	7,917,744,877	7,182,972,349	6,662,561,165	6,232,856,297	5,899,798,976
HOSPITAL UNIT (Excludes Separate Nursing Home Units)					
Utilization - Inpatient					
Beds..........................	12,413	13,124	13,069	13,455	14,210
Admissions.....................	576,456	575,849	555,586	549,946	550,790
Inpatient Days	2,653,543	2,656,174	2,587,690	2,596,699	2,611,012
Average Length of Stay...........	4.6	4.6	4.7	4.7	4.7
Personnel					
Total Full Time...............	53,066	50,535	47,736	49,158	48,254
Total Part Time	41,988	42,513	40,098	41,046	39,547
Revenue and Expenses - Totals					
(Includes Inpatient and Outpatient)					
Total Net Revenue...............	$8,402,275,478	$7,614,643,256	$7,003,452,628	$6,535,271,256	$6,247,192,029
Total Expenses.................	7,837,518,200	7,116,127,111	6,570,298,128	6,157,416,203	5,833,422,569
COMMUNITY HEALTH INDICATORS PER 1000 POPULATION					
Total Population (in thousands)	5,441	5,402	5,364	5,250	5,222
Inpatient					
Beds..........................	2.7	2.9	2.9	3.0	3.2
Admissions.....................	106.6	107.2	104.1	105.4	106.1
Inpatient Days	624.2	639.7	621.0	646.5	659.3
Inpatient Surgeries...............	33.4	34.2	33.8	34.2	34.6
Births..........................	12.1	12.5	12.4	12.6	12.6
Outpatient					
Emergency Outpatient Visits	336.9	345.5	332.9	328.3	308.0
Other Outpatient Visits...........	1,797.2	1,696.3	1,690.7	1,673.7	1,536.8
Total Outpatient Visits	2,134.1	2,041.7	2,023.7	2,001.9	1,844.8
Outpatient Surgeries	71.5	66.4	64.6	62.7	59.3
Expense per Capita (per person)....	$1,455.1	$1,329.7	$1,242.2	$1,187.1	$1,129.8

States

TABLE 6

WYOMING

U.S. Registered Community Hospitals
(Nonfederal, short-term general and other special hospitals)

Overview 1998–2002

	2002	2001	2000	1999	1998
Total U.S. Community Hospitals in Wyoming	24	24	24	23	25
Bed Size Category					
6-24	0	0	0	0	1
25-49	9	9	9	9	9
50-99	10	10	9	8	8
100-199	4	4	4	5	7
200-299	1	1	2	1	0
300-399	0	0	0	0	0
400-499	0	0	0	0	0
500 +	0	0	0	0	0
Location					
Hospitals Urban	2	2	2	2	2
Hospitals Rural	22	22	22	21	23
Control					
State and Local Government	16	16	16	15	17
Not for Profit	5	5	5	5	6
Investor owned	3	3	3	3	2
Physician Models					
Independent Practice Association	2	2	2	3	3
Group Practice without Walls	0	0	0	0	0
Open Physician-Hospital Organization	2	1	1	2	3
Closed Physician-Hospital Organization	1	1	1	1	1
Management Service Organization	1	1	1	1	2
Integrated Salary Model	7	5	4	3	3
Equity Model	0	0	0	0	0
Foundation	0	0	1	0	0
Insurance Products					
Health Maintenance Organization	1	0	1	1	3
Preferred Provider Organization	1	3	4	4	5
Indemnity Fee for Service	1	1	1	0	0
Managed Care Contracts					
Health Maintenance Organization	3	3	2	3	3
Preferred Provider Organization	12	10	10	10	8
Affiliations					
Hospitals in a System	5	6	5	6	7
Hospitals in a Network	2	2	2	0	1
Hospitals in a Group Purchasing Organization	21	22	20	17	17

TABLE 6

WYOMING

U.S. Registered Community Hospitals
(Nonfederal, short-term general and other special hospitals)

Utilization, Personnel, Revenue and Expenses, Community Health Indicators 1998–2002

	2002	2001	2000	1999	1998
TOTAL FACILITY (Includes Hospital and Nursing Home Units)					
Utilization - Inpatient					
Beds	1,882	1,920	1,920	1,830	1,935
Admissions	49,201	47,587	47,852	45,212	43,833
Inpatient Days	370,143	379,674	392,856	350,011	380,351
Average Length of Stay	7.5	8.0	8.2	7.7	8.7
Inpatient Surgeries	13,393	13,020	13,277	13,788	13,237
Births	5,945	5,779	5,668	5,376	5,396
Utilization - Outpatient					
Emergency Outpatient Visits	212,868	196,723	198,691	184,370	173,155
Other Outpatient Visits	676,043	621,299	679,917	681,309	676,373
Total Outpatient Visits	888,911	818,022	878,608	865,679	849,528
Outpatient Surgeries	28,197	27,168	26,600	24,333	23,230
Personnel					
Full Time RNs	1,424	1,385	1,250	1,346	1,255
Full Time LPNs	185	251	254	237	157
Part Time RNs	426	440	461	339	588
Part Time LPNs	47	86	78	56	53
Total Full Time	6,224	6,265	5,693	5,719	5,651
Total Part Time	1,798	1,905	2,075	1,532	2,085
Revenue - Inpatient					
Gross Inpatient Revenue	$539,374,103	$490,186,370	$459,146,586	$391,557,628	$373,737,424
Revenue - Outpatient					
Gross Outpatient Revenue	$429,084,211	$370,431,371	$341,692,739	$286,160,208	$265,896,402
Revenue and Expenses - Totals					
(Includes Inpatient and Outpatient)					
Total Gross Revenue	$968,458,314	$860,617,741	$800,839,325	$677,717,836	$639,633,826
Deductions from Revenue	371,291,521	307,942,802	270,948,291	213,650,230	197,412,034
Net Patient Revenue	597,166,793	552,674,939	529,891,034	464,067,606	442,221,792
Other Operating Revenue	28,889,946	26,930,485	26,084,236	23,737,455	23,324,074
Other Nonoperating Revenue	16,008,231	16,580,965	17,942,529	12,176,866	16,335,608
Total Net Revenue	642,064,970	596,186,389	573,917,799	499,981,927	481,881,474
Total Expenses	610,888,942	558,590,503	514,916,805	445,760,593	430,470,596
HOSPITAL UNIT (Excludes Separate Nursing Home Units)					
Utilization - Inpatient					
Beds	1,271	1,298	1,296	1,275	1,306
Admissions	47,931	46,489	46,687	44,283	43,021
Inpatient Days	178,227	183,768	194,293	175,560	186,006
Average Length of Stay	3.7	4.0	4.2	4.0	4.3
Personnel					
Total Full Time	5,750	5,740	5,248	5,351	5,233
Total Part Time	1,636	1,743	1,937	1,440	1,948
Revenue and Expenses - Totals					
(Includes Inpatient and Outpatient)					
Total Net Revenue	$617,051,893	$568,830,781	$548,439,718	$480,479,888	$451,481,646
Total Expenses	589,286,951	533,736,510	494,194,490	427,158,396	410,789,054
COMMUNITY HEALTH INDICATORS PER 1000 POPULATION					
Total Population (in thousands)	499	494	494	480	480
Inpatient					
Beds	3.8	3.9	3.9	3.8	4.0
Admissions	98.7	96.2	96.9	94.3	91.3
Inpatient Days	742.2	767.9	795.6	729.8	792.3
Inpatient Surgeries	26.9	26.3	26.9	28.7	27.6
Births	11.9	11.7	11.5	11.2	11.2
Outpatient					
Emergency Outpatient Visits	426.8	397.9	402.4	384.4	360.7
Other Outpatient Visits	1,355.6	1,256.6	1,377.0	1,420.6	1,409.0
Total Outpatient Visits	1,782.4	1,654.5	1,779.3	1,805.0	1,769.7
Outpatient Surgeries	56.5	54.9	53.9	50.7	48.4
Expense per Capita (per person)	$1,225.0	$1,129.8	$1,042.8	$929.4	$896.7

States

Table 7

The facilities and services presented in Table 7 are listed below in alphabetical order by major heading (where applicable).

Table 7

2002 Facilities and Services in the U.S. Census Divisions and States

These data include only hospital-based facilities and services as reported by responding hospitals in Section C of the 2002 AHA Annual Survey, beginning on page 197. All hospitals are represented with Community Hospitals listed separately under United States. No estimates have been made for nonresponding hospitals. Definitions of facilities and services are listed in the Glossary, page 187.

CLASSIFICATION	HOSPITALS REPORTING	GEN MED SURG ADULT No.	Pct	GEN MED SURG PEDIATRIC No.	Pct	OBSTETRICS INPATIENT No.	Pct	NEONATAL INTERMEDIATE No.	Pct	NEONATAL No.	Pct	IC PEDIATRIC No.	Pct	IC CARDIAC No.	Pct	IC MED SURG No.	Pct	OTHER No.	Pct
UNITED STATES	4,876	4,217	86.5	2,262	46.4	2,963	60.8	660	13.5	891	18.3	450	9.2	1,585	32.5	3,146	64.5	454	9.3
COMMUNITY HOSPITALS	4,275	4,013	93.9	2,217	51.9	2,923	68.4	650	15.2	879	20.6	442	10.3	1,536	35.9	3,019	70.6	434	10.2
CENSUS DIVISION 1, NEW ENGLAND	214	182	85.0	120	56.1	145	67.8	25	11.7	31	14.5	15	7.0	65	30.4	164	76.6	13	6.1
Connecticut	33	28	84.8	22	66.7	26	78.8	2	6.1	12	36.4	2	6.1	14	42.4	27	81.8	2	6.1
Maine	39	36	92.3	16	41.0	31	79.5	1	2.6	2	5.1	2	5.1	7	17.9	33	84.6	1	2.6
Massachusetts	83	68	81.9	52	62.7	47	56.6	16	19.3	12	14.5	6	7.2	28	33.7	60	72.3	6	7.2
New Hampshire	30	25	83.3	17	56.7	24	80.0	3	10.0	3	10.0	3	10.0	7	23.3	24	80.0	1	3.3
Rhode Island	15	12	80.0	6	40.0	6	40.0	2	13.3	1	6.7	1	6.7	4	26.7	8	53.3	3	20.0
Vermont	14	13	92.9	7	50.0	11	78.6	1	7.1	1	7.1	1	7.1	5	35.7	12	85.7	0	0.0
CENSUS DIVISION 2, MIDDLE ATLANTIC	455	391	85.9	250	54.9	295	64.8	109	24.0	109	24.0	50	11.0	207	45.5	352	77.4	49	10.8
New Jersey	78	68	87.2	51	65.4	54	69.2	39	50.0	19	24.4	11	14.1	42	53.8	66	84.6	10	12.8
New York	184	158	85.9	109	59.2	118	64.1	40	21.7	45	24.5	29	15.8	88	47.8	139	75.5	16	8.7
Pennsylvania	193	165	85.5	90	46.6	123	63.7	30	15.5	45	23.3	10	5.2	77	39.9	147	76.2	23	11.9
CENSUS DIVISION 3, SOUTH ATLANTIC	681	591	86.8	324	47.6	404	59.3	123	18.1	141	20.7	78	11.5	260	38.2	491	72.1	85	12.5
Delaware	8	6	75.0	4	50.0	5	62.5	1	12.5	4	50.0	3	37.5	4	50.0	6	75.0	2	25.0
District of Columbia	10	8	80.0	4	40.0	6	60.0	2	20.0	6	60.0	3	30.0	7	70.0	8	80.0	1	10.0
Florida	146	129	88.4	57	39.0	77	52.7	22	15.1	38	26.0	24	16.4	64	43.8	112	76.7	20	13.7
Georgia	133	113	85.0	55	41.4	72	54.1	25	18.8	25	18.8	8	6.0	37	27.8	81	60.9	10	7.5
Maryland	59	45	76.3	34	57.6	33	55.9	6	10.2	15	25.4	4	6.8	28	47.5	45	76.3	8	13.6
North Carolina	109	97	89.0	53	48.6	75	68.8	27	24.8	19	17.4	10	9.2	32	29.4	78	71.6	20	18.3
South Carolina	68	62	91.2	52	76.5	46	67.6	20	29.4	12	17.6	11	16.2	39	57.4	51	75.0	9	13.2
Virginia	84	75	89.3	39	46.4	58	69.0	12	14.3	16	19.0	9	10.7	28	33.3	70	83.3	9	10.7
West Virginia	64	56	87.5	26	40.6	32	50.0	8	12.5	6	9.4	6	9.4	21	32.8	40	62.5	6	9.4
CENSUS DIVISION 4, EAST NORTH CENTRAL	887	616	89.7	414	60.3	487	70.9	81	11.8	117	17.0	84	12.2	279	40.6	511	74.4	119	17.3
Illinois	169	155	91.7	106	62.7	118	69.8	34	20.1	30	17.8	19	11.2	54	32.0	135	79.9	6	3.6
Indiana	103	90	87.4	53	51.5	82	79.6	15	14.6	18	17.5	7	6.8	34	33.0	75	72.8	7	6.8
Michigan	142	129	90.8	80	56.3	91	64.1	12	8.5	22	15.5	13	9.2	55	38.7	96	67.6	14	9.9
Ohio	149	131	87.9	71	47.7	101	67.8	20	13.4	28	18.8	8	5.4	52	34.9	116	77.9	16	10.7
Wisconsin	124	111	89.5	104	83.9	95	76.6	0	0.0	19	15.3	37	29.8	84	67.7	89	71.8	76	61.3
CENSUS DIVISION 5, EAST SOUTH CENTRAL	447	391	87.5	221	49.4	228	51.0	60	13.4	68	15.2	38	8.5	143	32.0	260	58.2	49	11.0
Alabama	110	99	90.0	52	47.3	55	50.0	7	6.4	20	18.2	6	5.5	29	26.4	63	57.3	18	16.4
Kentucky	98	88	89.8	40	40.8	48	49.0	15	15.3	12	12.2	4	4.1	32	32.7	64	65.3	8	8.2
Mississippi	104	95	91.3	80	76.9	51	49.0	27	26.0	18	17.3	19	18.3	50	48.1	55	52.9	8	7.7
Tennessee	135	109	80.7	49	36.3	74	54.8	11	8.1	18	13.3	9	6.7	32	23.7	78	57.8	15	11.1
CENSUS DIVISION 6, WEST NORTH CENTRAL	680	625	91.9	281	41.3	410	60.3	62	9.1	75	11.0	40	5.9	164	24.1	356	52.4	29	4.3
Iowa	124	118	95.2	55	44.4	88	71.0	8	6.5	16	12.9	8	6.5	26	21.0	77	62.1	3	2.4
Kansas	142	130	91.5	42	29.6	69	48.6	11	7.7	9	6.3	5	3.5	16	11.3	55	38.7	3	2.1
Minnesota	109	102	93.6	54	49.5	84	77.1	11	10.1	10	9.2	8	7.3	39	35.8	57	52.3	7	6.4
Missouri	141	119	84.4	62	44.0	75	53.2	18	12.8	21	14.9	9	6.4	36	25.5	94	66.7	13	9.2
Nebraska	72	67	93.1	29	40.3	45	62.5	6	8.3	9	12.5	2	2.8	17	23.6	32	44.4	1	1.4
North Dakota	36	36	100.0	20	55.6	22	61.1	6	16.7	7	19.4	5	13.9	18	50.0	19	52.8	1	2.8
South Dakota	56	53	94.6	19	33.9	27	48.2	2	3.6	3	5.4	3	5.4	12	21.4	22	39.3	1	1.8
CENSUS DIVISION 7, WEST SOUTH CENTRAL	798	618	77.4	265	33.2	396	49.6	104	13.0	132	16.5	60	7.5	178	22.3	415	52.0	45	5.6
Arkansas	102	82	80.4	25	24.5	51	50.0	16	15.7	13	12.7	2	2.0	35	34.3	52	51.0	7	6.9
Louisiana	142	107	75.4	48	33.8	53	37.3	14	9.9	29	20.4	14	9.9	27	19.0	79	55.6	6	4.2
Oklahoma	87	74	85.1	39	44.8	49	56.3	11	12.6	13	14.9	9	10.3	23	26.4	46	52.9	8	9.2
Texas	467	355	76.0	153	32.8	243	52.0	63	13.5	77	16.5	35	7.5	93	19.9	238	51.0	24	5.1
CENSUS DIVISION 8, MOUNTAIN	339	304	89.7	142	41.9	217	64.0	41	12.1	50	14.7	26	7.7	86	25.4	196	57.8	23	6.8
Arizona	58	51	87.9	21	36.2	36	62.1	5	8.6	8	13.8	5	8.6	17	29.3	34	58.6	2	3.4
Colorado	59	52	88.1	30	50.8	42	71.2	10	16.9	16	27.1	5	8.5	14	23.7	38	64.4	6	10.2
Idaho	38	34	89.5	10	26.3	24	63.2	2	5.3	4	10.5	2	5.3	6	15.8	17	44.7	3	7.9
Montana	55	52	94.5	21	38.2	29	52.7	5	9.1	6	10.9	5	9.1	19	34.5	25	45.5	2	3.6
Nevada	26	23	88.5	12	46.2	15	57.7	0	0.0	4	15.4	3	11.5	6	23.1	18	69.2	3	11.5
New Mexico	38	33	86.8	18	47.4	24	63.2	7	18.4	4	10.5	4	10.5	6	15.8	22	57.9	5	13.2
Utah	38	33	86.8	20	52.6	30	78.9	9	23.7	8	21.1	1	2.6	14	36.8	24	63.2	2	5.3
Wyoming	27	26	96.3	10	37.0	17	63.0	3	11.1	0	0.0	1	3.7	4	14.8	18	66.7	0	0.0
CENSUS DIVISION 9, PACIFIC	575	499	86.8	245	42.6	381	66.3	55	9.6	168	29.2	59	10.3	203	35.3	401	69.7	42	7.3
Alaska	18	17	94.4	8	44.4	15	83.3	1	5.6	3	16.7	1	5.6	4	22.2	9	50.0	1	5.6
California	392	330	84.2	171	43.6	242	61.7	31	7.9	139	35.5	45	11.5	150	38.3	279	71.2	26	6.6
Hawaii	25	21	84.0	6	24.0	12	48.0	2	8.0	3	12.0	3	12.0	7	28.0	12	48.0	0	0.0
Oregon	58	58	100.0	24	41.4	51	87.9	6	10.3	6	10.3	3	5.2	18	31.0	47	81.0	6	10.3
Washington	82	73	89.0	36	43.9	61	74.4	15	18.3	17	20.7	7	8.5	24	29.3	54	65.9	9	11.0

Column groups: GENERAL MEDICAL SURGICAL CARE (ADULT UNITS, PEDIATRIC UNITS); OBSTETRICS INPATIENT CARE UNITS; NEONATAL INTERMEDIATE CARE UNITS; NEONATAL UNITS; INTENSIVE CARE (PEDIATRIC UNITS, CARDIAC UNITS, MEDICAL SURGICAL UNITS); OTHER UNITS.

Table 7 (Continued)

These data include only hospital-based facilities and services as reported by responding hospitals in Section C of the 2002 AHA Annual Survey, beginning on page 197. All hospitals are represented with Community Hospitals listed separately under United States. No estimates have been made for nonresponding hospitals. Definitions of facilities and services are listed in the Glossary, page 187.

CLASSIFICATION	HOSPITALS REPORTING	BURN CARE (UNITS)		ACUTE LONG-TERM CARE (UNITS)		LONG-TERM CARE SKILLED NURSING CARE (UNITS)		LONG-TERM CARE INTERMEDIATE CARE (UNITS)		LONG-TERM CARE OTHER LONG-TERM CARE (UNITS)		PSYCHIATRIC INPATIENT CARE (UNITS)		ALCOHOL/DRUG ABUSE OR DEPENDENCY INPATIENT CARE (UNITS)		OTHER SPECIAL CARE (UNITS)		PHYSICAL REHABILITATION INPATIENT CARE (UNITS)	
		Number	Percent	Number	Percent	Number	Percent	Number	Percent	Number	Percent	Number	Percent	Number	Percent	Number	Percent	Number	Percent
UNITED STATES	4,876	178	3.7	256	5.3	1,681	34.5	472	9.7	726	14.9	1,784	36.6	595	12.2	663	13.6	1,318	27.0
COMMUNITY HOSPITALS	4,275	172	4.0	167	3.9	1,588	37.1	415	9.7	632	14.8	1,400	32.7	445	10.4	621	14.5	1,243	29.1
CENSUS DIVISION 1, NEW ENGLAND	214	7	3.3	7	3.3	58	27.1	24	11.2	28	13.1	112	52.3	24	11.2	15	7.0	51	23.8
Connecticut	33	1	3.0	1	3.0	2	6.1	3	9.1	5	15.2	25	75.8	5	15.2	3	9.1	11	33.3
Maine	39	1	2.6	1	2.6	14	35.9	6	15.4	2	5.1	11	28.2	6	15.4	1	2.6	6	15.4
Massachusetts	83	3	3.6	4	4.8	25	30.1	4	4.8	14	16.9	46	55.4	8	9.6	7	8.4	15	18.1
New Hampshire	30	1	3.3	1	3.3	11	36.7	8	26.7	6	20.0	14	46.7	2	6.7	3	10.0	9	30.0
Rhode Island	15	0	0.0	0	0.0	3	20.0	1	6.7	0	0.0	10	66.7	1	6.7	1	6.7	6	40.0
Vermont	14	1	7.1	0	0.0	3	21.4	2	14.3	1	7.1	6	42.9	2	14.3	0	0.0	4	28.6
CENSUS DIVISION 2, MIDDLE ATLANTIC	455	20	4.4	13	2.9	150	33.0	26	5.7	72	15.8	261	57.4	88	19.3	59	13.0	148	32.5
New Jersey	78	2	2.6	1	1.3	15	19.2	6	7.7	14	17.9	47	60.3	11	14.1	7	9.0	12	15.4
New York	184	10	5.4	4	2.2	58	31.5	7	3.8	34	18.5	110	59.8	54	29.3	26	14.1	65	35.3
Pennsylvania	193	8	4.1	8	4.1	77	39.9	13	6.7	24	12.4	104	53.9	23	11.9	26	13.5	71	36.8
CENSUS DIVISION 3, SOUTH ATLANTIC	681	26	3.8	41	6.0	219	32.2	81	11.9	143	21.0	263	38.6	102	15.0	140	20.6	182	26.7
Delaware	8	0	0.0	0	0.0	5	62.5	4	50.0	3	37.5	4	50.0	1	12.5	3	25.0	4	50.0
District of Columbia	10	1	10.0	0	0.0	4	40.0	2	20.0	4	40.0	9	90.0	1	10.0	3	30.0	3	30.0
Florida	146	5	3.4	6	4.1	35	24.0	14	9.6	23	15.8	48	32.9	18	12.3	27	18.5	33	22.6
Georgia	133	3	2.3	12	9.0	40	30.1	13	9.8	27	20.3	37	27.8	18	13.5	20	15.0	33	24.8
Maryland	59	2	3.4	3	5.1	21	35.6	4	6.8	15	25.4	38	64.4	9	15.3	15	25.4	15	25.4
North Carolina	109	3	2.8	5	4.6	46	42.2	18	16.5	18	16.5	49	45.0	16	14.7	22	20.2	27	24.8
South Carolina	68	3	4.4	9	13.2	14	20.6	0	0.0	32	47.1	19	27.9	16	23.5	27	39.7	40	58.8
Virginia	84	6	7.1	5	6.0	20	23.8	17	20.2	11	13.1	40	47.6	16	19.0	16	19.0	19	22.6
West Virginia	64	3	4.7	1	1.6	34	53.1	9	14.1	10	15.6	19	29.7	7	10.9	8	12.5	8	12.5
CENSUS DIVISION 4, EAST NORTH CENTRAL	687	38	5.5	29	4.2	244	35.5	71	10.3	89	13.0	295	42.9	124	18.0	167	24.3	248	36.1
Illinois	169	4	2.4	7	4.1	70	41.4	13	7.7	14	8.3	79	46.7	24	14.2	16	9.5	49	29.0
Indiana	103	2	1.9	4	3.9	45	43.7	12	11.7	14	13.6	35	34.0	14	13.6	10	9.7	29	28.2
Michigan	142	9	6.3	5	3.5	35	24.6	9	6.3	20	14.1	57	40.1	15	10.6	16	11.3	52	36.6
Ohio	149	7	4.7	3	2.0	58	38.9	12	8.1	25	16.8	75	50.3	25	16.8	21	14.1	49	32.9
Wisconsin	124	16	12.9	10	8.1	36	29.0	25	20.2	16	12.9	49	39.5	46	37.1	104	83.9	69	55.6
CENSUS DIVISION 5, EAST SOUTH CENTRAL	447	14	3.1	15	3.4	133	29.8	20	4.5	86	19.2	166	37.1	49	11.0	65	14.5	109	24.4
Alabama	110	3	2.7	4	3.6	12	10.9	3	2.7	29	26.4	33	30.0	5	4.5	10	9.1	16	14.5
Kentucky	98	4	4.1	6	6.1	45	45.9	6	6.1	13	13.3	33	33.7	11	11.2	14	14.3	17	17.3
Mississippi	104	4	3.8	0	0.0	34	32.7	1	1.0	20	19.2	58	55.8	20	19.2	20	19.2	45	43.3
Tennessee	135	3	2.2	5	3.7	42	31.1	10	7.4	24	17.8	42	31.1	13	9.6	21	15.6	31	23.0
CENSUS DIVISION 6, WEST NORTH CENTRAL	680	20	2.9	28	4.1	340	50.0	136	20.0	117	17.2	176	25.9	50	7.4	58	8.5	137	20.1
Iowa	124	4	3.2	2	1.6	60	48.4	35	28.2	21	16.9	36	29.0	10	8.1	12	9.7	17	13.7
Kansas	142	2	1.4	5	3.5	73	51.4	43	30.3	15	10.6	29	20.4	1	0.7	4	2.8	21	14.8
Minnesota	109	3	2.8	6	5.5	56	51.4	6	5.5	14	12.8	26	23.9	11	10.1	10	9.2	18	16.5
Missouri	141	6	4.3	5	3.5	68	48.2	16	11.3	30	21.3	63	44.7	23	16.3	24	17.0	54	38.3
Nebraska	72	3	4.2	3	4.2	37	51.4	19	26.4	12	16.7	8	11.1	3	4.2	2	2.8	12	16.7
North Dakota	36	1	2.8	1	2.8	17	47.2	6	16.7	7	19.4	7	19.4	2	5.6	2	5.6	7	19.4
South Dakota	56	1	1.8	4	7.1	29	51.8	11	19.6	18	32.1	7	12.5	0	0.0	4	7.1	8	14.3
CENSUS DIVISION 7, WEST SOUTH CENTRAL	798	17	2.1	75	9.4	174	21.8	37	4.6	79	9.9	242	30.3	72	9.0	81	10.2	228	28.6
Arkansas	102	2	2.0	5	4.9	30	29.4	4	3.9	15	14.7	39	38.2	5	4.9	4	3.9	32	31.4
Louisiana	142	3	2.1	15	10.6	40	28.2	10	7.0	16	11.3	72	50.7	11	7.7	9	6.3	46	32.4
Oklahoma	87	5	5.7	8	9.2	27	31.0	11	12.6	17	19.5	30	34.5	6	6.9	10	11.5	29	33.3
Texas	467	7	1.5	47	10.1	77	16.5	12	2.6	31	6.6	101	21.6	50	10.7	58	12.4	121	25.9
CENSUS DIVISION 8, MOUNTAIN	339	14	4.1	18	5.3	150	44.2	38	11.2	43	12.7	89	26.3	34	10.0	23	6.8	91	26.8
Arizona	58	4	6.9	4	6.9	15	25.9	6	10.3	10	17.2	14	24.1	4	6.9	2	3.4	23	39.7
Colorado	59	4	6.8	4	6.8	27	45.8	4	6.8	9	15.3	20	33.9	8	13.6	8	13.6	25	42.4
Idaho	38	0	0.0	0	0.0	20	52.6	1	2.6	3	7.9	8	21.1	2	5.3	1	2.6	6	15.8
Montana	55	1	1.8	6	10.9	43	78.2	5	9.1	9	16.4	10	18.2	3	5.5	4	7.3	8	14.5
Nevada	26	1	3.8	2	7.7	5	19.2	2	7.7	4	15.4	7	26.9	1	3.8	1	3.8	6	23.1
New Mexico	38	2	5.3	2	5.3	9	23.7	6	15.8	5	13.2	12	31.6	7	18.4	5	13.2	9	23.7
Utah	38	2	5.3	0	0.0	21	55.3	7	18.4	1	2.6	12	31.6	4	10.5	1	2.6	9	23.7
Wyoming	27	0	0.0	0	0.0	10	37.0	7	25.9	2	7.4	6	22.2	4	14.8	1	3.7	5	18.5
CENSUS DIVISION 9, PACIFIC	575	22	3.8	30	5.2	213	37.0	39	6.8	69	12.0	180	31.3	52	9.0	55	9.6	124	21.6
Alaska	18	1	5.6	1	5.6	7	38.9	5	27.8	1	5.6	8	44.4	3	16.7	1	5.6	4	22.2
California	392	17	4.3	21	5.4	163	41.6	12	3.1	39	9.9	124	31.6	31	7.9	35	8.9	87	22.2
Hawaii	25	1	4.0	2	8.0	12	48.0	8	32.0	9	36.0	8	32.0	1	4.0	1	4.0	1	4.0
Oregon	58	2	3.4	3	5.2	12	20.7	8	13.8	5	8.6	16	27.6	4	6.9	7	12.1	8	13.8
Washington	82	1	1.2	3	3.7	19	23.2	6	7.3	15	18.3	24	29.3	13	15.9	11	13.4	24	29.3

Table 7 (Continued)

These data include only hospital-based facilities and services as reported by responding hospitals in Section C of the 2001 AHA Annual Survey, beginning on page 197. All hospitals are represented with Community Hospitals listed separately under United States. No estimates have been made for nonresponding hospitals. Definitions of facilities and services are listed in the Glossary, page 187.

CLASSIFICATION	HOSPITALS REPORTING	ADULT DAY CARE PROGRAM Number	Percent	ALCOHOL/DRUG ABUSE OR DEPENDENCY OUTPATIENT SERVICES Number	Percent	AMBULANCE SERVICES Number	Percent	ANGIOPLASTY Number	Percent	ARTHRITIS TREATMENT CENTER Number	Percent	ASSISTED LIVING Number	Percent	AUXILIARY Number	Percent	BIRTHING/LDR/LDRP ROOM Number	Percent	BREAST CANCER SCREENING Number	Percent
UNITED STATES	4,876	452	9.3	952	19.5	873	17.9	1,217	25.0	298	6.1	252	5.2	3,026	62.1	2,903	59.5	3,504	71.9
COMMUNITY HOSPITALS	4,275	396	9.3	726	17.0	819	19.2	1,165	27.3	268	6.3	225	5.3	2,946	68.9	2,873	67.2	3,408	79.7
CENSUS DIVISION 1, NEW ENGLAND	214	25	11.7	74	34.6	31	14.5	43	20.1	19	8.9	12	5.6	129	60.3	142	66.4	170	79.4
Connecticut	33	4	12.1	16	48.5	2	6.1	8	24.2	2	6.1	1	3.0	22	66.7	26	78.8	28	84.8
Maine	39	1	2.6	15	38.5	10	25.6	5	12.8	0	0.0	3	7.7	24	61.5	30	76.9	34	87.2
Massachusetts	83	9	10.8	32	38.6	7	8.4	17	20.5	9	10.8	2	2.4	49	59.0	46	55.4	64	77.1
New Hampshire	30	7	23.3	2	6.7	7	23.3	8	26.7	3	10.0	2	6.7	17	56.7	24	80.0	24	80.0
Rhode Island	15	2	13.3	5	33.3	2	13.3	3	20.0	3	20.0	2	13.3	8	53.3	6	40.0	10	66.7
Vermont	14	2	14.3	4	28.6	3	21.4	2	14.3	2	14.3	2	14.3	9	64.3	10	71.4	10	71.4
CENSUS DIVISION 2, MIDDLE ATLANTIC	455	69	15.2	140	30.8	81	17.8	121	26.6	49	10.8	22	4.8	303	66.6	286	62.9	371	81.5
New Jersey	78	21	26.9	32	41.0	10	12.8	21	26.9	9	11.5	4	5.1	59	75.6	52	66.7	67	85.9
New York	184	32	17.4	74	40.2	35	19.0	39	21.2	21	11.4	6	3.3	111	60.3	112	60.9	147	79.9
Pennsylvania	193	16	8.3	34	17.6	36	18.7	61	31.6	19	9.8	12	6.2	133	68.9	122	63.2	157	81.3
CENSUS DIVISION 3, SOUTH ATLANTIC	681	58	8.5	151	22.2	106	15.6	190	27.9	47	6.9	27	4.0	430	63.1	395	58.0	521	76.5
Delaware	8	2	25.0	3	37.5	1	12.5	4	50.0	2	25.0	1	12.5	7	87.5	5	62.5	6	75.0
District of Columbia	10	0	0.0	6	60.0	3	30.0	7	70.0	7	70.0	0	0.0	4	40.0	6	60.0	7	70.0
Florida	146	9	6.2	21	14.4	19	13.0	56	38.4	9	6.2	2	1.4	92	63.0	72	49.3	112	76.7
Georgia	133	7	5.3	29	21.8	33	24.8	21	15.8	3	2.3	9	6.8	79	59.4	71	53.4	100	75.2
Maryland	59	6	10.2	15	25.4	5	8.5	20	33.9	7	11.9	3	5.1	45	76.3	31	52.5	40	67.8
North Carolina	109	9	8.3	24	22.0	21	19.3	26	23.9	8	7.3	2	1.8	67	61.5	76	69.7	82	75.2
South Carolina	68	19	27.9	15	22.1	1	1.5	18	26.5	1	1.5	4	5.9	38	55.9	45	66.2	55	80.9
Virginia	84	6	7.1	28	33.3	14	16.7	29	34.5	5	6.0	5	6.0	62	73.8	57	67.9	72	85.7
West Virginia	64	0	0.0	10	15.6	9	14.1	9	14.1	5	7.8	1	1.6	36	56.3	32	50.0	47	73.4
CENSUS DIVISION 4, EAST NORTH CENTRAL	687	77	11.2	201	29.3	136	19.8	202	29.4	76	11.1	43	6.3	480	69.9	475	69.1	571	83.1
Illinois	169	25	14.8	52	30.8	39	23.1	68	40.2	23	13.6	12	7.1	114	67.5	114	67.5	147	87.0
Indiana	103	7	6.8	27	26.2	35	34.0	25	24.3	6	5.8	5	4.9	58	56.3	78	75.7	83	80.6
Michigan	142	12	8.5	36	25.4	20	14.1	33	23.2	10	7.0	8	5.6	109	76.8	88	62.0	121	85.2
Ohio	149	10	6.7	42	28.2	18	12.1	47	31.5	17	11.4	9	6.0	110	73.8	99	66.4	121	81.2
Wisconsin	124	23	18.5	44	35.5	24	19.4	29	23.4	20	16.1	9	7.3	89	71.8	96	77.4	99	79.8
CENSUS DIVISION 5, EAST SOUTH CENTRAL	447	19	4.3	50	11.2	73	16.3	77	17.2	19	4.3	12	2.7	215	48.1	213	47.7	308	68.9
Alabama	110	4	3.6	7	6.4	15	13.6	24	21.8	5	4.5	7	6.4	71	64.5	44	40.0	71	64.5
Kentucky	98	8	8.2	15	15.3	12	12.2	21	21.4	5	5.1	1	1.0	65	66.3	49	50.0	82	83.7
Mississippi	104	4	3.8	11	10.6	19	18.3	3	2.9	4	3.8	0	0.0	22	21.2	48	46.2	62	59.6
Tennessee	135	3	2.2	17	12.6	27	20.0	29	21.5	5	3.7	4	3.0	57	42.2	72	53.3	93	68.9
CENSUS DIVISION 6, WEST NORTH CENTRAL	680	89	13.1	100	14.7	184	27.1	119	17.5	29	4.3	81	11.9	489	71.9	422	62.1	477	70.1
Iowa	124	15	12.1	26	21.0	54	43.5	18	14.5	4	3.2	9	7.3	108	87.1	88	71.0	111	89.5
Kansas	142	18	12.7	8	5.6	24	16.9	16	11.3	2	1.4	13	9.2	83	58.5	79	55.6	76	53.5
Minnesota	109	26	23.9	22	20.2	35	32.1	14	12.8	2	1.8	18	16.5	81	74.3	84	77.1	82	75.2
Missouri	141	7	5.0	26	18.4	32	22.7	49	34.8	13	9.2	6	4.3	108	76.6	73	51.8	103	73.0
Nebraska	72	11	15.3	7	9.7	17	23.6	12	16.7	4	2.8	8	11.1	48	66.7	50	69.4	52	72.2
North Dakota	36	3	8.3	5	13.9	9	25.0	6	16.7	4	11.1	5	13.9	27	75.0	21	58.3	22	61.1
South Dakota	56	9	16.1	6	10.7	13	23.2	4	7.1	2	3.6	22	39.3	34	60.7	27	48.2	31	55.4
CENSUS DIVISION 7, WEST SOUTH CENTRAL	798	27	3.4	78	9.8	134	16.8	198	24.8	22	2.8	22	2.8	449	56.3	374	46.9	449	56.3
Arkansas	102	7	6.9	9	8.8	23	22.5	24	23.5	5	4.9	2	2.0	70	68.6	48	47.1	69	67.6
Louisiana	142	6	4.2	20	14.1	16	11.3	38	26.8	4	2.8	2	1.4	67	47.2	46	32.4	76	53.5
Oklahoma	87	7	8.0	7	8.0	19	21.8	20	23.0	2	2.3	4	4.6	57	65.5	47	54.0	51	58.6
Texas	467	7	1.5	42	9.0	76	16.3	116	24.8	11	2.4	14	3.0	255	54.6	233	49.9	253	54.2
CENSUS DIVISION 8, MOUNTAIN	339	40	11.8	64	18.9	62	18.3	88	26.0	12	3.5	17	5.0	201	59.3	226	66.7	241	71.1
Arizona	58	7	12.1	15	25.9	3	5.2	25	43.1	3	5.2	1	1.7	35	60.3	35	60.3	38	65.5
Colorado	59	4	6.8	14	23.7	15	25.4	19	32.2	4	6.8	2	3.4	39	66.1	43	72.9	47	79.7
Idaho	38	5	13.2	3	7.9	8	21.1	4	10.5	1	2.6	0	0.0	29	76.3	29	76.3	25	65.8
Montana	55	18	32.7	4	7.3	15	27.3	7	12.7	1	1.8	12	21.8	31	56.4	31	56.4	35	63.6
Nevada	26	1	3.8	5	19.2	3	11.5	10	38.5	0	0.0	0	0.0	11	42.3	16	61.5	18	69.2
New Mexico	38	1	2.6	9	23.7	5	13.2	8	21.1	0	0.0	0	0.0	19	50.0	20	52.6	27	71.1
Utah	38	3	7.9	7	18.4	4	10.5	11	28.9	2	5.3	0	0.0	21	55.3	32	84.2	30	78.9
Wyoming	27	1	3.7	7	25.9	9	33.3	4	14.8	0	0.0	2	7.4	16	59.3	20	74.1	21	77.8
CENSUS DIVISION 9, PACIFIC	575	48	8.3	94	16.3	66	11.5	179	31.1	25	4.3	16	2.8	330	57.4	370	64.3	396	68.9
Alaska	18	1	5.6	7	38.9	4	22.2	2	11.1	0	0.0	0	0.0	10	55.6	15	83.3	14	77.8
California	392	34	8.7	60	15.3	38	9.7	126	32.1	18	4.6	7	1.8	214	54.6	230	58.7	259	66.1
Hawaii	25	2	8.0	3	12.0	2	8.0	6	24.0	2	8.0	0	0.0	13	52.0	12	48.0	13	52.0
Oregon	58	7	12.1	7	12.1	7	12.1	17	29.3	3	5.2	3	5.2	46	79.3	51	87.9	48	82.8
Washington	82	4	4.9	17	20.7	15	18.3	28	34.1	2	2.4	6	7.3	47	57.3	62	75.6	62	75.6

Table 7 (Continued)

These data include only hospital-based facilities and services as reported by responding hospitals in Section C of the 2002 AHA Annual Survey, beginning on page 197. All hospitals are represented with Community Hospitals listed separately under United States. No estimates have been made for nonresponding hospitals. Definitions of facilities and services are listed in the Glossary, page 187.

Classification	Hospitals Reporting	Cardiac Catheterization Laboratory No.	%	Case Management No.	%	Children Wellness Program No.	%	Chiropractic Services No.	%	Community Outreach No.	%	Complementary Medicine Services No.	%	Crisis Prevention No.	%	CT Scanner No.	%	Dental Services No.	%	Diagnostic Radioisotope Facility No.	%	Emergency Department No.	%
UNITED STATES	4,876	1,728	35.4	3,594	73.7	895	18.4	108	2.2	3,047	62.5	797	16.3	948	19.4	3,889	79.8	1,164	23.9	2,757	56.5	4,037	82.8
COMMUNITY HOSPITALS	4,275	1,663	38.9	3,254	76.1	849	19.9	88	2.1	2,833	66.3	738	17.3	802	18.8	3,733	87.3	940	22.0	2,652	62.0	3,867	90.5
CENSUS DIVISION 1, NEW ENGLAND	214	79	36.9	179	83.6	63	29.4	10	4.7	173	80.8	65	30.4	64	29.9	178	83.2	60	28.0	143	66.8	171	79.9
Connecticut	33	16	48.5	29	87.9	14	42.4	1	3.0	30	90.9	13	39.4	17	51.5	27	81.8	16	48.5	27	81.8	27	81.8
Maine	39	10	25.6	32	82.1	8	20.5	1	2.6	29	74.4	8	20.5	3	7.7	35	89.7	4	10.3	24	61.5	35	89.7
Massachusetts	83	32	38.6	71	85.5	22	26.5	5	6.0	64	77.1	27	32.5	30	36.1	67	80.7	21	25.3	54	65.1	63	75.9
New Hampshire	30	13	43.3	25	83.3	13	43.3	2	6.7	27	90.0	9	30.0	8	26.7	26	86.7	12	40.0	18	60.0	26	86.7
Rhode Island	15	6	40.0	12	80.0	2	13.3	1	6.7	11	73.3	3	20.0	3	20.0	11	73.3	5	33.3	10	66.7	8	53.3
Vermont	14	2	14.3	10	71.4	4	28.6	0	0.0	12	85.7	5	35.7	3	21.4	12	85.7	2	14.3	10	71.4	12	85.7
CENSUS DIVISION 2, MIDDLE ATLANTIC	455	193	42.4	393	86.4	151	33.2	17	3.7	364	80.0	126	27.7	154	33.8	385	84.6	204	44.8	329	72.3	377	82.9
New Jersey	78	44	56.4	70	89.7	37	47.4	5	6.4	67	85.9	26	33.3	38	48.7	67	85.9	37	47.4	62	79.5	66	84.6
New York	184	58	31.5	157	85.3	57	31.0	6	3.3	145	78.8	51	27.7	71	38.6	156	84.8	93	50.5	126	68.5	149	81.0
Pennsylvania	193	91	47.2	166	86.0	57	29.5	6	3.1	152	78.8	49	25.4	45	23.3	162	83.9	74	38.3	141	73.1	162	83.9
CENSUS DIVISION 3, SOUTH ATLANTIC	681	313	46.0	539	79.1	136	20.0	14	2.1	473	69.5	118	17.3	151	22.2	577	84.7	191	28.0	452	66.4	568	83.4
Delaware	8	6	75.0	7	87.5	4	50.0	0	0.0	7	87.5	4	50.0	3	37.5	7	87.5	3	37.5	5	62.5	7	87.5
District of Columbia	10	9	90.0	10	100.0	3	30.0	2	20.0	8	80.0	5	50.0	6	60.0	9	90.0	5	50.0	8	80.0	9	90.0
Florida	146	87	59.6	130	89.0	23	15.8	0	0.0	93	63.7	22	15.1	27	18.5	125	85.6	32	21.9	106	72.6	128	87.7
Georgia	133	44	33.1	99	74.4	16	12.0	4	3.0	83	62.4	16	12.0	25	18.8	112	84.2	33	24.8	75	56.4	108	81.2
Maryland	59	35	59.3	48	81.4	15	25.4	2	3.4	48	81.4	17	28.8	23	39.0	44	74.6	17	28.8	38	64.4	43	72.9
North Carolina	109	46	42.2	88	80.7	19	17.4	3	2.8	74	67.9	20	18.3	23	21.1	93	85.3	39	35.8	74	67.9	90	82.6
South Carolina	68	30	44.1	37	54.4	21	30.9	1	1.5	60	88.2	4	5.9	5	7.4	58	85.3	14	20.6	45	66.2	55	80.9
Virginia	84	41	48.8	74	88.1	18	21.4	2	2.4	62	73.8	20	23.8	30	35.7	74	88.1	31	36.9	60	71.4	72	85.7
West Virginia	64	15	23.4	46	71.9	17	26.6	0	0.0	38	59.4	10	15.6	9	14.1	55	85.9	17	26.6	41	64.1	56	87.5
CENSUS DIVISION 4, EAST NORTH CENTRAL	687	279	40.6	536	78.0	156	22.7	22	3.2	476	69.3	175	25.5	174	25.3	601	87.5	178	25.9	458	66.7	595	86.6
Illinois	169	79	46.7	141	83.4	46	27.2	9	5.3	126	74.6	37	21.9	55	32.5	155	91.7	49	29.0	121	71.6	147	87.0
Indiana	103	38	36.9	80	77.7	21	20.4	2	1.9	76	73.8	20	19.4	17	16.5	88	85.4	28	27.2	68	66.0	80	77.7
Michigan	142	55	38.7	106	74.6	32	22.5	3	2.1	102	71.8	42	29.6	37	26.1	123	86.6	41	28.9	99	69.7	126	88.7
Ohio	149	69	46.3	123	82.6	32	21.5	5	3.4	112	75.2	46	30.9	35	23.5	131	87.9	43	28.9	105	70.5	131	87.9
Wisconsin	124	38	30.6	86	69.4	25	20.2	3	2.4	60	48.4	30	24.2	30	24.2	104	83.9	17	13.7	65	52.4	111	89.5
CENSUS DIVISION 5, EAST SOUTH CENTRAL	447	148	33.1	296	66.2	45	10.1	3	0.7	236	52.8	32	7.2	52	11.6	353	79.0	96	21.5	250	55.9	353	79.0
Alabama	110	43	39.1	64	58.2	7	6.4	0	0.0	48	43.6	3	2.7	7	6.4	74	67.3	14	12.7	73	66.4	76	69.1
Kentucky	98	40	40.8	75	76.5	16	16.3	1	1.0	57	58.2	16	16.3	15	15.3	88	89.8	23	23.5	52	53.1	86	87.8
Mississippi	104	24	23.1	56	53.8	8	7.7	1	1.0	60	57.7	5	4.8	10	9.6	83	79.8	35	33.7	52	50.0	85	81.7
Tennessee	135	41	30.4	101	74.8	14	10.4	1	0.7	71	52.6	8	5.9	20	14.8	108	80.0	24	17.8	73	54.1	106	78.5
CENSUS DIVISION 6, WEST NORTH CENTRAL	680	144	21.2	392	57.6	89	13.1	17	2.5	396	58.2	102	15.0	118	17.4	498	73.2	133	19.6	261	38.4	606	89.1
Iowa	124	22	17.7	85	68.5	25	20.2	4	3.2	83	66.9	26	21.0	22	17.7	105	84.7	28	22.6	51	41.1	118	95.2
Kansas	142	21	14.8	69	48.6	10	7.0	1	0.7	47	33.1	7	4.9	11	7.7	92	64.8	16	11.3	47	33.1	127	89.4
Minnesota	109	17	15.6	55	50.5	11	10.1	2	1.8	80	73.4	19	17.4	15	13.8	82	75.2	16	14.7	40	36.7	90	82.6
Missouri	141	58	41.1	108	76.6	16	11.3	5	3.5	86	61.0	28	19.9	46	32.6	117	83.0	50	35.5	77	54.6	122	86.5
Nebraska	72	13	18.1	33	45.8	11	15.3	2	2.8	43	59.7	9	12.5	13	18.1	48	66.7	13	18.1	18	25.0	62	86.1
North Dakota	36	6	16.7	14	38.9	7	19.4	1	2.8	22	61.1	7	19.4	6	16.7	23	63.9	2	5.6	13	36.1	34	94.4
South Dakota	56	7	12.5	28	50.0	9	16.1	2	3.6	35	62.5	6	10.7	5	8.9	31	55.4	8	14.3	15	26.8	53	94.6
CENSUS DIVISION 7, WEST SOUTH CENTRAL	798	250	31.3	593	74.3	99	12.4	9	1.1	373	46.7	48	6.0	78	9.8	568	71.2	149	18.7	372	46.6	612	76.7
Arkansas	102	35	34.3	85	83.3	6	5.9	1	1.0	57	55.9	8	7.8	11	10.8	82	80.4	17	16.7	57	55.9	83	81.4
Louisiana	142	45	31.7	108	76.1	25	17.6	1	0.7	59	41.5	13	9.2	13	9.2	96	67.6	25	17.6	58	40.8	94	66.2
Oklahoma	87	27	31.0	63	72.4	9	10.3	2	2.3	46	52.9	5	5.7	13	14.9	68	78.2	22	25.3	42	48.3	74	85.1
Texas	467	143	30.6	337	72.2	59	12.6	5	1.1	211	45.2	22	4.7	41	8.8	322	69.0	85	18.2	215	46.0	361	77.3
CENSUS DIVISION 8, MOUNTAIN	339	104	30.7	236	69.6	60	17.7	5	1.5	204	60.2	53	15.6	60	17.7	266	78.5	65	19.2	162	47.8	290	85.5
Arizona	58	32	55.2	50	86.2	14	24.1	2	3.4	35	60.3	11	19.0	13	22.4	47	81.0	14	24.1	31	53.4	51	87.9
Colorado	59	23	39.0	46	78.0	6	10.2	1	1.7	42	71.2	24	40.7	13	22.0	52	88.1	13	22.0	31	52.5	49	83.1
Idaho	38	4	10.5	20	52.6	6	15.8	1	2.6	25	65.8	3	7.9	4	10.5	30	78.9	8	21.1	13	34.2	28	73.7
Montana	55	9	16.4	24	43.6	12	21.8	0	0.0	30	54.5	6	10.9	8	14.5	33	60.0	5	9.1	23	41.8	52	94.5
Nevada	26	10	38.5	20	76.9	6	23.1	0	0.0	14	53.8	1	3.8	0	0.0	21	80.8	5	19.2	15	57.7	21	80.8
New Mexico	38	8	21.1	28	73.7	8	21.1	0	0.0	22	57.9	2	5.3	8	21.1	28	73.7	9	23.7	16	42.1	31	81.6
Utah	38	15	39.5	30	78.9	7	18.4	1	2.6	23	60.5	3	7.9	12	31.6	33	86.8	9	23.7	18	47.4	33	86.8
Wyoming	27	3	11.1	18	66.7	1	3.7	0	0.0	13	48.1	3	11.1	2	7.4	22	81.5	2	7.4	15	55.6	25	92.6
CENSUS DIVISION 9, PACIFIC	575	218	37.9	430	74.8	96	16.7	11	1.9	352	61.2	78	13.6	97	16.9	463	80.5	88	15.3	330	57.4	465	80.9
Alaska	18	2	11.1	12	66.7	3	16.7	1	5.6	10	55.6	2	11.1	1	5.6	13	72.2	5	27.8	5	27.8	15	83.3
California	392	158	40.3	313	79.8	61	15.6	8	2.0	243	62.0	47	12.0	63	16.1	310	79.1	63	16.1	230	58.7	299	76.3
Hawaii	25	8	32.0	15	60.0	5	20.0	0	0.0	8	32.0	3	12.0	4	16.0	14	56.0	4	16.0	13	52.0	18	72.0
Oregon	58	17	29.3	34	58.6	13	22.4	1	1.7	39	67.2	12	20.7	9	15.5	57	98.3	7	12.1	37	63.8	58	100.0
Washington	82	33	40.2	56	68.3	14	17.1	1	1.2	52	63.4	14	17.1	18	22.0	69	84.1	9	11.0	45	54.9	75	91.5

Table 7 (Continued)

These data include only hospital-based facilities and services as reported by responding hospitals in Section C of the 2002 AHA Annual Survey, beginning on page 197. All hospitals are represented with Community Hospitals listed separately under United States. No estimates have been made for nonresponding hospitals. Definitions of facilities and services are listed in the Glossary, page 187.

CLASSIFICATION	HOSPITALS REPORTING	ENABLING SERVICES Number	Percent	ENROLLMENT ASSISTANCE SERVICES Number	Percent	EXTRACORPOREAL SHOCK WAVE LITHOTRIPTER (ESWL) Number	Percent	FITNESS CENTER Number	Percent	GERIATRIC SERVICES Number	Percent	HEALTH FAIR Number	Percent	HEALTH INFORMATION CENTER Number	Percent	HEALTH SCREENINGS Number	Percent
UNITED STATES	4,876	853	17.5	1,507	30.9	945	19.4	1,278	26.2	2,035	41.7	3,425	70.2	2,146	44.0	3,459	70.9
COMMUNITY HOSPITALS	4,275	788	18.4	1,371	32.1	914	21.4	1,185	27.7	1,815	42.5	3,245	75.9	1,989	46.5	3,241	75.8
CENSUS DIVISION 1, NEW ENGLAND	214	53	24.8	97	45.3	75	35.0	46	21.5	115	53.7	161	75.2	136	63.6	182	85.0
Connecticut	33	10	30.3	16	48.5	17	51.5	11	33.3	22	66.7	28	84.8	25	75.8	27	81.8
Maine	39	3	7.7	12	30.8	11	28.2	10	25.6	18	46.2	25	64.1	18	46.2	35	89.7
Massachusetts	83	22	26.5	39	47.0	22	26.5	7	8.4	40	48.2	58	69.9	51	61.4	68	81.9
New Hampshire	30	11	36.7	20	66.7	13	43.3	13	43.3	17	56.7	27	90.0	21	70.0	26	86.7
Rhode Island	15	3	20.0	5	33.3	9	60.0	1	6.7	11	73.3	12	80.0	11	73.3	13	86.7
Vermont	14	4	28.6	5	35.7	3	21.4	4	28.6	7	50.0	11	78.6	10	71.4	13	92.9
CENSUS DIVISION 2, MIDDLE ATLANTIC	455	108	23.7	200	44.0	114	25.1	123	27.0	262	57.6	356	78.2	256	56.7	382	84.0
New Jersey	78	23	29.5	35	44.9	12	15.4	26	33.3	52	66.7	68	87.2	51	65.4	70	89.7
New York	184	32	17.4	83	45.1	48	26.1	39	21.2	108	58.7	143	77.7	104	56.5	153	83.2
Pennsylvania	193	53	27.5	82	42.5	54	28.0	58	30.1	102	52.8	145	75.1	103	53.4	159	82.4
CENSUS DIVISION 3, SOUTH ATLANTIC	681	146	21.4	217	31.9	173	25.4	190	27.9	293	43.0	525	77.1	330	48.5	540	79.3
Delaware	8	5	62.5	5	62.5	3	37.5	4	50.0	3	37.5	7	87.5	5	62.5	6	75.0
District of Columbia	10	6	60.0	7	70.0	2	20.0	4	40.0	7	70.0	9	90.0	9	90.0	9	90.0
Florida	146	32	21.9	40	27.4	44	30.1	50	34.2	73	50.0	103	70.5	67	45.9	110	75.3
Georgia	133	30	22.6	42	31.6	30	22.6	31	23.3	39	29.3	94	70.7	54	40.6	101	75.9
Maryland	59	19	32.2	24	40.7	15	25.4	13	22.0	33	55.9	48	81.4	42	71.2	45	76.3
North Carolina	109	21	19.3	37	33.9	17	15.6	32	29.4	48	44.0	83	76.1	54	49.5	90	82.6
South Carolina	68	0	0.0	1	1.5	16	23.5	20	29.4	30	44.1	60	88.2	24	35.3	55	80.9
Virginia	84	26	31.0	41	48.8	29	34.5	18	21.4	37	44.0	67	79.8	47	56.0	72	85.7
West Virginia	64	7	10.9	20	31.3	17	26.6	18	28.1	23	35.9	54	84.4	28	43.8	52	81.3
CENSUS DIVISION 4, EAST NORTH CENTRAL	687	176	25.6	250	36.4	131	19.1	236	34.4	378	55.0	518	75.4	424	61.7	550	80.1
Illinois	169	40	23.7	60	35.5	27	16.0	51	30.2	83	49.1	141	83.4	95	56.2	144	85.2
Indiana	103	16	15.5	31	30.1	27	26.2	30	29.1	40	38.8	84	81.6	54	52.4	87	84.5
Michigan	142	44	31.0	62	43.7	24	16.9	53	37.3	73	51.4	109	76.8	78	54.9	120	84.5
Ohio	149	45	30.2	63	42.3	30	20.1	54	36.2	73	49.0	125	83.9	79	53.0	129	86.6
Wisconsin	124	31	25.0	34	27.4	23	18.5	48	38.7	109	87.9	59	47.6	118	95.2	70	56.5
CENSUS DIVISION 5, EAST SOUTH CENTRAL	447	45	10.1	102	22.8	81	18.1	99	22.1	146	32.7	269	60.2	121	27.1	216	48.3
Alabama	110	9	8.2	21	19.1	13	11.8	22	20.0	28	25.5	65	59.1	30	27.3	53	48.2
Kentucky	98	15	15.3	34	34.7	20	20.4	21	21.4	42	42.9	75	76.5	44	44.9	72	73.5
Mississippi	104	3	2.9	14	13.5	20	19.2	28	26.9	24	23.1	35	33.7	15	14.4	5	4.8
Tennessee	135	18	13.3	33	24.4	28	20.7	28	20.7	52	38.5	94	69.6	32	23.7	86	63.7
CENSUS DIVISION 6, WEST NORTH CENTRAL	680	121	17.8	159	23.4	77	11.3	229	33.7	253	37.2	476	70.0	257	37.8	498	73.2
Iowa	124	24	19.4	39	31.5	12	9.7	48	38.7	50	39.5	96	77.4	61	49.2	113	91.1
Kansas	142	16	11.3	18	12.7	17	12.0	42	29.6	39	35.2	87	61.3	31	21.8	70	49.3
Minnesota	109	10	9.2	20	18.3	12	11.0	30	27.5	39	35.8	65	59.6	36	33.0	71	65.1
Missouri	141	53	37.6	54	38.3	22	15.6	50	35.5	61	43.3	110	78.0	76	53.9	117	83.0
Nebraska	72	8	11.1	8	11.1	6	8.3	27	37.5	16	22.2	53	73.6	20	27.8	48	66.7
North Dakota	36	6	16.7	8	22.2	5	13.9	12	33.3	17	47.2	26	72.2	16	44.4	31	86.1
South Dakota	56	4	7.1	12	21.4	3	5.4	20	35.7	21	37.5	39	69.6	17	30.4	48	85.7
CENSUS DIVISION 7, WEST SOUTH CENTRAL	798	82	10.3	209	26.2	132	16.5	176	22.1	274	34.3	516	64.7	251	31.5	496	62.2
Arkansas	102	5	4.9	28	27.5	17	16.7	19	18.6	36	35.3	77	75.5	32	31.4	78	76.5
Louisiana	142	9	6.3	39	27.5	15	10.6	33	23.2	52	36.6	80	56.3	43	30.3	77	54.2
Oklahoma	87	5	5.7	16	18.4	15	17.2	15	17.2	33	37.9	59	67.8	29	33.3	54	62.1
Texas	467	63	13.5	126	27.0	85	18.2	109	23.3	153	32.8	300	64.2	147	31.5	287	61.5
CENSUS DIVISION 8, MOUNTAIN	339	44	13.0	98	28.9	52	15.3	79	23.3	122	36.0	241	71.1	132	38.9	228	67.3
Arizona	58	10	17.2	22	37.9	10	17.2	15	25.9	22	37.9	39	67.2	26	44.8	38	65.5
Colorado	59	10	16.9	22	37.3	12	20.3	22	37.3	23	39.0	38	64.4	30	50.8	38	64.4
Idaho	38	6	15.8	9	23.7	6	15.8	5	13.2	10	26.3	28	73.7	14	36.8	24	63.2
Montana	55	4	7.3	17	30.9	6	10.9	12	21.8	25	45.5	43	78.2	15	27.3	44	80.0
Nevada	26	2	7.7	5	19.2	3	11.5	1	3.8	8	30.8	18	69.2	11	42.3	17	65.4
New Mexico	38	3	7.9	11	28.9	7	18.4	6	15.8	8	21.1	19	50.0	9	23.7	22	57.9
Utah	38	9	23.7	9	23.7	4	10.5	13	34.2	17	44.7	34	89.5	21	55.3	27	71.1
Wyoming	27	0	0.0	3	11.1	4	14.8	5	18.5	9	33.3	22	81.5	6	22.2	18	66.7
CENSUS DIVISION 9, PACIFIC	575	78	13.6	175	30.4	110	19.1	100	17.4	192	33.4	363	63.1	237	41.2	367	63.8
Alaska	18	0	0.0	5	27.8	2	11.1	4	22.2	2	11.1	13	72.2	3	16.7	11	61.1
California	392	45	11.5	112	28.6	77	19.6	55	14.0	130	33.2	240	61.2	156	39.8	235	59.9
Hawaii	25	3	12.0	5	20.0	3	12.0	4	16.0	8	32.0	10	40.0	7	28.0	10	40.0
Oregon	58	15	25.9	25	43.1	9	15.5	19	32.8	24	41.4	44	75.9	31	53.4	50	86.2
Washington	82	15	18.3	28	34.1	19	23.2	18	22.0	28	34.1	56	68.3	40	48.8	61	74.4

Table 7 (Continued)

These data include only hospital-based facilities and services as reported by responding hospitals in Section C of the 2002 AHA Annual Survey, beginning on page 197. All hospitals are represented with Community Hospitals listed separately under United States. No estimates have been made for nonresponding hospitals. Definitions of facilities and services are listed in the Glossary, page 187.

CLASSIFICATION	HOSPITALS REPORTING	HEMODIALYSIS		HIV/AIDS SERVICES		HOME HEALTH SERVICES		HOSPICE		MAGNETIC RESONANCE IMAGING (MRI)		MEALS ON WHEELS		NUTRITION PROGRAMS CENTER		OCCUPATIONAL HEALTH SERVICES	
		Number	Percent	Number	Percent	Number	Percent	Number	Percent	Number	Percent	Number	Percent	Number	Percent	Number	Percent
UNITED STATES	4,876	1,292	26.5	1,398	28.7	1,924	39.5	1,134	23.3	2,541	52.1	650	13.3	3,347	68.6	3,035	62.2
COMMUNITY HOSPITALS	4,275	1,210	28.3	1,258	29.4	1,831	42.8	1,057	24.7	2,452	57.4	639	14.9	3,045	71.2	2,821	66.0
CENSUS DIVISION 1. NEW ENGLAND	214	67	31.3	103	48.1	61	28.5	61	28.5	112	52.3	25	11.7	183	85.5	163	76.2
Connecticut	33	15	45.5	23	69.7	8	24.2	17	51.5	25	75.8	8	24.2	30	90.9	23	69.7
Maine	39	6	15.4	12	30.8	14	35.9	6	15.4	11	28.2	5	12.8	31	79.5	30	76.9
Massachusetts	83	28	33.7	41	49.4	25	30.1	20	24.1	43	51.8	9	10.8	72	86.7	61	73.5
New Hampshire	30	7	23.3	15	50.0	7	23.3	9	30.0	15	50.0	1	3.3	28	93.3	28	93.3
Rhode Island	15	9	60.0	6	40.0	6	40.0	4	26.7	9	60.0	1	6.7	11	73.3	9	60.0
Vermont	14	2	14.3	6	42.9	1	7.1	5	35.7	9	64.3	1	7.1	11	78.6	12	85.7
CENSUS DIVISION 2. MIDDLE ATLANTIC	455	176	38.7	210	46.2	162	35.6	116	25.5	252	55.4	60	13.2	378	83.1	331	72.7
New Jersey	78	36	46.2	47	60.3	25	32.1	20	25.6	44	56.4	18	23.1	69	88.5	55	70.5
New York	184	92	50.0	85	46.2	49	26.6	37	20.1	107	58.2	25	13.6	148	80.4	134	72.8
Pennsylvania	193	48	24.9	78	40.4	88	45.6	59	30.6	101	52.3	17	8.8	161	83.4	142	73.6
CENSUS DIVISION 3. SOUTH ATLANTIC	681	249	36.6	257	37.7	233	34.2	135	19.8	404	59.3	46	6.8	487	71.5	444	65.2
Delaware	8	6	75.0	6	75.0	5	62.5	0	0.0	6	75.0	0	0.0	7	87.5	5	62.5
District of Columbia	10	8	80.0	8	80.0	3	30.0	2	20.0	9	90.0	1	10.0	9	90.0	10	100.0
Florida	146	66	45.2	57	39.0	51	34.9	24	16.4	103	70.5	6	4.1	108	74.0	97	66.4
Georgia	133	37	27.8	35	26.3	29	21.8	25	18.8	62	46.6	4	3.0	88	66.2	85	63.9
Maryland	59	30	50.8	23	39.0	13	22.0	10	16.9	32	54.2	5	8.5	46	78.0	40	67.8
North Carolina	109	33	30.3	29	26.6	45	41.3	24	22.0	64	58.7	10	9.2	75	68.8	74	67.9
South Carolina	68	24	35.3	45	66.2	14	20.6	10	14.7	33	48.5	6	8.8	39	57.4	37	54.4
Virginia	84	33	39.3	39	46.4	41	48.8	30	35.7	62	73.8	10	11.9	70	83.3	60	71.4
West Virginia	64	12	18.8	15	23.4	32	50.0	10	15.6	33	51.6	4	6.3	45	70.3	36	56.3
CENSUS DIVISION 4. EAST NORTH CENTRAL	687	203	29.5	199	29.0	303	44.1	216	31.4	396	57.6	180	26.2	568	82.7	505	73.5
Illinois	169	55	32.5	66	39.1	78	46.2	58	34.3	100	59.2	48	28.4	139	82.2	115	68.0
Indiana	103	21	20.4	23	22.3	59	57.3	37	35.9	71	68.9	32	31.1	80	77.7	75	72.8
Michigan	142	44	31.0	52	36.6	65	45.8	52	36.6	69	48.6	19	13.4	121	85.2	114	80.3
Ohio	149	51	34.2	48	32.2	72	48.3	45	30.2	102	68.5	37	24.8	122	81.9	112	75.2
Wisconsin	124	32	25.8	10	8.1	29	23.4	24	19.4	54	43.5	44	35.5	106	85.5	89	71.8
CENSUS DIVISION 5. EAST SOUTH CENTRAL	447	78	17.4	96	21.5	152	34.0	63	14.1	219	49.0	14	3.1	238	53.2	226	50.6
Alabama	110	24	21.8	17	15.5	42	38.2	17	15.5	65	59.1	6	5.5	45	40.9	56	50.9
Kentucky	98	20	20.4	23	23.5	44	44.9	19	19.4	36	36.7	6	6.1	66	67.3	56	57.1
Mississippi	104	2	1.9	28	26.9	23	22.1	5	4.8	40	38.5	1	1.0	42	40.4	31	29.8
Tennessee	135	32	23.7	28	20.7	43	31.9	22	16.3	78	57.8	1	0.7	85	63.0	83	61.5
CENSUS DIVISION 6. WEST NORTH CENTRAL	680	121	17.8	155	22.8	365	53.7	223	32.8	282	41.5	197	29.0	463	68.1	432	63.5
Iowa	124	28	22.6	33	26.6	74	59.7	58	46.8	58	46.8	56	45.2	102	82.3	94	75.8
Kansas	142	9	6.3	21	14.8	65	45.8	24	16.9	46	32.4	43	30.3	73	51.4	64	45.1
Minnesota	109	18	16.5	18	16.5	69	63.3	51	46.8	46	42.2	38	34.9	72	66.1	80	73.4
Missouri	141	36	25.5	59	41.8	65	46.1	32	22.7	83	58.9	26	18.4	114	80.9	99	70.2
Nebraska	72	12	16.7	9	12.5	41	56.9	24	33.3	23	31.9	13	18.1	47	65.3	40	55.6
North Dakota	36	7	19.4	6	16.7	19	52.8	13	36.1	11	30.6	7	19.4	26	72.2	23	63.9
South Dakota	56	11	19.6	9	16.1	32	57.1	21	37.5	15	26.8	14	25.0	29	51.8	32	57.1
CENSUS DIVISION 7. WEST SOUTH CENTRAL	798	157	19.7	140	17.5	288	36.1	105	13.2	366	46.1	48	6.0	456	57.1	387	48.5
Arkansas	102	21	20.6	18	17.6	66	64.7	24	23.5	51	50.0	7	6.9	59	57.8	51	50.0
Louisiana	142	35	24.6	26	18.3	37	26.1	14	9.9	54	38.0	3	2.1	73	51.4	71	50.0
Oklahoma	87	14	16.1	15	17.2	51	58.6	18	20.7	38	43.7	16	18.4	48	55.2	42	48.3
Texas	467	87	18.6	81	17.3	134	28.7	49	10.5	225	48.2	22	4.7	276	59.1	223	47.8
CENSUS DIVISION 8. MOUNTAIN	339	73	21.5	70	20.6	146	43.1	92	27.1	183	54.0	34	10.0	214	63.1	191	56.3
Arizona	58	19	32.8	17	29.3	19	32.8	17	29.3	34	58.6	7	12.1	43	74.1	40	69.0
Colorado	59	17	28.8	17	28.8	29	49.2	12	20.3	39	66.1	8	13.6	46	78.0	44	74.6
Idaho	38	3	7.9	5	13.2	20	52.6	13	34.2	18	47.4	4	10.5	24	63.2	23	60.5
Montana	55	8	14.5	7	12.7	30	54.5	22	40.0	18	32.7	10	18.2	24	43.6	26	47.3
Nevada	26	6	23.1	8	30.8	7	26.9	2	7.7	18	69.2	1	3.8	16	61.5	14	53.8
New Mexico	38	7	18.4	4	10.5	11	28.9	7	18.4	16	42.1	2	5.3	19	50.0	14	36.8
Utah	38	8	21.1	8	21.1	16	42.1	9	23.7	24	63.2	1	2.6	25	65.8	15	39.5
Wyoming	27	5	18.5	4	14.8	14	51.9	10	37.0	16	59.3	1	3.7	17	63.0	15	55.6
CENSUS DIVISION 9. PACIFIC	575	168	29.2	168	29.2	214	37.2	123	21.4	325	56.5	46	8.0	360	62.6	356	61.9
Alaska	18	3	16.7	3	16.7	9	50.0	0	0.0	8	44.4	1	5.6	11	61.1	8	44.4
California	392	125	31.9	121	30.9	131	33.4	70	17.9	234	59.7	37	9.4	231	58.9	237	60.5
Hawaii	25	6	24.0	7	28.0	4	16.0	2	8.0	12	48.0	2	8.0	15	60.0	19	76.0
Oregon	58	13	22.4	14	24.1	42	72.4	29	50.0	35	60.3	2	3.4	46	79.3	39	67.2
Washington	82	21	25.6	23	28.0	28	34.1	22	26.8	36	43.9	4	4.9	57	69.5	53	64.6

Table 7 (Continued)

These data include only hospital-based facilities and services as reported by responding hospitals in Section C of the 2002 AHA Annual Survey, beginning on page 197. All hospitals are represented with Community Hospitals listed separately under United States. No estimates have been made for nonresponding hospitals. Definitions of facilities and services are listed in the Glossary; page 187.

CLASSIFICATION	HOSPITALS REPORTING	ONCOLOGY SERVICES Number	ONCOLOGY SERVICES Percent	OPEN HEART SURGERY Number	OPEN HEART SURGERY Percent	OUTPATIENT CARE CENTER (FREESTANDING) Number	OUTPATIENT CARE CENTER (FREESTANDING) Percent	OUTPATIENT CARE CENTER SERVICES (HOSPITAL BASED) Number	OUTPATIENT CARE CENTER SERVICES (HOSPITAL BASED) Percent	OUTPATIENT SURGERY Number	OUTPATIENT SURGERY Percent	PAIN MANAGEMENT PROGRAM Number	PAIN MANAGEMENT PROGRAM Percent	PALLIATIVE CARE PROGRAM Number	PALLIATIVE CARE PROGRAM Percent	PATIENT EDUCATION CENTER Number	PATIENT EDUCATION CENTER Percent	PATIENT REPRESENTATIVE SERVICES Number	PATIENT REPRESENTATIVE SERVICES Percent
UNITED STATES	4,876	2,580	52.9	987	20.2	1,263	25.7	3,452	70.8	3,953	81.1	2,256	46.3	951	19.5	2,708	55.5	2,990	61.3
COMMUNITY HOSPITALS	4,275	2,477	57.9	953	22.3	1,110	26.0	3,231	75.6	3,796	88.8	2,070	48.4	844	19.7	2,462	57.6	2,685	62.8
CENSUS DIVISION 1, NEW ENGLAND	214	170	79.4	29	13.6	69	32.2	170	79.4	180	84.1	138	64.5	73	34.1	132	61.7	153	71.5
Connecticut	33	25	75.8	7	21.2	14	42.4	27	81.8	27	81.8	25	75.8	15	45.5	26	78.8	27	81.8
Maine	39	32	82.1	2	5.1	10	25.6	30	76.9	36	92.3	20	51.3	12	30.8	20	51.3	20	51.3
Massachusetts	83	68	81.9	12	14.5	25	30.1	65	78.3	67	80.7	55	66.3	22	26.5	48	57.8	63	75.9
New Hampshire	30	24	80.0	5	16.7	11	36.7	24	80.0	26	86.7	20	66.7	12	40.0	19	63.3	24	80.0
Rhode Island	15	11	73.3	2	13.3	5	33.3	12	80.0	11	73.3	8	53.3	3	20.0	9	60.0	9	60.0
Vermont	14	10	71.4	1	7.1	4	28.6	12	85.7	13	92.9	10	71.4	9	64.3	10	71.4	10	71.4
CENSUS DIVISION 2, MIDDLE ATLANTIC	455	319	70.1	98	21.5	186	40.9	356	78.2	380	83.5	302	66.4	126	27.7	317	69.7	354	77.8
New Jersey	78	64	82.1	13	16.7	26	33.3	59	75.6	68	87.2	59	75.6	25	32.1	61	78.2	67	85.9
New York	184	125	67.9	28	15.2	98	53.3	146	79.3	147	79.9	123	66.8	50	27.2	130	70.7	149	81.0
Pennsylvania	193	130	67.4	57	29.5	62	32.1	151	78.2	165	85.5	120	62.2	51	26.4	126	65.3	138	71.5
CENSUS DIVISION 3, SOUTH ATLANTIC	681	378	55.5	142	20.9	218	32.0	508	74.6	577	84.7	349	51.2	151	22.2	445	65.3	454	66.7
Delaware	8	6	75.0	3	37.5	5	62.5	7	87.5	7	87.5	5	62.5	2	25.0	6	75.0	7	87.5
District of Columbia	10	9	90.0	7	70.0	6	60.0	10	100.0	9	90.0	10	100.0	7	70.0	10	100.0	10	100.0
Florida	146	94	64.4	47	32.2	51	34.9	113	77.4	127	87.0	84	57.5	35	24.0	80	54.8	88	60.3
Georgia	133	49	36.8	18	13.5	40	30.1	89	66.9	109	82.0	55	41.4	21	15.8	77	57.9	85	63.9
Maryland	59	41	69.5	9	15.3	21	35.6	46	78.0	45	76.3	39	66.1	18	30.5	37	62.7	46	78.0
North Carolina	109	70	64.2	21	19.3	32	29.4	77	70.6	93	85.3	56	51.4	27	24.8	66	60.6	69	63.3
South Carolina	68	22	32.4	16	23.5	22	32.4	53	77.9	58	85.3	32	47.1	0	0.0	66	97.1	43	63.2
Virginia	84	54	64.3	16	19.0	27	32.1	64	76.2	76	90.5	50	59.5	26	31.0	64	76.2	70	83.3
West Virginia	64	33	51.6	5	7.8	14	21.9	49	76.6	53	82.8	18	28.1	15	23.4	39	60.9	36	56.3
CENSUS DIVISION 4, EAST NORTH CENTRAL	687	476	69.3	163	23.7	236	34.4	574	83.6	610	88.8	404	58.8	148	21.5	483	70.3	476	69.3
Illinois	169	123	72.8	51	30.2	57	33.7	141	83.4	156	92.3	104	61.5	41	24.3	107	63.3	111	65.7
Indiana	103	68	66.0	20	19.4	33	32.0	79	76.7	89	86.4	55	53.4	22	21.4	60	58.3	62	60.2
Michigan	142	94	66.2	28	19.7	49	34.5	113	79.6	124	87.3	84	59.2	41	28.9	100	70.4	103	72.5
Ohio	149	111	74.5	40	26.8	51	34.2	122	81.9	131	87.9	82	55.0	44	29.5	100	67.1	110	73.8
Wisconsin	124	80	64.5	24	19.4	46	37.1	119	96.0	110	88.7	79	63.7	0	0.0	116	93.5	90	72.6
CENSUS DIVISION 5, EAST SOUTH CENTRAL	447	174	38.9	76	17.0	58	13.0	237	53.0	332	74.3	165	36.9	43	9.6	212	47.4	262	58.6
Alabama	110	43	39.1	21	19.1	15	13.6	59	53.6	67	60.9	34	30.9	12	10.9	44	40.0	43	39.1
Kentucky	98	46	46.9	16	16.3	17	17.3	69	70.4	85	86.7	42	42.9	13	13.3	51	52.0	63	64.3
Mississippi	104	29	27.9	16	15.4	3	2.9	32	30.8	74	71.2	42	40.4	1	1.0	54	51.9	69	66.3
Tennessee	135	56	41.5	23	17.0	23	17.0	77	57.0	106	78.5	47	34.8	17	12.6	63	46.7	87	64.4
CENSUS DIVISION 6, WEST NORTH CENTRAL	680	325	47.8	90	13.2	96	14.1	501	73.7	593	87.2	249	36.6	136	20.0	347	51.0	348	51.2
Iowa	124	77	62.1	13	10.5	11	10.5	105	84.7	116	93.5	43	34.7	21	16.9	70	56.5	60	48.4
Kansas	142	50	35.2	13	9.2	11	7.7	82	57.7	113	79.6	37	26.1	23	16.2	50	35.2	55	38.7
Minnesota	109	56	51.4	10	9.2	13	11.9	88	80.7	105	96.3	40	36.7	28	25.7	55	50.5	56	51.4
Missouri	141	72	51.1	35	24.8	39	27.7	116	82.3	118	83.7	71	50.4	40	28.4	92	65.2	111	78.7
Nebraska	72	37	51.4	9	12.5	9	12.5	53	73.6	64	88.9	26	36.1	6	8.3	32	44.4	30	41.7
North Dakota	36	15	41.7	6	16.7	3	8.3	19	52.8	32	88.9	13	36.1	11	30.6	18	50.0	19	52.8
South Dakota	56	18	32.1	4	7.1	8	14.3	38	67.9	45	80.4	19	33.9	7	12.5	30	53.6	17	30.4
CENSUS DIVISION 7, WEST SOUTH CENTRAL	798	281	35.2	179	22.4	162	20.3	501	62.8	570	71.4	261	32.7	81	10.2	344	43.1	436	54.6
Arkansas	102	42	41.2	23	22.5	17	16.7	76	74.5	80	78.4	32	31.4	8	7.8	40	39.2	52	51.0
Louisiana	142	50	35.2	34	23.9	29	20.4	69	48.6	85	59.9	39	27.5	15	10.6	64	45.1	78	54.9
Oklahoma	87	32	36.8	17	19.5	15	17.2	58	66.7	73	83.9	30	34.5	13	14.9	32	36.8	40	46.0
Texas	467	157	33.6	105	22.5	101	21.6	298	63.8	332	71.1	160	34.3	45	9.6	208	44.5	266	57.0
CENSUS DIVISION 8, MOUNTAIN	339	145	42.8	57	16.8	78	23.0	217	64.0	265	78.2	147	43.4	77	22.7	157	46.3	187	55.2
Arizona	58	31	53.4	14	24.1	18	31.0	42	72.4	48	82.8	32	55.2	16	27.6	31	53.4	37	63.8
Colorado	59	36	61.0	14	23.7	21	35.6	46	78.0	52	88.1	33	55.9	15	25.4	36	61.0	45	76.3
Idaho	38	14	36.8	5	10.5	6	15.8	19	50.0	28	73.7	15	39.5	7	18.4	17	44.7	18	47.4
Montana	55	17	30.9	5	9.1	4	7.3	34	61.8	37	67.3	18	32.7	14	25.5	16	29.1	20	36.4
Nevada	26	13	50.0	7	26.9	10	38.5	17	65.4	19	73.1	12	46.2	3	11.5	10	38.5	16	61.5
New Mexico	38	12	31.6	4	10.5	5	13.2	18	47.4	29	76.3	13	34.2	11	28.9	11	28.9	17	44.7
Utah	38	13	34.2	7	18.4	11	28.9	24	63.2	30	78.9	17	44.7	8	21.1	23	60.5	21	55.3
Wyoming	27	9	33.3	2	7.4	3	11.1	17	63.0	22	81.5	7	25.9	3	11.1	13	48.1	13	48.1
CENSUS DIVISION 9, PACIFIC	575	312	54.3	153	26.6	150	26.1	388	67.5	446	77.6	241	41.9	116	20.2	271	47.1	320	55.7
Alaska	18	8	44.4	2	11.1	2	11.1	12	66.7	14	77.8	7	38.9	3	16.7	5	27.8	9	50.0
California	392	215	54.8	114	29.1	104	26.5	258	65.8	289	73.7	157	40.1	68	17.3	177	45.2	213	54.3
Hawaii	25	12	48.0	6	24.0	5	20.0	12	48.0	14	56.0	9	36.0	3	12.0	8	32.0	10	40.0
Oregon	58	31	53.4	11	19.0	17	29.3	49	84.5	56	96.6	29	50.0	18	31.0	36	62.1	37	63.8
Washington	82	46	56.1	20	24.4	22	26.8	57	69.5	73	89.0	39	47.6	24	29.3	45	54.9	51	62.2

Table 7 (Continued)

These data include only hospital-based facilities and services as reported by responding hospitals in Section C of the 2002 AHA Annual Survey, beginning on page 197. All hospitals are represented with Community Hospitals listed separately under United States. No estimates have been made for nonresponding hospitals. Definitions of facilities and services are listed in the Glossary, page 187.

CLASSIFICATION	HOSPITALS REPORTING	PHYSICAL REHABILITATION OUTPATIENT SERVICES		POSITRON EMISSION TOMOGRAPHY (PET)		PRIMARY CARE DEPARTMENT		PSYCHIATRIC CHILD/ADOLESCENT SERVICES		PSYCHIATRIC CONSULTATION/ LIAISON SERVICES		PSYCHIATRIC EDUCATION SERVICES		PSYCHIATRIC EMERGENCY SERVICES		PSYCHIATRIC GERIATRIC SERVICES	
		Number	Percent	Number	Percent	Number	Percent	Number	Percent	Number	Percent	Number	Percent	Number	Percent	Number	Percent
UNITED STATES	4,876	3,746	76.8	581	11.9	1,749	35.9	924	18.9	1,559	32.0	1,228	25.2	1,627	33.4	1,497	30.7
COMMUNITY HOSPITALS	4,275	3,554	83.1	560	13.1	1,592	37.2	688	16.1	1,261	29.5	926	21.7	1,373	32.1	1,197	28.0
CENSUS DIVISION 1, NEW ENGLAND	214	178	83.2	37	17.3	100	46.7	72	33.6	112	52.3	85	39.7	107	50.0	106	49.5
Connecticut	33	23	69.7	16	48.5	18	54.5	20	60.6	26	78.8	24	72.7	26	78.8	25	75.8
Maine	39	34	87.2	2	5.1	15	38.5	8	20.5	10	25.6	6	15.4	12	30.8	9	23.1
Massachusetts	83	70	84.3	13	15.7	33	39.8	30	36.1	43	51.8	35	42.2	39	47.0	43	51.8
New Hampshire	30	28	93.3	5	16.7	16	53.3	8	26.7	14	46.7	8	26.7	14	46.7	14	46.7
Rhode Island	15	10	66.7			9	60.0	2	13.3	11	73.3	6	40.0	11	73.3	9	60.0
Vermont	14	13	92.9	1	7.1	9	64.3	4	28.6	8	57.1	6	42.9	5	35.7	6	42.9
CENSUS DIVISION 2, MIDDLE ATLANTIC	455	380	83.5	82	18.0	240	52.7	156	34.3	249	54.7	187	41.1	237	52.1	222	48.8
New Jersey	78	69	88.5	14	17.9	47	60.3	31	39.7	48	61.5	36	46.2	46	59.0	38	48.7
New York	184	151	82.1	31	16.8	121	65.8	71	38.6	105	57.1	77	41.8	102	55.4	88	47.8
Pennsylvania	193	160	82.9	37	19.2	72	37.3	54	28.0	96	49.7	74	38.3	89	46.1	96	49.7
CENSUS DIVISION 3, SOUTH ATLANTIC	681	546	80.2	122	17.9	233	34.2	138	20.3	249	36.6	202	29.7	263	38.6	224	32.9
Delaware	8	7	87.5	0	0.0	5	62.5	4	50.0	5	62.5	2	25.0	6	75.0	5	62.5
District of Columbia	10	10	100.0	6	60.0	8	80.0	5	50.0	9	90.0	6	60.0	9	90.0	7	70.0
Florida	146	123	84.2	36	24.7	55	37.7	23	15.8	41	28.1	33	22.6	46	31.5	41	28.1
Georgia	133	99	74.4	21	15.8	35	26.3	18	13.5	34	25.6	31	23.3	36	27.1	29	21.8
Maryland	59	45	76.3	14	23.7	23	39.0	25	42.4	40	67.8	28	47.5	38	64.4	28	47.5
North Carolina	109	92	84.4	9	8.3	35	32.1	25	22.9	41	37.6	38	34.9	46	42.2	46	42.2
South Carolina	68	46	67.6	5	7.4	13	19.1	15	22.1	25	36.8	20	29.4	24	35.3	19	27.9
Virginia	84	75	89.3	18	21.4	31	36.9	15	17.9	35	41.7	26	31.0	40	47.6	30	35.7
West Virginia	64	49	76.6	13	20.3	28	43.8	8	12.5	19	29.7	18	28.1	18	28.1	19	29.7
CENSUS DIVISION 4, EAST NORTH CENTRAL	687	598	87.0	100	14.6	328	47.7	165	24.0	273	39.7	226	32.9	297	43.2	249	36.2
Illinois	169	157	92.9	36	21.3	74	43.8	48	28.4	75	44.4	59	34.9	78	46.2	65	38.5
Indiana	103	89	86.4	19	18.4	43	41.7	20	19.4	31	30.1	26	25.2	33	32.0	28	27.2
Michigan	142	123	86.6	9	6.3	91	64.1	23	16.2	57	40.1	49	34.5	64	45.1	47	33.1
Ohio	149	126	84.6	27	18.1	68	45.6	35	23.5	63	42.3	55	36.9	72	48.3	60	40.3
Wisconsin	124	103	83.1	9	7.3	52	41.9	39	31.5	47	37.9	37	29.8	50	40.3	49	39.5
CENSUS DIVISION 5, EAST SOUTH CENTRAL	447	301	67.3	41	9.2	106	23.7	48	10.7	102	22.8	81	18.1	96	21.5	130	29.1
Alabama	110	62	56.4	9	8.2	21	19.1	8	7.3	19	17.3	16	14.5	21	19.1	23	20.9
Kentucky	98	78	79.6	12	12.2	30	30.6	10	10.2	26	26.5	20	20.4	26	26.5	24	24.5
Mississippi	104	56	53.8	8	7.7	21	20.2	13	12.5	22	21.2	19	18.3	19	18.3	39	37.5
Tennessee	135	105	77.8	12	8.9	34	25.2	17	12.6	35	25.9	26	19.3	30	22.2	44	32.6
CENSUS DIVISION 6, WEST NORTH CENTRAL	680	541	79.6	48	7.1	236	34.7	111	16.3	171	25.1	135	19.9	182	26.8	162	23.8
Iowa	124	102	82.3	10	8.1	54	43.5	32	25.8	36	29.0	33	26.6	47	37.9	30	24.2
Kansas	142	113	79.6	8	5.6	36	25.4	10	7.0	14	9.9	13	9.2	20	14.1	28	19.7
Minnesota	109	93	85.3	8	7.3	33	30.3	22	20.2	34	31.2	25	22.9	33	30.3	29	26.6
Missouri	141	112	79.4	11	7.8	57	40.4	27	19.1	62	44.0	45	31.9	55	39.0	50	35.5
Nebraska	72	51	70.8	5	6.9	19	26.4	8	11.1	12	16.7	8	11.1	12	16.7	10	13.9
North Dakota	36	29	80.6	2	5.6	17	47.2	7	19.4	6	16.7	6	16.7	7	19.4	8	22.2
South Dakota	56	41	73.2	4	7.1	20	35.7	5	8.9	7	12.5	5	8.9	8	14.3	7	12.5
CENSUS DIVISION 7, WEST SOUTH CENTRAL	798	546	68.4	54	6.8	207	25.9	88	11.0	156	19.5	133	16.7	170	21.3	205	25.7
Arkansas	102	76	74.5	3	2.9	29	28.4	13	12.7	24	23.5	17	16.7	21	20.6	35	34.3
Louisiana	142	81	57.0	9	6.3	37	26.1	16	11.3	36	25.4	31	21.8	42	29.6	55	38.7
Oklahoma	87	65	74.7	7	8.0	28	32.2	11	12.6	23	26.4	20	23.0	26	29.9	28	32.2
Texas	467	324	69.4	35	7.5	113	24.2	48	10.3	73	15.6	65	13.9	81	17.3	87	18.6
CENSUS DIVISION 8, MOUNTAIN	339	255	75.2	31	9.1	123	36.3	62	18.3	98	28.9	70	20.6	102	30.1	75	22.1
Arizona	58	48	82.8	8	13.8	21	36.2	11	19.0	21	36.2	12	20.7	17	29.3	16	27.6
Colorado	59	54	91.5	7	11.9	31	52.5	12	20.3	21	35.6	14	23.7	22	37.3	16	27.1
Idaho	38	26	68.4	2	5.3	8	21.1	5	13.2	7	18.4	6	15.8	8	21.1	6	15.8
Montana	55	37	67.3	3	5.5	23	41.8	6	10.9	9	16.4	8	14.5	14	25.5	8	14.5
Nevada	26	20	76.9	1	3.8	13	50.0	4	15.4	6	23.1	6	23.1	5	19.2	4	15.4
New Mexico	38	27	71.1	2	5.3	8	21.1	12	31.6	17	44.7	10	26.3	14	36.8	8	21.1
Utah	38	24	63.2	6	15.8	13	34.2	6	15.8	11	28.9	7	18.4	13	34.2	10	26.3
Wyoming	27	19	70.4	2	7.4	6	22.2	6	22.2	6	22.2	7	25.9	9	33.3	7	25.9
CENSUS DIVISION 9, PACIFIC	575	401	69.7	66	11.5	176	30.6	84	14.6	149	25.9	109	19.0	173	30.1	124	21.6
Alaska	18	13	72.2	0	0.0	3	16.7	4	22.2	6	33.3	2	11.1	9	50.0	2	11.1
California	392	265	67.6	45	11.5	105	26.8	56	14.3	100	25.5	75	19.1	107	27.3	92	23.5
Hawaii	25	15	60.0	1	4.0	4	16.0	5	20.0	6	24.0	5	20.0	6	24.0	5	20.0
Oregon	58	48	82.8	4	6.9	24	41.4	6	10.3	15	25.9	10	17.2	26	44.8	6	10.3
Washington	82	60	73.2	16	19.5	40	48.8	13	15.9	22	26.8	17	20.7	25	30.5	19	23.2

Table 7 (Continued)

These data include only hospital-based facilities and services as reported by responding hospitals in Section C of the 2002 AHA Annual Survey, beginning on page 197. All hospitals are represented with Community Hospitals listed separately under United States. No estimates have been made for nonresponding hospitals. Definitions of facilities and services are listed in the Glossary, page 187.

CLASSIFICATION	HOSPITALS REPORTING	PSYCHIATRIC OUTPATIENT SERVICES		PSYCHIATRIC PARTIAL HOSPITALIZATION PROGRAM		RADIATION THERAPY		REPRODUCTIVE HEALTH		RETIREMENT HOUSING		SLEEP CENTER		SINGLE PHOTON EMISSION COMPUTED TOMOGRAPHY (SPECT)		SOCIAL WORK SERVICES		SPORTS MEDICINE	
		Number	Percent	Number	Percent	Number	Percent	Number	Percent	Number	Percent	Number	Percent	Number	Percent	Number	Percent	Number	Percent
UNITED STATES	4,876	1,340	27.5	1,002	20.5	1,190	24.4	836	17.1	182	3.7	1,702	34.9	1,523	31.2	4,171	85.5	1,648	33.8
COMMUNITY HOSPITALS	4,275	1,055	24.7	791	18.5	1,155	27.0	770	18.0	179	4.2	1,631	38.2	1,470	34.4	3,682	86.1	1,617	37.8
CENSUS DIVISION 1, NEW ENGLAND	214	106	49.5	78	36.4	67	31.3	70	32.7	9	4.2	104	48.6	100	46.7	206	96.3	93	43.5
Connecticut	33	22	66.7	18	54.5	18	54.5	17	51.5	2	6.1	21	63.6	23	69.7	33	100.0	17	51.5
Maine	39	11	28.2	9	23.1	6	15.4	8	20.5	2	5.1	13	33.3	13	33.3	37	94.9	13	33.3
Massachusetts	83	43	51.8	32	38.6	30	36.1	26	31.3	1	1.2	39	47.0	36	43.4	78	94.0	39	47.0
New Hampshire	30	12	40.0	8	26.7	7	23.3	11	36.7	2	6.7	15	50.0	14	46.7	29	96.7	14	46.7
Rhode Island	15	7	46.7	5	33.3	3	20.0	3	20.0	1	6.7	10	66.7	8	53.3	15	100.0	4	26.7
Vermont	14	11	78.6	6	42.9	3	21.4	5	35.7	1	7.1	6	42.9	6	42.9	14	100.0	6	42.9
CENSUS DIVISION 2, MIDDLE ATLANTIC	455	188	41.3	130	28.6	179	39.3	144	31.6	11	2.4	196	43.1	199	43.7	438	96.3	179	39.3
New Jersey	78	34	43.6	33	42.3	37	47.4	27	34.6	2	2.6	35	44.9	46	59.0	76	97.4	31	39.7
New York	184	88	47.8	51	27.7	70	38.0	73	39.7	4	2.2	66	35.9	66	35.9	177	96.2	65	35.3
Pennsylvania	193	66	34.2	46	23.8	72	37.3	44	22.8	5	2.6	95	49.2	87	45.1	185	95.9	83	43.0
CENSUS DIVISION 3, SOUTH ATLANTIC	681	197	28.9	164	24.1	217	31.9	122	17.9	11	1.6	281	41.3	269	39.5	601	88.3	234	34.4
Delaware	8	5	62.5	4	50.0	2	25.0	2	25.0	0	0.0	5	62.5	5	62.5	7	87.5	4	50.0
District of Columbia	10	7	70.0	7	70.0	7	70.0	5	50.0	0	0.0	8	80.0	8	80.0	10	100.0	8	80.0
Florida	146	36	24.7	28	19.2	55	37.7	29	19.9	1	0.7	65	44.5	63	43.2	116	79.5	47	32.2
Georgia	133	31	23.3	25	18.8	27	20.3	15	11.3	4	3.0	60	45.1	30	22.6	109	82.0	38	28.6
Maryland	59	27	45.8	23	39.0	20	33.9	18	30.5	0	0.0	34	57.6	27	45.8	58	98.3	17	28.8
North Carolina	109	32	29.4	24	22.0	39	35.8	18	16.5	2	1.8	57	52.3	46	42.2	102	93.6	36	33.0
South Carolina	68	14	20.6	15	22.1	21	30.9	9	13.2	2	2.9	0	0.0	15	22.1	61	89.7	22	32.4
Virginia	84	31	36.9	32	38.1	34	40.5	16	19.0	1	1.2	30	35.7	46	54.8	78	92.9	36	42.9
West Virginia	64	14	21.9	6	9.4	12	18.8	10	15.6	1	1.6	22	34.4	29	45.3	60	93.8	26	40.6
CENSUS DIVISION 4, EAST NORTH CENTRAL	687	248	36.1	181	26.3	202	29.4	136	19.8	30	4.4	331	48.2	306	44.5	631	91.8	352	51.2
Illinois	169	69	40.8	63	37.3	56	33.1	36	21.3	8	4.7	87	51.5	73	43.2	155	91.7	78	46.2
Indiana	103	32	31.1	18	17.5	31	30.1	18	17.5	1	1.0	51	49.5	44	42.7	86	83.5	46	44.7
Michigan	142	46	32.4	29	20.4	41	28.9	41	28.9	6	4.2	72	50.7	64	45.1	132	93.0	71	50.0
Ohio	149	57	38.3	44	29.5	48	32.2	26	17.4	5	3.4	81	54.4	79	53.0	142	95.3	80	53.7
Wisconsin	124	44	35.5	27	21.8	26	21.0	15	12.1	10	8.1	40	32.3	46	37.1	116	93.5	77	62.1
CENSUS DIVISION 5, EAST SOUTH CENTRAL	447	87	19.5	66	14.8	79	17.7	48	10.7	8	1.8	118	26.4	107	23.9	383	85.7	136	30.4
Alabama	110	17	15.5	17	15.5	24	21.8	10	9.1	3	2.7	31	28.2	15	13.6	87	79.1	33	30.0
Kentucky	98	23	23.5	15	15.3	18	18.4	12	12.2	2	2.0	26	26.5	29	29.6	84	85.7	30	30.6
Mississippi	104	22	21.2	14	13.5	3	2.9	6	5.8	2	1.9	17	16.3	29	27.9	99	95.2	23	22.1
Tennessee	135	25	18.5	20	14.8	34	25.2	20	14.8	1	0.7	44	32.6	34	25.2	113	83.7	50	37.0
CENSUS DIVISION 6, WEST NORTH CENTRAL	680	163	24.0	102	15.0	99	14.6	90	13.2	87	12.8	234	34.4	153	22.5	544	80.0	261	38.4
Iowa	124	40	32.3	28	22.6	20	16.1	18	14.5	19	15.3	48	38.7	31	25.0	102	82.3	59	47.6
Kansas	142	14	9.9	7	4.9	12	8.5	15	10.6	15	10.6	49	34.5	21	14.8	94	66.2	34	23.9
Minnesota	109	32	29.4	16	14.7	13	11.9	13	11.9	18	16.5	30	27.5	18	16.5	94	86.2	37	33.9
Missouri	141	47	33.3	30	21.3	29	20.6	22	15.6	3	2.1	68	48.2	56	39.7	130	92.2	65	46.1
Nebraska	72	13	18.1	8	11.1	13	18.1	7	9.7	6	8.3	19	26.4	15	20.8	52	72.2	32	44.4
North Dakota	36	10	27.8	7	19.4	5	13.9	6	16.7	13	36.1	6	16.7	7	19.4	34	94.4	16	44.4
South Dakota	56	7	12.5	6	10.7	7	12.5	9	16.1	13	23.2	14	25.0	5	8.9	38	67.9	18	32.1
CENSUS DIVISION 7, WEST SOUTH CENTRAL	798	130	16.3	113	14.2	126	15.8	78	9.8	13	1.6	221	27.7	169	21.2	639	80.1	186	23.3
Arkansas	102	15	14.7	10	9.8	12	11.8	12	11.8	3	2.9	31	30.4	31	30.4	80	78.4	22	21.6
Louisiana	142	30	21.1	30	21.1	23	16.2	15	10.6	2	1.4	39	27.5	31	21.8	113	79.6	28	19.7
Oklahoma	87	20	23.0	12	13.8	20	23.0	6	6.9	2	2.3	27	31.0	23	26.4	68	78.2	25	28.7
Texas	467	65	13.9	61	13.1	71	15.2	45	9.6	6	1.3	124	26.6	96	20.6	378	80.9	111	23.8
CENSUS DIVISION 8, MOUNTAIN	339	87	25.7	50	14.7	67	19.8	51	15.0	4	1.2	98	28.9	74	21.8	270	79.6	84	24.8
Arizona	58	23	39.7	8	13.8	17	29.3	9	15.5	0	0.0	16	27.6	18	31.0	50	86.2	8	13.8
Colorado	59	17	28.8	13	22.0	15	25.4	10	16.9	2	3.4	26	44.1	21	35.6	47	79.7	24	40.7
Idaho	38	5	13.2	2	5.3	6	15.8	2	5.3	0	0.0	9	23.7	4	10.5	29	76.3	11	28.9
Montana	55	8	14.5	9	16.4	5	9.1	8	14.5	2	3.6	9	16.4	10	18.2	45	81.8	17	30.9
Nevada	26	7	26.9	3	11.5	5	19.2	4	15.4	0	0.0	5	19.2	6	23.1	20	76.9	5	19.2
New Mexico	38	14	36.8	5	13.2	6	15.8	5	13.2	0	0.0	9	23.7	4	10.5	29	76.3	4	10.5
Utah	38	6	15.8	8	21.1	8	21.1	10	26.3	0	0.0	16	42.1	6	15.8	30	78.9	10	26.3
Wyoming	27	7	25.9	2	7.4	5	18.5	3	11.1	0	0.0	8	29.6	5	18.5	20	74.1	5	18.5
CENSUS DIVISION 9, PACIFIC	575	134	23.3	118	20.5	154	26.8	97	16.9	9	1.6	119	20.7	146	25.4	459	79.8	123	21.4
Alaska	18	8	44.4	3	16.7	2	11.1	3	16.7	0	0.0	5	27.8	2	11.1	14	77.8	3	16.7
California	392	89	22.7	86	21.9	106	27.0	65	16.6	6	1.5	61	15.6	103	26.3	317	80.9	72	18.4
Hawaii	25	6	24.0	6	24.0	4	16.0	5	20.0	0	0.0	5	20.0	3	12.0	22	88.0	6	24.0
Oregon	58	9	15.5	7	12.1	15	25.9	8	13.8	3	5.2	18	31.0	23	39.7	44	75.9	15	25.9
Washington	82	22	26.8	16	19.5	27	32.9	16	19.5	0	0.0	30	36.6	15	18.3	62	75.6	27	32.9

Table 7 (Continued)

These data include only hospital-based facilities and services as reported by responding hospitals in Section C of the 2001 AHA Annual Survey, beginning on page 197. All hospitals are represented with Community Hospitals listed separately under United States. No estimates have been made for nonresponding hospitals. Definitions of facilities and services are listed in the Glossary, page 187.

CLASSIFICATION	HOSPITALS REPORTING	SUPPORT GROUPS		TEEN OUTREACH SERVICES		TOBACCO TREATMENT		TRANSPLANT SERVICES		TRANSPORTATION TO HEALTH FACILITIES		TRAUMA CENTER (CERTIFIED)		ULTRASOUND		URGENT CARE CENTER		VOLUNTEER SERVICES DEPARTMENT		WOMEN'S HEALTH SERVICES	
		Number	Percent	Number	Percent	Number	Percent	Number	Percent	Number	Percent	Number	Percent	Number	Percent	Number	Percent	Number	Percent	Number	Percent
UNITED STATES	4,876	2,959	60.7	670	13.7	1,642	33.7	409	8.4	1,356	27.8	1,436	29.5	3,842	78.8	1,151	23.6	3,643	74.7	2,104	43.2
COMMUNITY HOSPITALS	4,275	2,687	62.9	644	15.1	1,482	34.7	391	9.1	1,151	26.9	1,409	33.0	3,667	85.8	1,056	24.7	3,341	78.2	1,968	46.0
CENSUS DIVISION 1, NEW ENGLAND	214	183	85.5	61	28.5	136	63.6	22	10.3	65	30.4	66	30.8	179	83.6	90	42.1	202	94.4	135	63.1
Connecticut	33	32	97.0	17	51.5	23	69.7	5	15.2	8	24.2	15	45.5	28	84.8	21	63.6	32	97.0	23	69.7
Maine	39	32	82.1	5	12.8	31	79.5	1	2.6	7	17.9	11	28.2	33	84.6	9	23.1	34	87.2	21	53.8
Massachusetts	83	67	80.7	28	33.7	39	47.0	10	12.0	26	31.3	20	24.1	68	81.9	34	41.0	81	97.6	52	62.7
New Hampshire	30	26	86.7	7	23.3	23	76.7	3	10.0	11	36.7	15	50.0	26	86.7	13	43.3	28	93.3	22	73.3
Rhode Island	15	13	86.7	3	20.0	8	53.3	2	13.3	7	46.7	1	6.7	12	80.0	6	40.0	14	93.3	9	60.0
Vermont	14	13	92.9	1	7.1	12	85.7	1	7.1	6	42.9	4	28.6	12	85.7	7	50.0	13	92.9	8	57.1
CENSUS DIVISION 2, MIDDLE ATLANTIC	455	349	76.7	124	27.3	226	49.7	52	11.4	181	39.8	105	23.1	390	85.7	107	23.5	415	91.2	276	60.7
New Jersey	78	69	88.5	37	47.4	35	44.9	8	10.3	51	65.4	17	21.8	67	85.9	19	24.4	76	97.4	53	67.9
New York	184	133	72.3	46	25.0	88	47.8	23	12.5	67	36.4	51	27.7	159	86.4	54	29.3	167	90.8	119	64.7
Pennsylvania	193	147	76.2	41	21.2	103	53.4	21	10.9	63	32.6	37	19.2	164	85.0	34	17.6	172	89.1	104	53.9
CENSUS DIVISION 3, SOUTH ATLANTIC	681	450	66.1	96	14.1	236	34.7	112	16.4	193	28.3	150	22.0	576	84.6	164	24.1	577	84.7	356	52.3
Delaware	8	7	87.5	2	25.0	3	37.5	3	37.5	2	25.0	6	75.0	7	87.5	1	12.5	7	87.5	6	75.0
District of Columbia	10	10	100.0	4	40.0	5	50.0	6	60.0	7	70.0	5	50.0	10	100.0	4	40.0	10	100.0	9	90.0
Florida	146	100	68.5	18	12.3	44	30.1	16	11.0	43	29.5	24	16.4	127	87.0	39	26.7	124	84.9	76	52.1
Georgia	133	71	53.4	19	14.3	49	36.8	11	8.3	32	24.1	18	13.5	112	84.2	27	20.3	103	77.4	57	42.9
Maryland	59	50	84.7	13	22.0	33	55.9	4	6.8	16	27.1	16	27.1	44	74.6	15	25.4	56	94.9	33	55.9
North Carolina	109	72	66.1	16	14.7	42	38.5	7	6.4	39	35.8	21	19.3	93	85.3	31	28.4	94	86.2	48	44.0
South Carolina	68	40	58.8	9	13.2	0	0.0	52	76.5	17	25.0	22	32.4	57	83.8	13	19.1	53	77.9	47	69.1
Virginia	84	63	75.0	10	11.9	31	36.9	9	10.7	22	26.2	18	21.4	75	89.3	21	25.0	77	91.7	49	58.3
West Virginia	64	37	57.8	5	7.8	29	45.3	4	6.3	15	23.4	20	31.3	51	79.7	13	20.3	53	82.8	31	48.4
CENSUS DIVISION 4, EAST NORTH CENTRAL	687	517	75.3	114	16.6	330	48.0	53	7.7	234	34.1	229	33.3	588	85.6	256	37.3	582	84.7	351	51.1
Illinois	169	132	78.1	26	15.4	81	47.9	13	7.7	74	43.8	73	43.2	152	89.9	42	24.9	148	87.6	90	53.3
Indiana	103	78	75.7	16	15.5	64	62.1	5	4.9	27	26.2	18	17.5	88	85.4	32	31.1	92	89.3	55	53.4
Michigan	142	120	84.5	23	16.2	66	46.5	13	9.2	50	35.2	46	32.4	126	88.7	71	50.0	128	90.1	76	53.5
Ohio	149	118	79.2	30	20.1	74	49.7	16	10.7	56	37.6	39	26.2	130	87.2	43	28.9	139	93.3	79	53.0
Wisconsin	124	69	55.6	19	15.3	45	36.3	6	4.8	27	21.8	53	42.7	92	74.2	68	54.8	75	60.5	51	41.1
CENSUS DIVISION 5, EAST SOUTH CENTRAL	447	211	47.2	41	9.2	112	25.1	28	6.3	85	19.0	135	30.2	296	66.2	46	10.3	262	58.6	158	35.3
Alabama	110	43	39.1	10	9.1	15	13.6	6	5.5	19	17.3	27	24.5	87	79.1	9	8.2	82	74.5	35	31.8
Kentucky	98	58	59.2	12	12.2	48	49.0	6	6.1	17	17.3	26	26.5	87	88.8	19	19.4	75	76.5	43	43.9
Mississippi	104	41	39.4	8	7.7	12	11.5	3	2.9	24	23.1	64	61.5	13	12.5	8	7.7	4	3.8	30	28.8
Tennessee	135	69	51.1	11	8.1	37	27.4	15	11.1	25	18.5	18	13.3	109	80.7	10	7.4	101	74.8	50	37.0
CENSUS DIVISION 6, WEST NORTH CENTRAL	680	389	57.2	71	10.4	212	31.2	31	4.6	190	27.9	172	25.3	495	72.8	122	17.9	456	67.1	192	28.2
Iowa	124	89	71.8	20	16.1	49	39.5	7	5.6	36	29.0	78	62.9	104	83.9	26	21.0	93	75.0	36	29.0
Kansas	142	50	35.2	7	4.9	21	14.8	3	2.1	31	21.8	12	8.5	80	56.3	8	5.6	79	55.6	25	17.6
Minnesota	109	76	69.7	8	7.3	36	33.0	3	2.8	26	23.9	28	25.7	83	76.1	31	28.4	79	72.5	25	22.9
Missouri	141	99	70.2	22	15.6	58	41.1	9	6.4	55	39.0	32	22.7	112	79.4	36	25.5	119	84.4	60	42.6
Nebraska	72	36	50.0	7	9.7	23	31.9	4	5.6	16	22.2	12	16.7	53	73.6	9	12.5	38	52.8	16	22.2
North Dakota	36	20	55.6	5	13.9	7	19.4	2	5.6	11	30.6	2	5.6	20	55.6	2	5.6	24	66.7	16	44.4
South Dakota	56	19	33.9	2	3.6	18	32.1	3	5.4	15	27.4	8	14.3	43	76.8	8	14.3	24	42.9	14	25.0
CENSUS DIVISION 7, WEST SOUTH CENTRAL	798	374	46.9	39	4.9	143	17.9	45	5.6	170	21.3	274	34.3	568	71.2	112	14.0	491	61.5	264	33.1
Arkansas	102	57	55.9	6	5.9	25	24.5	4	3.9	25	24.5	14	13.7	81	79.4	13	12.7	65	63.7	37	36.3
Louisiana	142	52	36.6	5	3.5	26	18.3	7	4.9	30	21.1	24	16.9	100	70.4	26	18.3	75	52.8	42	29.6
Oklahoma	87	40	46.0	2	2.3	20	23.0	8	9.2	16	18.4	38	43.7	66	75.9	16	18.4	61	70.1	28	32.2
Texas	467	225	48.2	26	5.6	72	15.4	26	5.6	99	21.2	198	42.4	321	68.7	57	12.2	290	62.1	157	33.6
CENSUS DIVISION 8, MOUNTAIN	339	162	47.8	51	15.0	115	33.9	20	5.9	80	23.6	116	34.2	276	81.4	88	26.0	231	68.1	132	38.9
Arizona	58	37	63.8	8	13.8	21	36.2	5	8.6	11	19.0	17	29.3	52	89.7	17	29.3	45	77.6	26	44.8
Colorado	59	33	55.9	11	18.6	25	42.4	3	5.1	16	27.1	47	79.7	49	83.1	15	25.4	44	74.6	27	45.8
Idaho	38	17	44.7	8	21.1	12	31.6	4	10.5	9	23.7	5	13.2	30	78.9	9	23.7	25	65.8	13	34.2
Montana	55	19	34.5	8	14.5	20	36.4	1	1.8	23	41.8	14	25.5	36	65.5	10	18.2	34	61.8	15	27.3
Nevada	26	9	34.6	2	7.7	6	23.1	2	7.7	6	23.1	3	11.5	20	76.9	10	38.5	17	65.4	12	46.2
New Mexico	38	10	26.3	6	15.8	12	31.6	2	5.3	4	10.5	5	13.2	31	81.6	12	31.6	16	42.1	10	26.3
Utah	38	22	57.9	6	15.8	10	26.3	3	7.9	5	13.2	11	28.9	33	86.8	13	34.2	32	84.2	22	57.9
Wyoming	27	15	55.6	2	7.4	9	33.3	0	0.0	6	22.2	14	51.9	25	92.6	2	7.4	18	66.7	7	25.9
CENSUS DIVISION 9, PACIFIC	575	324	56.3	73	12.7	132	23.0	46	8.0	158	27.5	171	29.7	474	82.4	166	28.9	427	74.3	240	41.7
Alaska	18	10	55.6	2	11.1	6	33.3	0	0.0	3	16.7	1	5.6	17	94.4	3	16.7	9	50.0	6	33.3
California	392	206	52.6	56	14.3	64	16.3	31	7.9	123	31.4	65	16.6	317	80.9	118	30.1	291	74.2	159	40.6
Hawaii	25	13	52.0	3	12.0	4	16.0	1	4.0	4	16.3	4	16.0	14	56.0	4	16.0	17	68.0	7	28.0
Oregon	58	46	79.3	5	8.6	29	50.0	6	10.3	14	24.1	43	74.1	57	98.3	13	22.4	47	81.0	30	51.7
Washington	82	49	59.8	7	8.5	29	35.4	8	9.8	13	15.9	59	72.0	69	84.1	28	34.1	63	76.8	38	46.3

Table 8

Metropolitan Statistical Areas

According to the U.S. Office of Management and Budget, an MSA is a geographical designation that represents an integrated social and economic unit with a large population nucleus. Under these standards, an area qualifies for recognition as an MSA if there is a city within the area of at least 50,000 population or an urban area of at least 50,000 with a total metropolitan population of at least 100,000. MSAs are defined as entire counties. In addition to the county containing the main city, an MSA also includes additional counties having strong economic and social ties to the central county. Such counties must have a specified level of commuting to the central counties and must meet certain standards regarding metropolitan character, such as population density.

When an MSA encompasses two or more central cities, up to three cities may be specified in the MSA title. They will be listed in order of population size. When a single central city exists, the MSA is named for that particular city. The official MSA title will also include a list of each of the states it covers. A MSA may extend beyond a single state.

This publication includes the most current MSAs as defined by the Office of Management and Budget.

TABLE 8

U.S. CENSUS DIVISION 1, NEW ENGLAND

U.S. Community Hospitals
(Nonfederal, short-term general and other special hospitals)

2002 Utilization, Personnel and Finances

MSAs

CLASSIFICATION	Hospitals	Beds	Admissions	Inpatient Days	Adjusted Patient Days	Average Daily Census	Adjusted Average Daily Census	Average Stay (days)	Surgical Operations	NEWBORNS Bassinets	Births	OUTPATIENT VISITS Emergency	Total
UNITED STATES	4,927	820,653	34,478,280	196,690,099	322,970,965	539,685	885,994	5.7	27,576,675	59,974	3,870,191	109,951,738	556,404,212
Nonmetropolitan	2,178	171,591	5,382,463	35,210,002	72,269,855	96,579	198,275	6.5	4,598,958	13,757	531,940	23,038,926	114,101,059
Metropolitan	2,749	649,062	29,095,817	161,480,097	250,701,110	443,106	687,719	5.5	22,977,717	46,217	3,338,251	86,912,812	442,303,153
CENSUS DIVISION 1, NEW ENGLAND	203	34,324	1,580,396	9,120,976	17,060,235	24,988	46,743	5.8	1,464,040	2,635	168,792	6,233,520	36,102,917
Nonmetropolitan	77	6,638	265,073	1,561,232	3,584,185	4,274	9,821	5.9	268,679	702	29,007	1,373,491	7,634,488
Metropolitan	126	27,686	1,315,323	7,559,744	13,476,050	20,714	36,922	5.7	1,195,361	1,933	139,785	4,860,029	28,468,429
Connecticut	35	7,714	375,686	2,239,055	3,538,511	6,135	9,693	6.0	299,309	543	42,607	1,392,274	6,641,745
Nonmetropolitan	6	447	26,291	115,989	251,431	317	688	4.4	24,233	61	2,718	143,468	812,030
Metropolitan	29	7,267	349,395	2,123,066	3,287,080	5,818	9,005	6.1	275,076	482	39,889	1,248,806	5,829,715
Bridgeport	4	845	45,673	238,050	363,559	652	996	5.2	31,267	72	5,251	182,477	541,496
Danbury	2	340	19,293	85,071	154,985	233	425	4.4	17,392	36	2,723	83,484	311,307
Hartford	10	2,524	125,068	783,721	1,284,964	2,148	3,520	6.3	109,266	140	12,806	409,500	2,636,906
New Haven-Meriden	6	1,945	74,985	595,646	769,148	1,633	2,107	7.9	50,401	64	7,016	224,509	819,996
New London-Norwich	2	433	23,712	113,510	205,835	311	564	4.8	22,750	46	2,861	131,361	404,066
Stamford-Norwalk	3	740	36,641	190,302	313,116	521	858	5.2	27,946	59	6,497	116,989	728,988
Waterbury	2	440	24,023	116,766	195,473	320	535	4.9	16,054	65	2,735	100,486	386,956
Maine	37	3,694	145,917	889,005	1,644,149	2,434	4,505	6.1	157,687	325	13,072	709,091	3,731,261
Nonmetropolitan	29	2,062	68,968	451,737	958,823	1,237	2,626	6.5	88,321	219	6,320	441,115	2,385,482
Metropolitan	8	1,632	76,949	437,268	685,326	1,197	1,879	5.7	69,366	106	6,752	267,976	1,345,779
Bangor	2	417	19,381	107,891	170,501	295	467	5.6	22,542	20	1,623	69,502	448,770
Lewiston-Auburn	2	332	13,948	78,183	135,747	214	372	5.6	10,777	38	1,360	69,354	372,842
Portland	3	804	39,531	229,679	331,759	629	910	5.8	31,829	41	3,375	108,115	425,560
Portsmouth-Rochester	1	79	4,089	21,515	47,319	59	130	5.3	4,218	7	394	21,005	98,607
Massachusetts	78	16,033	765,820	4,348,099	8,437,917	11,913	23,122	5.7	691,220	1,137	80,034	2,882,602	19,024,487
Nonmetropolitan	11	1,482	73,483	378,893	857,960	1,038	2,352	5.2	58,747	169	10,435	331,708	1,663,690
Metropolitan	67	14,551	692,337	3,969,206	7,579,957	10,875	20,770	5.7	632,473	968	69,599	2,550,894	17,360,797
Barnstable-Yarmouth	1	226	15,039	66,319	143,096	182	392	4.4	20,830	10	986	79,208	391,326
Boston	36	8,283	400,762	2,348,111	4,512,121	6,433	12,362	5.9	362,954	506	40,313	1,265,323	10,728,339
Brockton	2	481	25,211	119,030	233,533	326	639	4.7	22,674	40	2,130	116,604	383,225
Fitchburg-Leominster	2	236	14,606	65,721	132,399	180	363	4.5	9,969	13	625	84,983	297,521
Lawrence	5	625	26,116	143,415	284,077	393	778	5.5	19,647	53	3,126	133,208	543,516
Lowell	2	339	16,356	71,150	193,028	195	529	4.4	20,686	39	2,761	90,043	516,404
Pittsfield	1	296	13,429	76,986	150,712	211	413	5.7	10,943	20	822	53,797	70,239
Providence-Fall River-Warwick	3	1,012	46,121	276,375	550,454	758	1,509	6.0	55,260	95	4,880	237,809	1,141,761
Springfield	9	1,770	70,385	461,238	794,566	1,263	2,178	6.6	61,741	96	7,289	272,690	1,797,861
Worcester	6	1,283	64,312	340,861	585,971	934	1,607	5.3	47,769	96	6,667	217,229	1,490,605
New Hampshire	28	2,879	117,996	646,838	1,409,067	1,770	3,861	5.5	118,609	320	13,748	550,380	3,022,907
Nonmetropolitan	18	1,505	60,575	360,602	829,192	986	2,273	6.0	56,917	161	5,460	255,166	1,715,672
Metropolitan	10	1,374	57,421	286,236	579,875	784	1,588	5.0	61,692	159	8,288	295,214	1,307,235
Lawrence	2	162	4,313	34,561	73,268	95	200	8.0	5,331	10	539	26,468	252,778
Manchester	2	456	19,460	99,577	164,447	273	451	5.1	14,470	34	2,659	73,401	300,959
Nashua	2	308	13,785	62,244	152,077	171	416	4.5	10,361	65	2,296	76,829	372,437
Portsmouth-Rochester	4	448	19,863	89,854	190,083	245	521	4.5	31,530	50	2,794	118,516	381,061
Rhode Island	11	2,428	122,741	649,451	1,206,212	1,781	3,303	5.3	142,776	176	13,328	468,530	2,211,989
Nonmetropolitan	1	148	6,217	33,868	79,977	93	219	5.4	8,701	9	640	31,451	86,578
Metropolitan	10	2,280	116,524	615,583	1,126,235	1,688	3,084	5.3	134,075	167	12,688	437,079	2,125,411
New London-Norwich	1	125	4,590	18,994	47,043	52	129	4.1	14,268	18	405	23,258	466,900
Providence-Fall River-Warwick	9	2,155	111,934	596,589	1,079,192	1,636	2,955	5.3	119,807	149	12,283	413,821	1,658,511
Vermont	14	1,576	52,236	348,528	824,379	955	2,259	6.7	54,439	134	6,003	230,643	1,470,528
Nonmetropolitan	12	994	29,539	220,143	606,802	603	1,663	7.5	31,760	83	3,434	170,583	971,036
Metropolitan	2	582	22,697	128,385	217,577	352	596	5.7	22,679	51	2,569	60,060	499,492
Burlington	2	582	22,697	128,385	217,577	352	596	5.7	22,679	51	2,569	60,060	499,492

TABLE 8

U.S. CENSUS DIVISION 1, NEW ENGLAND

U.S. Community Hospitals
(Nonfederal, short-term general and other special hospitals)

2002 Utilization, Personnel and Finances

FULL-TIME EQUIVALENT PERSONNEL					FULL-TIME EQUIV. TRAINEES			EXPENSES						
								LABOR				TOTAL		
Physicians and Dentists	Registered Nurses	Licensed Practical Nurses	Other Salaried Personnel	Total Personnel	Medical and Dental Residents	Other Trainees	Total Trainees	Payroll (in thousands)	Employee Benefits (in thousands)	Total (in thousands)	Percent of Total	Amount (in thousands)	Adjusted per Admission	Adjusted per Inpatient Day
72,823	988,139	125,865	2,882,668	4,069,495	78,715	5,463	84,178	$175,961,479	$40,049,573	$216,011,067	51.9	$416,591,059	$7,354.60	$1,289.87
8,448	145,133	36,374	479,821	669,776	1,763	161	1,924	24,016,766	5,768,570	29,785,337	53.7	55,454,326	5,047.87	767.32
64,375	843,006	89,491	2,402,847	3,399,719	76,952	5,302	82,254	151,944,713	34,281,003	186,225,730	51.6	361,136,733	7,909.61	1,440.51
8,635	50,231	3,483	169,834	232,183	6,828	606	7,434	10,636,919	2,307,696	12,944,612	52.3	24,762,701	8,126.92	1,451.49
716	9,377	805	29,015	39,913	426	1	427	1,720,320	389,131	2,109,452	55.7	3,787,607	6,217.35	1,056.76
7,919	40,854	2,678	140,819	192,270	6,402	605	7,007	8,916,599	1,918,565	10,835,160	51.7	20,975,094	8,604.12	1,556.47
825	10,749	617	34,011	46,202	1,151	79	1,230	2,423,379	548,645	2,972,022	56.7	5,243,316	8,403.50	1,481.79
58	637	55	2,208	2,958	0	0	0	156,461	40,612	197,073	56.8	347,095	6,054.65	1,380.48
767	10,112	562	31,803	43,244	1,151	79	1,230	2,266,918	508,033	2,774,949	56.7	4,896,222	8,641.15	1,489.54
104	1,081	104	3,370	4,659	105	3	108	246,179	56,845	303,025	55.0	550,959	7,834.69	1,515.46
9	522	23	1,874	2,428	55	0	55	130,879	34,580	165,458	55.4	298,787	8,514.14	1,927.84
286	3,844	190	12,947	17,267	122	23	145	843,260	174,815	1,018,074	57.5	1,769,193	8,358.03	1,376.84
116	2,486	109	5,710	8,421	652	26	678	492,554	117,751	610,305	56.1	1,087,372	10,363.23	1,413.74
49	541	62	2,192	2,844	0	0	0	148,537	34,140	182,677	58.2	313,847	7,271.88	1,524.75
127	978	21	3,618	4,744	143	2	145	260,027	56,030	316,057	56.1	563,586	9,207.11	1,799.93
76	660	53	2,092	2,881	74	25	99	145,481	33,872	179,353	57.4	312,477	7,767.66	1,598.57
529	5,478	336	15,791	22,134	242	1	243	909,268	210,174	1,119,443	53.2	2,105,062	7,640.96	1,280.34
199	2,674	231	8,425	11,529	0	1	1	426,583	97,324	523,909	55.3	947,086	6,164.48	987.76
330	2,804	105	7,366	10,605	242	0	242	482,685	112,850	595,534	51.4	1,157,977	9,502.44	1,689.67
96	959	35	1,874	2,964	27	0	27	143,596	32,797	176,393	51.8	340,254	11,045.77	1,995.61
57	487	10	1,070	1,624	16	0	16	67,468	15,784	83,252	42.3	196,704	8,124.55	1,449.05
157	1,145	60	4,016	5,378	198	0	198	243,438	56,964	300,402	54.0	556,280	9,615.40	1,676.76
20	213	0	406	639	1	0	1	28,183	7,304	35,487	54.8	64,739	7,198.87	1,368.15
6,032	24,725	1,686	87,645	120,088	4,043	507	4,550	5,323,769	1,075,878	6,399,646	49.3	12,979,805	8,484.83	1,538.27
153	2,386	163	6,615	9,317	94	0	94	459,960	95,351	555,312	56.8	977,975	6,422.34	1,139.88
5,879	22,339	1,523	81,030	110,771	3,949	507	4,456	4,863,808	980,527	5,844,334	48.7	12,001,829	8,712.83	1,583.36
30	362	15	1,422	1,829	0	0	0	88,909	24,698	113,607	44.0	258,315	7,960.65	1,805.19
5,163	14,628	897	55,083	75,771	3,362	498	3,860	3,181,922	614,202	3,796,124	46.2	8,222,723	10,220.61	1,822.36
40	534	6	1,735	2,315	0	0	0	122,784	18,600	141,384	60.6	233,119	4,715.68	998.23
18	307	36	1,080	1,441	5	0	5	67,372	12,510	79,883	58.6	136,280	4,753.58	1,029.32
40	706	69	2,094	2,909	7	0	7	139,550	25,629	165,179	57.5	287,033	5,509.90	1,010.40
6	423	46	1,488	1,963	0	0	0	86,461	14,381	100,841	53.6	188,206	4,243.94	975.02
59	360	44	1,025	1,488	62	0	62	82,540	18,076	100,616	56.7	177,577	6,754.82	1,178.26
50	1,282	99	4,317	5,748	0	0	0	273,664	65,453	339,117	61.6	550,852	5,938.27	1,000.72
309	1,991	145	7,356	9,801	273	2	275	418,838	87,175	506,012	53.1	952,304	7,055.15	1,198.52
164	1,746	166	5,430	7,506	240	7	247	401,768	99,803	501,571	50.4	995,419	8,892.52	1,698.75
210	4,411	226	13,742	18,589	328	0	328	811,810	197,214	1,009,023	55.1	1,830,377	7,164.86	1,299.00
169	2,562	156	7,791	10,678	328	0	328	453,987	102,576	556,562	55.0	1,011,336	7,376.25	1,219.66
41	1,849	70	5,951	7,911	0	0	0	357,823	94,638	452,461	55.2	819,041	6,919.98	1,412.44
0	156	3	645	804	0	0	0	37,158	7,110	44,269	55.9	79,240	8,023.48	1,081.51
7	646	23	1,894	2,570	0	0	0	122,260	42,448	164,708	56.8	289,844	8,925.68	1,762.54
18	343	25	1,483	1,869	0	0	0	85,651	18,412	104,063	59.6	174,734	5,202.13	1,148.99
16	704	19	1,929	2,668	0	0	0	112,754	26,668	139,421	50.7	275,223	6,487.91	1,447.91
493	2,943	283	11,034	14,753	721	2	723	809,548	185,852	995,399	55.6	1,791,384	7,811.21	1,485.13
0	121	9	431	561	0	0	0	31,185	4,959	36,144	47.9	75,419	5,137.17	943.01
493	2,822	274	10,603	14,192	721	2	723	778,363	180,894	959,255	55.9	1,715,965	7,994.10	1,523.63
11	79	6	357	453	0	0	0	27,714	8,523	36,236	59.9	60,487	5,320.83	1,285.78
482	2,743	268	10,246	13,739	721	2	723	750,649	172,371	923,019	55.8	1,655,478	8,143.59	1,534.00
546	1,925	335	7,611	10,417	343	17	360	359,146	89,933	449,079	55.3	812,757	6,111.46	985.90
137	997	191	3,545	4,870	4	0	4	192,143	48,309	240,452	56.1	428,697	4,552.27	706.49
409	928	144	4,066	5,547	339	17	356	167,003	41,624	208,627	54.3	384,060	9,894.12	1,765.17
409	928	144	4,066	5,547	339	17	356	167,003	41,624	208,627	54.3	384,060	9,894.12	1,765.17

MSAs

TABLE **8**

U.S. CENSUS DIVISION 2, MIDDLE ATLANTIC

U.S. Community Hospitals
(Nonfederal, short-term general and other special hospitals)

2002 Utilization, Personnel and Finances

CLASSIFICATION	Hospitals	Beds	Admissions	Inpatient Days	Adjusted Patient Days	Average Daily Census	Adjusted Average Daily Census	Average Stay (days)	Surgical Operations	NEWBORNS Bassinets	Births	OUTPATIENT VISITS Emergency	Total
UNITED STATES	4,927	820,653	34,478,280	196,690,099	322,970,965	539,685	885,994	5.7	27,576,675	59,974	3,870,191	109,951,738	556,404,212
Nonmetropolitan	2,178	171,591	5,382,463	35,210,002	72,269,855	96,579	198,275	6.5	4,598,958	13,757	531,940	23,038,926	114,101,059
Metropolitan	2,749	649,062	29,095,817	161,480,097	250,701,110	443,106	687,719	5.5	22,977,717	46,217	3,338,251	86,912,812	442,303,153
CENSUS DIVISION 2, MIDDLE ATLANTIC	493	130,198	5,356,471	34,925,191	53,868,224	95,706	147,574	6.5	4,319,935	8,084	503,700	15,474,182	95,067,572
Nonmetropolitan	81	10,548	342,970	2,440,319	5,088,422	6,687	13,933	7.1	339,662	790	28,133	1,406,282	9,331,856
Metropolitan	412	119,650	5,013,501	32,484,872	48,779,802	89,019	133,641	6.5	3,980,273	7,294	475,567	14,067,900	85,735,716
New Jersey	81	24,094	1,094,781	6,190,443	8,567,858	16,971	23,477	5.7	720,160	1,803	112,900	2,940,592	15,898,001
Metropolitan	81	24,094	1,094,781	6,190,443	8,567,858	16,971	23,477	5.7	720,160	1,803	112,900	2,940,592	15,898,001
Atlantic-Cape May	5	1,002	47,163	262,395	389,814	720	1,068	5.6	27,793	73	4,231	176,753	572,159
Bergen-Passaic	10	3,759	197,854	941,383	1,300,596	2,580	3,564	4.8	109,163	274	17,995	370,886	4,332,452
Jersey City	8	1,957	66,406	398,797	549,698	1,095	1,507	6.0	53,623	144	6,851	219,902	1,049,233
Middlesex-Somerset-Hunterdon	7	2,158	113,138	656,417	984,012	1,799	2,696	5.8	60,907	222	14,975	251,670	1,448,007
Monmouth-Ocean	10	2,901	146,657	803,285	1,073,815	2,201	2,944	5.5	99,300	241	13,629	432,430	1,851,833
Newark	23	7,744	307,639	1,994,605	2,685,332	5,468	7,359	6.5	209,425	514	32,181	797,735	3,568,910
Philadelphia	11	2,694	142,131	714,253	950,008	1,959	2,600	5.0	98,602	178	14,599	392,248	1,452,690
Trenton	6	1,456	53,826	313,003	478,384	858	1,311	5.8	43,173	103	6,406	211,334	1,393,205
Vineland-Millville-Bridgeton	1	423	19,967	106,305	156,199	291	428	5.3	18,174	54	2,033	87,634	229,512
New York	211	65,570	2,463,447	18,394,472	28,128,614	50,400	77,058	7.5	2,078,441	3,704	251,311	7,474,440	46,760,534
Nonmetropolitan	38	5,185	135,082	1,199,041	2,424,731	3,285	6,642	8.9	123,613	367	12,270	611,361	4,374,822
Metropolitan	173	60,385	2,328,365	17,195,431	25,703,883	47,115	70,416	7.4	1,954,828	3,337	239,041	6,863,079	42,385,712
Albany-Schenectady-Troy	13	2,916	109,104	750,275	1,259,520	2,057	3,451	6.9	103,507	142	9,705	371,529	2,239,862
Binghamton	2	656	28,243	162,501	374,560	446	1,026	5.8	32,840	36	2,684	86,644	1,232,284
Buffalo-Niagara Falls	14	5,127	158,182	1,207,756	1,817,246	3,309	4,980	7.6	166,344	295	16,100	466,638	2,648,216
Dutchess County	3	650	28,088	173,389	255,883	475	701	6.2	20,753	46	3,126	88,015	599,185
Elmira	2	489	14,717	130,709	230,777	358	632	8.9	11,153	20	1,428	52,530	353,375
Glens Falls	1	332	13,593	78,423	175,313	215	480	5.8	14,346	25	1,418	43,787	454,888
Jamestown	4	586	15,342	123,505	229,022	337	628	8.1	22,345	68	1,325	61,968	436,267
Nassau-Suffolk	26	8,764	387,921	2,738,491	3,822,872	7,503	10,471	7.1	342,662	581	41,645	953,954	4,630,351
New York	77	33,428	1,303,420	9,884,548	14,168,947	27,085	38,816	7.6	981,518	1,594	133,631	3,827,726	22,905,195
Newburgh	5	871	39,966	221,536	371,635	607	1,018	5.5	47,723	46	3,889	146,501	412,155
Rochester	12	3,216	105,969	798,313	1,457,587	2,187	3,991	7.5	105,408	254	11,590	418,212	4,109,720
Syracuse	9	2,160	87,117	586,098	949,153	1,606	2,601	6.7	77,576	158	9,483	232,900	1,456,423
Utica-Rome	5	1,190	36,703	339,887	591,368	930	1,621	9.3	28,653	72	3,017	112,675	907,791
Pennsylvania	201	40,534	1,798,243	10,340,276	17,171,752	28,335	47,039	5.8	1,521,334	2,577	139,489	5,059,150	32,409,037
Nonmetropolitan	43	5,363	207,888	1,241,278	2,663,691	3,402	7,291	6.0	216,049	423	15,863	794,921	4,957,034
Metropolitan	158	35,171	1,590,355	9,098,998	14,508,061	24,933	39,748	5.7	1,305,285	2,154	123,626	4,264,229	27,452,003
Allentown-Bethlehem-Easton	8	2,073	98,254	557,212	873,400	1,527	2,392	5.7	80,413	110	8,045	287,258	1,685,201
Altoona	5	508	24,473	131,251	252,917	360	693	5.4	32,078	29	2,048	73,371	713,553
Erie	7	1,152	43,023	221,454	334,799	606	917	5.1	20,591	73	3,647	137,381	445,209
Harrisburg-Lebanon-Carlisle	7	1,667	88,843	506,962	775,544	1,390	2,124	5.7	81,647	92	7,042	236,629	1,656,478
Johnstown	6	828	36,533	187,478	362,822	514	993	5.1	43,173	44	2,025	107,623	829,037
Lancaster	5	1,063	46,740	227,641	394,358	623	1,080	4.9	55,540	100	5,747	133,293	1,354,304
Philadelphia	53	13,670	639,688	3,695,613	5,529,068	10,127	15,150	5.8	457,733	919	51,706	1,646,446	9,384,057
Pittsburgh	39	8,682	393,268	2,270,073	3,673,539	6,221	10,066	5.8	342,114	439	24,847	953,706	5,931,028
Reading	3	978	40,786	250,155	424,413	686	1,163	6.1	34,712	62	3,967	118,551	1,021,518
Scranton--Wilkes-Barre--Hazleton	15	2,634	92,488	588,483	980,462	1,611	2,685	6.4	67,231	165	6,457	266,876	2,000,774
Sharon	3	559	24,153	124,667	255,083	342	699	5.2	19,618	43	1,561	82,068	622,037
State College	2	285	10,475	58,250	96,166	160	263	5.6	12,708	3	1,175	36,644	217,226
Williamsport	2	434	14,543	105,245	234,745	288	644	7.2	30,782	22	1,255	71,008	549,272
York	3	638	37,088	174,514	320,745	478	879	4.7	26,945	53	4,104	113,375	1,042,309

TABLE 8

U.S. CENSUS DIVISION 2, MIDDLE ATLANTIC

U.S. Community Hospitals
(Nonfederal, short-term general and other special hospitals)

2002 Utilization, Personnel and Finances

FULL-TIME EQUIVALENT PERSONNEL					FULL-TIME EQUIV. TRAINEES			EXPENSES						
								LABOR				TOTAL		
Physicians and Dentists	Registered Nurses	Licensed Practical Nurses	Other Salaried Personnel	Total Personnel	Medical and Dental Residents	Other Trainees	Total Trainees	Payroll (in thousands)	Employee Benefits (in thousands)	Total (in thousands)	Percent of Total	Amount (in thousands)	Adjusted per Admission	Adjusted per Inpatient Day
72,823	988,139	125,865	2,882,668	4,069,495	78,715	5,463	84,178	$175,961,479	$40,049,573	$216,011,067	51.9	$416,591,059	$7,354.60	$1,289.87
8,448	145,133	36,374	479,821	669,776	1,763	161	1,924	24,016,766	5,768,570	29,785,337	53.7	55,454,326	5,047.87	767.32
64,375	843,006	89,491	2,402,847	3,399,719	76,952	5,302	82,254	151,944,713	34,281,003	186,225,730	51.6	361,136,733	7,909.61	1,440.51
17,235	153,859	16,983	472,530	660,607	21,680	535	22,215	30,797,469	7,021,771	37,819,237	54.0	70,060,853	8,406.60	1,300.60
1,035	9,170	2,259	31,237	43,701	364	15	379	1,620,279	369,610	1,989,889	54.2	3,670,094	5,069.38	721.26
16,200	144,689	14,724	441,293	616,906	21,316	520	21,836	29,177,190	6,652,161	35,829,348	54.0	66,390,759	8,724.09	1,361.03
2,242	27,455	2,313	83,410	115,420	2,015	58	2,073	5,676,363	1,249,158	6,925,518	53.9	12,841,554	8,445.62	1,498.81
2,242	27,455	2,313	83,410	115,420	2,015	58	2,073	5,676,363	1,249,158	6,925,518	53.9	12,841,554	8,445.62	1,498.81
47	1,519	124	3,767	5,457	32	0	32	237,898	71,607	309,505	57.7	536,138	7,780.15	1,375.37
397	4,896	147	13,698	19,138	319	7	326	967,169	199,256	1,166,425	53.9	2,163,968	7,971.21	1,663.83
215	1,462	95	4,410	6,182	134	0	134	324,715	70,470	395,185	53.0	745,458	8,126.21	1,356.12
289	3,128	274	8,791	12,482	187	11	198	659,034	131,622	790,655	52.8	1,498,771	8,923.75	1,523.12
164	3,304	371	9,805	13,644	127	3	130	670,500	158,671	829,171	52.9	1,568,663	7,973.20	1,460.83
601	7,388	610	25,184	33,783	866	11	877	1,759,683	382,955	2,142,635	54.7	3,920,609	9,247.66	1,460.01
405	3,553	353	10,971	15,282	282	24	306	653,110	139,310	792,420	53.1	1,491,574	7,882.00	1,570.06
112	1,715	169	5,181	7,177	68	2	70	313,456	68,976	382,432	53.1	720,582	8,879.52	1,506.28
12	490	170	1,603	2,275	0	0	0	90,798	26,291	117,090	59.8	195,791	6,673.40	1,253.47
10,338	73,280	8,482	236,494	328,594	13,298	336	13,634	16,621,546	3,968,522	20,590,069	56.3	36,549,754	9,626.77	1,299.38
486	3,578	935	13,811	18,810	73	0	73	736,164	160,048	896,212	57.0	1,573,607	5,654.50	648.98
9,852	69,702	7,547	222,683	309,784	13,225	336	13,561	15,885,382	3,808,475	19,693,857	56.3	34,976,147	9,940.97	1,360.73
264	3,082	370	9,975	13,691	246	11	257	559,424	119,894	679,317	54.8	1,239,256	6,964.50	983.91
77	792	85	2,911	3,865	66	0	66	156,188	42,611	198,798	52.5	378,469	5,716.71	1,010.44
377	4,363	592	14,111	19,443	120	17	137	810,143	195,845	1,005,988	52.7	1,907,339	7,616.32	1,049.58
25	842	57	2,185	3,109	11	1	12	141,251	30,056	171,308	53.2	321,913	7,914.28	1,258.05
50	549	75	1,559	2,233	8	0	8	80,628	19,543	100,170	57.3	174,731	6,554.29	757.14
38	499	232	1,250	2,019	0	0	0	74,814	15,603	90,418	59.8	151,262	4,977.84	862.81
15	466	111	1,491	2,083	3	0	3	67,794	16,391	84,186	57.3	146,940	4,791.33	641.60
1,586	10,977	827	31,005	44,395	1,731	81	1,812	2,595,959	631,052	3,227,011	59.9	5,388,461	9,878.89	1,409.53
6,533	39,553	3,534	130,524	180,144	10,108	223	10,331	9,855,373	2,365,614	12,220,988	56.0	21,820,289	11,559.91	1,540.01
27	904	84	2,886	3,901	0	0	0	184,895	48,034	232,928	60.1	387,682	5,802.58	1,043.18
661	3,947	667	13,645	18,920	544	0	544	717,696	170,431	888,127	56.0	1,587,343	8,239.52	1,089.02
128	2,672	639	7,483	10,922	358	3	361	462,686	111,501	574,187	53.1	1,081,106	7,741.60	1,139.02
71	1,056	274	3,658	5,059	30	0	30	178,531	41,900	220,431	56.3	391,355	6,184.69	661.78
4,655	53,124	6,188	152,626	216,593	6,367	141	6,508	8,499,560	1,804,091	10,303,650	49.8	20,669,545	6,851.36	1,203.69
549	5,592	1,324	17,426	24,891	291	15	306	884,116	209,563	1,093,677	52.2	2,096,487	4,704.02	787.06
4,106	47,532	4,864	135,200	191,702	6,076	126	6,202	7,615,445	1,594,528	9,209,973	49.6	18,573,058	7,223.58	1,280.19
249	3,079	242	8,013	11,583	285	0	285	433,767	102,884	536,652	50.0	1,072,681	6,983.42	1,228.17
28	752	130	1,819	2,729	14	0	14	108,963	25,033	133,997	50.8	263,787	5,447.45	1,042.98
107	1,479	120	3,364	5,070	79	3	82	160,273	37,046	197,319	47.2	418,046	6,437.52	1,248.65
518	2,389	385	8,547	11,839	437	17	454	457,271	92,339	549,610	52.8	1,041,734	7,649.46	1,343.23
47	1,040	208	3,238	4,533	64	0	64	145,438	33,345	178,783	46.9	381,097	5,304.07	1,050.37
102	1,351	233	4,272	5,958	49	0	49	246,362	50,251	296,612	52.9	560,831	6,875.37	1,422.14
1,930	19,375	1,414	53,000	75,719	3,395	52	3,447	3,317,286	680,047	3,997,333	49.5	8,072,026	8,324.45	1,459.93
865	11,910	961	34,227	47,963	1,383	41	1,424	1,752,341	341,743	2,094,082	46.9	4,467,030	6,924.15	1,216.00
76	1,121	177	3,322	4,696	75	0	75	195,192	41,298	236,489	54.3	435,260	6,211.52	1,025.56
58	2,574	524	7,177	10,333	109	0	109	380,059	94,497	474,556	51.8	916,016	5,725.35	934.27
46	684	103	2,131	2,964	12	0	12	101,626	21,326	122,953	53.9	228,202	4,606.33	894.62
2	244	58	675	979	0	0	0	40,122	9,591	49,713	57.3	86,751	4,784.69	902.10
6	517	68	1,865	2,456	20	0	20	75,215	19,675	94,890	50.9	186,529	5,606.52	794.60
72	1,017	241	3,550	4,880	154	13	167	201,530	45,453	246,984	55.7	443,068	6,442.19	1,381.37

TABLE 8

U.S. CENSUS DIVISION 3, SOUTH ATLANTIC

U.S. Community Hospitals
(Nonfederal, short-term general and other special hospitals)

2002 Utilization, Personnel and Finances

CLASSIFICATION	Hospitals	Beds	Admissions	Inpatient Days	Adjusted Patient Days	Average Daily Census	Adjusted Average Daily Census	Average Stay (days)	Surgical Operations	NEWBORNS Bassinets	Births	OUTPATIENT VISITS Emergency	Total
UNITED STATES	4,927	820,653	34,478,280	196,690,099	322,970,965	539,685	885,994	5.7	27,576,675	59,974	3,870,191	109,951,738	556,404,212
Nonmetropolitan	2,178	171,591	5,382,463	35,210,002	72,269,855	96,579	198,275	6.5	4,598,958	13,757	531,940	23,038,926	114,101,059
Metropolitan	2,749	649,062	29,095,817	161,480,097	250,701,110	443,106	687,719	5.5	22,977,717	46,217	3,338,251	86,912,812	442,303,153
CENSUS DIVISION 3, SOUTH ATLANTIC	731	152,236	6,587,288	37,509,493	60,428,149	102,781	165,583	5.7	5,427,764	10,324	695,805	21,281,267	82,476,854
Nonmetropolitan	289	32,472	1,125,010	7,291,923	13,823,939	19,986	37,887	6.5	967,976	2,308	103,113	4,813,987	18,997,592
Metropolitan	442	119,764	5,462,278	30,217,570	46,604,210	82,795	127,696	5.5	4,459,788	8,016	592,692	16,467,280	63,479,262
Delaware	6	2,014	93,275	546,058	861,231	1,496	2,360	5.9	96,683	106	11,350	305,634	1,947,818
Nonmetropolitan	2	437	12,612	122,846	230,777	336	632	9.7	15,750	27	1,499	58,161	409,910
Metropolitan	4	1,577	80,663	423,212	630,454	1,160	1,728	5.2	80,933	79	9,851	247,473	1,537,908
Dover	1	329	17,478	81,224	143,608	223	393	4.6	20,164	29	2,020	61,372	349,250
Wilmington-Newark	3	1,248	63,185	341,988	486,846	937	1,335	5.4	60,769	50	7,831	186,101	1,188,658
District of Columbia	10	3,352	137,172	936,124	1,323,580	2,564	3,626	6.8	105,917	190	13,843	352,942	1,526,061
Metropolitan	10	3,352	137,172	936,124	1,323,580	2,564	3,626	6.8	105,917	190	13,843	352,942	1,526,061
Washington	10	3,352	137,172	936,124	1,323,580	2,564	3,626	6.8	105,917	190	13,843	352,942	1,526,061
Florida	202	51,201	2,315,230	12,303,559	18,351,481	33,707	50,287	5.3	1,600,616	2,750	208,996	6,623,448	22,490,291
Nonmetropolitan	32	2,521	104,825	505,009	880,217	1,385	2,413	4.8	81,952	119	6,590	421,009	1,502,951
Metropolitan	170	48,680	2,210,405	11,798,550	17,471,264	32,322	47,874	5.3	1,518,664	2,631	202,406	6,202,439	20,987,340
Daytona Beach	7	1,265	62,058	284,137	455,068	779	1,247	4.6	42,507	60	4,009	285,917	895,932
Fort Lauderdale	17	4,948	219,232	1,150,201	1,693,262	3,152	4,639	5.2	125,307	207	20,977	649,513	1,989,827
Fort Myers-Cape Coral	5	1,788	74,386	369,600	555,435	1,017	1,529	5.0	52,600	124	7,582	190,875	637,903
Fort Pierce-Port St. Lucie	3	827	41,157	204,484	287,385	560	787	5.0	33,185	66	3,272	118,217	201,449
Fort Walton Beach	3	422	19,613	96,587	141,043	265	386	4.9	17,941	32	1,764	81,529	203,994
Gainesville	4	1,129	55,183	313,922	442,394	861	1,211	5.7	39,756	45	5,257	120,760	814,722
Jacksonville	11	3,231	154,128	799,077	1,249,579	2,188	3,423	5.2	143,372	240	15,082	483,063	1,695,546
Lakeland-Winter Haven	4	1,367	63,295	358,288	523,131	982	1,433	5.7	37,636	70	5,765	228,159	554,912
Melbourne-Titusville-Palm Bay	5	1,192	63,746	301,749	451,500	826	1,237	4.7	29,482	98	5,041	180,475	572,429
Miami	26	8,118	340,301	2,148,742	3,213,782	5,887	8,806	6.3	206,697	418	31,641	830,138	2,994,967
Naples	1	482	31,231	140,265	178,120	384	488	4.5	12,809	24	3,519	114,598	271,995
Ocala	2	593	35,749	161,777	227,814	443	624	4.5	23,024	38	2,465	117,787	200,601
Orlando	12	5,421	272,349	1,414,190	2,070,830	3,874	5,673	5.2	173,699	340	28,917	771,022	2,390,269
Panama City	2	547	24,779	121,681	196,961	333	540	4.9	19,429	38	2,444	77,359	261,391
Pensacola	6	1,634	62,224	340,142	509,392	931	1,396	5.5	46,487	67	5,536	210,945	930,650
Punta Gorda	3	722	27,778	141,255	204,114	387	560	5.1	25,273	10	1,145	53,878	171,091
Sarasota-Bradenton	7	2,115	87,465	486,684	668,429	1,331	1,830	5.6	54,884	70	5,781	240,059	876,243
Tallahassee	4	865	36,000	213,504	322,775	585	885	5.9	25,308	54	4,742	98,628	361,328
Tampa-St. Petersburg-Clearwater	33	8,385	373,580	1,897,938	2,783,592	5,197	7,628	5.1	266,688	439	32,219	933,460	3,608,375
West Palm Beach-Boca Raton	15	3,629	166,151	854,327	1,296,658	2,340	3,552	5.1	142,580	191	15,248	416,057	1,353,716
Georgia	146	24,500	885,142	5,774,911	10,225,875	15,827	28,021	6.5	800,479	1,993	128,981	3,227,698	12,483,943
Nonmetropolitan	83	9,386	251,614	2,069,148	4,165,953	5,673	11,418	8.2	213,591	654	30,471	1,090,569	3,780,713
Metropolitan	63	15,114	633,528	3,705,763	6,059,922	10,154	16,603	5.8	586,888	1,339	98,510	2,137,129	8,703,230
Albany	2	617	22,993	124,087	252,831	340	693	5.4	19,247	66	2,763	80,636	628,045
Athens	2	617	24,058	147,516	276,024	404	756	6.1	34,224	36	3,257	86,444	330,461
Atlanta	36	8,744	395,295	2,255,754	3,606,336	6,181	9,880	5.7	347,881	831	70,318	1,337,240	4,932,360
Augusta-Aiken	6	1,494	55,399	313,964	485,773	861	1,330	5.7	59,003	97	6,777	191,897	1,009,175
Chattanooga	2	307	6,818	79,323	154,726	217	424	11.6	8,437	15	875	36,015	117,979
Columbus	4	1,073	31,711	195,877	338,656	537	928	6.2	27,760	76	3,686	122,961	325,264
Macon	7	1,097	49,830	269,887	429,332	739	1,177	5.4	55,061	135	5,876	152,605	742,818
Savannah	4	1,165	47,424	319,355	516,244	875	1,415	6.7	35,275	83	4,958	129,331	617,128

Table continues

MSAs

TABLE **8**

U.S. CENSUS DIVISION 3, SOUTH ATLANTIC

U.S. Community Hospitals
(Nonfederal, short-term general and other special hospitals)

2002 Utilization, Personnel and Finances

	FULL-TIME EQUIVALENT PERSONNEL				FULL-TIME EQUIV. TRAINEES			EXPENSES						
								LABOR				TOTAL		
Physicians and Dentists	Registered Nurses	Licensed Practical Nurses	Other Salaried Personnel	Total Personnel	Medical and Dental Residents	Other Trainees	Total Trainees	Payroll (in thousands)	Employee Benefits (in thousands)	Total (in thousands)	Percent of Total	Amount (in thousands)	Adjusted per Admission	Adjusted per Inpatient Day
72,823	988,139	125,865	2,882,668	4,069,495	78,715	5,463	84,178	$175,961,479	$40,049,573	$216,011,067	51.9	$416,591,059	$7,354.60	$1,289.87
8,448	145,133	36,374	479,821	669,776	1,763	161	1,924	24,016,766	5,768,570	29,785,337	53.7	55,454,326	5,047.87	767.32
64,375	843,006	89,491	2,402,847	3,399,719	76,952	5,302	82,254	151,944,713	34,281,003	186,225,730	51.6	361,136,733	7,909.61	1,440.51
8,918	188,587	22,536	512,792	732,833	11,583	668	12,251	30,777,799	6,715,369	37,493,172	51.0	73,497,911	6,982.09	1,216.29
1,145	29,599	7,091	91,047	128,882	482	17	499	4,602,159	1,111,294	5,713,463	53.0	10,773,954	5,139.53	779.37
7,773	158,988	15,445	421,745	603,951	11,101	651	11,752	26,175,640	5,604,075	31,779,709	50.7	62,723,957	7,440.26	1,345.89
458	3,445	242	10,042	14,187	236	0	236	577,382	143,078	720,460	59.9	1,201,883	8,270.71	1,395.54
18	384	33	1,539	1,974	6	0	6	77,677	16,764	94,441	73.1	129,250	5,317.84	560.06
440	3,061	209	8,503	12,213	230	0	230	499,705	126,314	626,019	58.4	1,072,633	8,863.78	1,701.37
10	530	62	1,510	2,112	0	0	0	80,210	25,519	105,729	57.7	183,364	5,933.73	1,276.84
430	2,531	147	6,993	10,101	230	0	230	419,495	100,795	520,290	58.5	889,269	9,868.60	1,826.59
1,037	4,618	322	14,510	20,487	1,065	47	1,112	1,110,442	172,146	1,282,589	55.4	2,313,103	11,805.04	1,747.61
1,037	4,618	322	14,510	20,487	1,065	47	1,112	1,110,442	172,146	1,282,589	55.4	2,313,103	11,805.04	1,747.61
1,037	4,618	322	14,510	20,487	1,065	47	1,112	1,110,442	172,146	1,282,589	55.4	2,313,103	11,805.04	1,747.61
1,993	57,491	6,927	158,422	224,833	2,737	231	2,968	9,436,303	2,123,747	11,560,048	49.8	23,194,125	6,717.23	1,263.88
61	2,199	582	6,727	9,569	4	0	4	347,217	86,728	433,945	50.1	865,772	4,767.76	983.59
1,932	55,292	6,345	151,695	215,264	2,733	231	2,964	9,089,086	2,037,020	11,126,103	49.8	22,328,353	6,825.44	1,278.00
41	1,569	222	4,461	6,293	35	15	50	231,507	58,888	290,396	45.3	640,619	6,424.11	1,407.74
184	5,607	609	13,081	19,481	69	8	77	848,179	179,695	1,027,874	49.9	2,060,182	6,341.34	1,216.69
117	1,509	200	5,583	7,409	17	11	28	321,875	56,758	378,633	54.3	697,455	6,236.24	1,255.69
54	829	71	2,952	3,906	0	0	0	153,575	39,262	192,837	49.4	390,175	6,681.65	1,357.67
1	459	72	888	1,420	1	0	1	53,195	13,438	66,634	51.4	129,716	4,451.92	919.69
22	1,553	195	5,268	7,038	13	14	27	257,494	59,535	317,030	48.1	659,583	8,533.77	1,490.94
37	4,069	224	10,603	14,933	31	15	46	618,995	159,489	778,484	47.7	1,630,848	6,665.36	1,305.12
24	1,411	278	4,183	5,896	0	22	22	222,933	44,083	267,016	51.9	514,792	5,596.66	984.06
121	1,479	173	4,501	6,274	125	5	130	266,639	57,123	323,761	51.8	625,302	6,529.68	1,384.94
332	9,398	939	24,685	35,354	1,250	98	1,348	1,736,259	384,238	2,120,494	50.0	4,241,097	8,495.06	1,319.66
2	713	74	2,108	2,897	0	0	0	113,818	24,026	137,844	49.2	279,990	7,059.76	1,571.92
0	897	39	2,072	3,008	0	0	0	118,838	28,019	146,857	47.9	306,617	6,082.35	1,345.91
403	7,031	616	21,169	29,219	576	19	595	1,177,700	292,144	1,469,844	52.5	2,801,700	7,009.37	1,352.94
3	560	124	1,731	2,418	0	0	0	83,998	22,018	106,016	48.7	217,845	5,479.81	1,106.03
64	1,964	218	4,380	6,626	5	7	12	215,549	41,501	257,051	46.1	557,609	5,960.42	1,094.66
17	591	101	1,527	2,236	13	1	14	90,266	20,887	111,153	47.5	234,012	5,817.42	1,146.48
28	1,998	354	6,295	8,675	10	0	10	314,534	68,489	383,022	47.9	799,361	6,618.60	1,195.88
44	846	169	2,973	4,032	30	0	30	167,991	32,350	200,342	53.4	374,939	6,914.24	1,161.61
356	9,310	1,219	24,350	35,235	476	12	488	1,493,869	328,882	1,822,749	49.5	3,682,202	6,703.87	1,322.82
82	3,499	448	8,885	12,914	82	4	86	601,872	126,194	728,066	49.1	1,484,309	5,917.45	1,144.72
1,307	28,863	4,657	78,292	113,119	1,328	58	1,386	4,490,225	1,011,899	5,502,129	52.0	10,576,055	6,951.87	1,034.24
285	7,138	2,364	23,363	33,150	138	6	144	1,102,648	262,136	1,364,789	53.3	2,558,342	5,253.99	614.11
1,022	21,725	2,293	54,929	79,969	1,190	52	1,242	3,387,578	749,763	4,137,340	51.6	8,017,713	7,751.13	1,323.07
53	574	150	2,418	3,195	16	0	16	123,077	21,972	145,049	51.0	284,143	6,033.91	1,123.84
5	836	55	2,394	3,290	0	0	0	136,990	32,081	169,071	57.0	296,663	6,892.41	1,074.77
424	13,913	1,128	32,965	48,430	474	49	523	2,151,076	461,198	2,612,275	51.8	5,044,582	7,910.76	1,398.81
356	2,096	341	5,230	8,023	421	0	421	301,564	81,894	383,459	50.3	761,822	8,741.40	1,568.27
1	222	94	905	1,222	0	0	0	39,211	10,078	49,289	57.9	85,192	6,395.78	550.60
0	939	194	3,043	4,176	39	0	39	133,872	31,226	165,097	47.2	349,767	6,496.53	1,032.81
42	1,602	189	3,889	5,722	120	0	120	252,206	57,265	309,471	52.8	586,482	7,223.84	1,366.03
141	1,543	142	4,085	5,911	120	3	123	249,581	54,049	303,629	49.9	609,062	8,569.05	1,179.79

Table continues

MSAs

TABLE **8**

U.S. CENSUS DIVISION 3, SOUTH ATLANTIC CONTINUED

U.S. Community Hospitals
(Nonfederal, short-term general and other special hospitals)

2002 Utilization, Personnel and Finances

CLASSIFICATION	Hospitals	Beds	Admissions	Inpatient Days	Adjusted Patient Days	Average Daily Census	Adjusted Average Daily Census	Average Stay (days)	Surgical Operations	NEWBORNS Bassinets	Births	OUTPATIENT VISITS Emergency	Total
Maryland.	49	11,417	634,914	3,049,647	4,622,969	8,359	12,666	4.8	533,799	924	63,744	1,943,614	6,464,183
Nonmetropolitan	9	865	50,216	217,056	385,485	595	1,055	4.3	49,036	74	4,353	200,901	1,285,159
Metropolitan	40	10,552	584,698	2,832,591	4,237,484	7,764	11,611	4.8	484,763	850	59,391	1,742,713	5,179,024
Baltimore	22	6,826	380,491	1,841,281	2,700,963	5,046	7,400	4.8	316,991	470	33,650	1,080,771	3,156,135
Cumberland	2	424	16,762	108,576	212,307	298	581	6.5	9,093	12	1,024	58,687	307,954
Hagerstown	1	301	15,664	72,338	136,871	198	375	4.6	10,231	41	1,720	63,701	216,035
Washington.	14	2,879	163,709	782,728	1,143,632	2,146	3,135	4.8	141,533	315	22,302	508,664	1,361,637
Wilmington-Newark	1	122	8,072	27,668	43,711	76	120	3.4	6,915	12	695	30,890	137,263
North Carolina	113	23,583	966,722	5,929,916	10,111,575	16,246	27,716	6.1	811,408	1,608	108,967	3,322,226	13,822,808
Nonmetropolitan	62	7,736	286,570	1,856,502	3,509,526	5,086	9,625	6.5	228,896	602	26,969	1,230,962	4,642,893
Metropolitan	51	15,847	680,152	4,073,414	6,602,049	11,160	18,091	6.0	582,512	1,006	81,998	2,091,264	9,179,915
Asheville	2	801	36,513	208,398	315,889	571	866	5.7	42,037	30	3,603	86,452	468,795
Charlotte-Gastonia-Rock Hill	12	3,558	155,588	926,940	1,532,010	2,540	4,197	6.0	142,867	278	21,045	530,084	2,185,242
Fayetteville	1	546	28,245	164,159	244,866	450	671	5.8	28,690	48	3,933	99,858	399,793
Goldsboro	1	270	11,667	60,215	92,594	165	254	5.2	12,216	30	1,229	45,021	136,888
Greensboro—Winston-Salem— High Point.	12	4,054	158,596	1,000,136	1,648,583	2,740	4,518	6.3	109,831	202	17,345	446,399	1,418,692
Greenville.	1	745	33,409	199,986	265,157	548	726	6.0	18,412	42	3,470	60,785	266,101
Hickory-Morganton-Lenoir	5	1,101	36,823	272,285	482,800	745	1,324	7.4	36,191	82	4,084	186,949	629,081
Jacksonville	1	133	7,801	32,249	60,067	88	165	4.1	6,182	23	1,441	32,953	115,975
Raleigh-Durham-Chapel Hill	11	3,427	154,534	916,386	1,485,309	2,511	4,069	5.9	138,871	196	20,233	422,911	2,962,564
Rocky Mount.	2	440	19,209	98,792	159,296	271	437	5.1	12,925	30	1,945	74,711	235,541
Wilmington	3	772	37,767	193,868	315,478	531	864	5.1	34,290	45	3,670	105,141	361,243
South Carolina	62	11,107	513,136	2,914,964	4,587,140	7,987	12,565	5.7	457,995	853	48,864	1,799,127	7,266,845
Nonmetropolitan	27	3,275	125,944	760,525	1,314,741	2,083	3,602	6.0	111,136	295	11,690	535,448	1,365,353
Metropolitan	35	7,832	387,192	2,154,439	3,272,399	5,904	8,963	5.6	346,859	558	37,174	1,263,679	5,901,492
Augusta-Aiken	2	291	12,039	58,976	89,316	162	245	4.9	8,358	18	872	55,929	65,901
Charleston-North Charleston	7	1,535	79,981	440,286	656,110	1,207	1,796	5.5	79,894	112	8,332	260,584	1,300,231
Charlotte-Gastonia-Rock Hill	1	233	15,296	69,681	96,754	191	265	4.6	13,288	33	1,738	46,642	139,747
Columbia	5	1,595	82,233	468,979	685,542	1,284	1,878	5.7	59,534	105	8,273	197,496	1,612,874
Florence	4	788	42,047	223,817	321,078	613	879	5.3	40,574	24	2,139	110,242	359,690
Greenville-Spartanburg-Anderson .	12	2,512	121,520	662,861	1,024,109	1,818	2,805	5.5	105,833	183	12,369	422,132	1,881,011
Myrtle Beach.	3	661	26,413	165,445	285,283	453	782	6.3	24,344	48	2,434	123,453	359,150
Sumter	1	217	7,663	64,394	114,207	176	313	8.4	15,034	35	1,017	47,201	182,888
Virginia.	86	17,241	746,686	4,278,445	7,057,976	11,729	19,339	5.7	739,868	1,408	90,401	2,606,320	10,789,497
Nonmetropolitan	35	4,136	151,179	836,307	1,492,098	2,295	4,089	5.5	139,764	314	12,332	665,097	3,026,528
Metropolitan	51	13,105	595,507	3,442,138	5,565,878	9,434	15,250	5.8	600,104	1,094	78,069	1,941,223	7,762,969
Charlottesville	2	694	36,053	180,790	327,161	496	896	5.0	50,098	45	3,009	93,034	1,303,630
Danville	1	350	12,254	73,660	122,858	202	337	6.0	9,233	20	1,104	39,272	119,385
Johnson City-Kingsport-Bristol . . .	1	135	5,161	22,301	49,119	61	135	4.3	8,879	12	700	29,104	93,314
Lynchburg	2	954	27,048	272,425	405,337	746	1,110	10.1	24,000	48	2,594	85,022	151,308
Norfolk-Virginia Beach-Newport News.	16	3,370	153,104	923,205	1,617,991	2,531	4,432	6.0	149,683	289	18,838	625,733	2,426,906
Richmond-Petersburg	12	3,471	139,598	838,507	1,272,424	2,298	3,486	6.0	148,818	221	14,728	404,372	1,808,266
Roanoke	2	1,106	49,758	303,348	437,629	831	1,199	6.1	51,293	107	3,851	152,329	399,416
Washington.	15	3,025	172,531	827,902	1,333,359	2,269	3,655	4.8	158,100	352	33,245	512,357	1,460,724
West Virginia	57	7,821	295,011	1,775,869	3,286,322	4,866	9,003	6.0	280,999	492	20,659	1,100,258	5,685,408
Nonmetropolitan	39	4,116	142,050	924,530	1,845,142	2,533	5,053	6.5	127,851	223	9,209	611,840	2,984,085
Metropolitan	18	3,705	152,961	851,339	1,441,180	2,333	3,950	5.6	153,148	269	11,450	488,418	2,701,323
Charleston	5	1,240	55,452	298,961	479,815	819	1,315	5.4	64,421	66	3,981	151,210	813,893
Cumberland	1	32	1,246	4,415	12,455	12	34	3.5	1,897	0	0	10,059	46,912
Huntington-Ashland.	3	729	34,293	176,269	258,043	483	707	5.1	28,449	55	2,985	108,157	456,761
Parkersburg-Marietta	3	483	22,141	121,033	209,250	332	573	5.5	18,123	50	1,567	75,998	437,309
Steubenville-Weirton	1	238	8,079	42,324	91,519	116	251	5.2	5,637	21	377	27,795	192,516
Washington.	2	204	9,551	44,940	91,948	124	252	4.7	11,044	21	1,089	50,893	187,463
Wheeling	3	779	22,199	163,397	298,150	447	818	7.4	23,577	56	1,451	64,306	566,469

MSAs

FULL-TIME EQUIVALENT PERSONNEL					FULL-TIME EQUIV. TRAINEES			EXPENSES						
								LABOR				TOTAL		
Physicians and Dentists	Registered Nurses	Licensed Practical Nurses	Other Salaried Personnel	Total Personnel	Medical and Dental Residents	Other Trainees	Total Trainees	Payroll (in thousands)	Employee Benefits (in thousands)	Total (in thousands)	Percent of Total	Amount (in thousands)	Adjusted per Admission	Adjusted per Inpatient Day
1,628	16,185	885	48,435	67,133	1,204	186	1,390	2,958,323	559,139	3,517,459	50.5	6,971,694	7,207.08	1,508.06
42	1,197	122	3,765	5,126	0	2	2	200,315	47,269	247,584	50.6	489,037	5,439.85	1,268.63
1,586	14,988	763	44,670	62,007	1,204	184	1,388	2,758,008	511,870	3,269,875	50.4	6,482,657	7,388.14	1,529.84
1,439	10,568	417	30,796	43,220	1,113	180	1,293	1,912,611	336,534	2,249,142	49.5	4,546,578	8,098.86	1,683.32
13	472	35	1,377	1,897	0	0	0	71,183	19,721	90,904	56.5	160,873	4,932.17	757.74
10	421	50	1,234	1,715	0	0	0	71,662	19,617	91,279	60.1	151,827	5,122.70	1,109.27
117	3,384	244	10,704	14,449	91	4	95	675,786	129,800	805,586	51.6	1,560,077	6,472.03	1,364.14
7	143	17	559	726	0	0	0	26,766	6,198	32,964	52.1	63,302	4,964.10	1,448.20
805	32,741	2,588	84,931	121,065	2,112	77	2,189	5,053,457	1,105,506	6,158,963	53.3	11,563,648	7,009.82	1,143.61
228	8,069	1,215	23,742	33,254	27	0	27	1,193,050	270,353	1,463,406	54.3	2,695,287	4,983.03	767.99
577	24,672	1,373	61,189	87,811	2,085	77	2,162	3,860,407	835,153	4,695,557	52.9	8,868,361	7,998.58	1,343.27
28	1,338	79	3,381	4,826	0	0	0	226,217	50,476	276,693	55.5	498,610	9,306.07	1,578.43
242	5,625	206	14,400	20,473	224	0	224	918,723	205,876	1,124,598	51.6	2,179,691	8,133.33	1,422.77
41	877	159	2,837	3,914	0	0	0	151,062	39,644	190,706	54.2	351,760	8,349.19	1,436.54
0	279	36	898	1,213	0	0	0	48,230	12,329	60,558	58.0	104,322	5,814.73	1,126.66
135	5,688	382	14,661	20,866	621	68	689	817,548	180,644	998,193	54.3	1,838,195	7,032.38	1,115.01
0	1,098	34	3,312	4,444	283	0	283	191,190	46,862	238,052	51.4	463,289	10,458.94	1,747.23
45	1,114	119	3,018	4,296	7	0	7	168,839	38,000	206,839	53.3	388,403	5,893.47	804.48
5	176	22	569	772	0	0	0	28,351	6,544	34,895	52.2	66,795	4,597.04	1,112.01
75	6,793	210	13,417	20,495	894	9	903	1,047,586	195,811	1,243,398	52.7	2,357,450	9,503.97	1,587.18
2	477	31	1,430	1,940	0	0	0	80,655	20,619	101,273	58.2	173,980	5,610.45	1,092.18
4	1,207	95	3,266	4,572	56	0	56	182,005	38,347	220,352	49.4	445,867	7,201.04	1,413.31
773	14,723	1,868	37,970	55,334	1,005	0	1,005	2,265,153	518,049	2,783,201	47.7	5,829,537	7,251.71	1,270.84
114	2,750	662	8,780	12,306	27	0	27	460,526	118,101	578,625	51.3	1,127,324	5,235.67	857.45
659	11,973	1,206	29,190	43,028	978	0	978	1,804,627	399,948	2,204,576	46.9	4,702,213	7,989.23	1,436.93
1	258	49	548	856	0	0	0	47,002	4,402	51,404	40.8	126,033	6,777.44	1,411.09
5	2,689	234	5,163	8,091	545	0	545	382,493	87,237	469,730	44.0	1,068,292	8,890.87	1,628.22
4	454	13	1,347	1,818	0	0	0	49,020	13,244	62,264	38.5	161,787	7,617.44	1,672.14
98	2,715	231	6,765	9,809	215	0	215	382,274	81,507	463,781	47.9	968,150	7,988.63	1,412.24
25	1,169	164	2,995	4,353	24	0	24	169,878	36,294	206,172	45.6	452,340	7,515.20	1,408.82
517	3,626	357	9,682	14,182	194	0	194	630,842	140,228	771,069	49.2	1,567,053	8,224.57	1,530.16
9	782	124	1,698	2,613	0	0	0	89,857	24,858	114,715	49.1	233,780	5,427.52	819.47
0	280	34	992	1,306	0	0	0	53,262	12,179	65,441	52.4	124,779	9,181.02	1,092.57
593	22,090	3,181	56,670	82,534	1,466	61	1,527	3,637,436	737,698	4,375,139	49.8	8,779,481	7,041.53	1,243.91
185	4,153	930	11,645	16,913	29	2	31	638,908	148,149	787,062	52.8	1,491,738	5,388.93	999.76
408	17,937	2,251	45,025	65,621	1,437	59	1,496	2,998,528	589,550	3,588,077	49.2	7,287,743	7,513.14	1,309.36
26	1,678	160	3,872	5,736	658	0	658	282,632	63,889	346,522	50.1	691,675	10,196.43	2,114.17
2	289	68	900	1,259	0	0	0	53,001	9,506	62,506	52.1	120,008	5,871.79	976.80
11	203	50	374	638	0	0	0	20,748	5,532	26,280	52.5	50,018	4,400.28	1,018.30
31	994	149	2,441	3,615	13	0	13	138,462	29,088	167,550	58.7	285,269	7,321.54	703.78
81	4,308	645	12,475	17,509	58	2	60	752,445	135,489	887,933	48.6	1,826,781	6,810.04	1,129.04
60	4,402	688	9,730	14,880	535	45	580	670,312	130,299	800,611	48.4	1,654,877	7,862.17	1,300.57
99	1,574	210	3,914	5,797	131	0	131	263,517	50,274	313,791	46.2	678,986	9,391.36	1,551.51
98	4,489	281	11,319	16,187	42	12	54	817,411	165,473	982,884	49.6	1,980,130	7,062.71	1,485.07
324	8,431	1,866	23,520	34,141	430	8	438	1,249,079	344,107	1,593,184	51.9	3,068,385	5,646.18	933.68
212	3,709	1,183	11,486	16,590	251	7	258	581,819	161,794	743,611	52.5	1,417,204	5,051.68	768.07
112	4,722	683	12,034	17,551	179	1	180	667,260	182,313	849,573	51.5	1,651,181	6,280.57	1,145.71
37	1,983	179	4,620	6,819	140	0	140	263,091	69,520	332,611	49.3	674,604	7,482.71	1,405.97
0	35	10	147	192	0	0	0	5,244	1,001	6,245	46.5	13,441	3,823.92	1,079.17
1	942	166	2,118	3,227	0	0	0	133,332	44,054	177,386	52.6	336,923	6,586.45	1,305.69
2	490	117	1,581	2,190	0	0	0	77,483	21,479	98,962	51.0	194,148	4,947.57	927.83
9	249	31	642	931	0	0	0	32,999	7,255	40,254	54.6	73,756	4,221.87	805.91
9	227	45	811	1,092	0	0	0	42,735	11,549	54,284	55.8	97,314	4,911.63	1,058.36
54	796	135	2,115	3,100	39	1	40	112,376	27,455	139,831	53.6	260,996	6,280.73	875.38

MSAs

TABLE 8

U.S. CENSUS DIVISION 4, EAST NORTH CENTRAL

U.S. Community Hospitals
(Nonfederal, short-term general and other special hospitals)

2002 Utilization, Personnel and Finances

CLASSIFICATION	Hospitals	Beds	Admissions	Inpatient Days	Adjusted Patient Days	Average Daily Census	Adjusted Average Daily Census	Average Stay (days)	Surgical Operations	NEWBORNS Bassinets	NEWBORNS Births	OUTPATIENT VISITS Emergency	OUTPATIENT VISITS Total
UNITED STATES	4,927	820,653	34,478,280	196,690,099	322,970,965	539,685	885,994	5.7	27,576,675	59,974	3,870,191	109,951,738	556,404,212
Nonmetropolitan	2,178	171,591	5,382,463	35,210,002	72,269,855	96,579	198,275	6.5	4,598,958	13,757	531,940	23,038,926	114,101,059
Metropolitan	2,749	649,062	29,095,817	161,480,097	250,701,110	443,106	687,719	5.5	22,977,717	46,217	3,338,251	86,912,812	442,303,153
CENSUS DIVISION 4, EAST NORTH CENTRAL	737	129,716	5,549,822	29,754,022	52,987,790	81,610	145,316	5.4	4,689,519	10,297	594,899	18,125,078	106,432,740
Nonmetropolitan	293	24,596	797,187	4,812,741	11,461,518	13,189	31,420	6.0	758,927	2,155	80,891	3,623,702	20,831,845
Metropolitan	444	105,120	4,752,635	24,941,281	41,526,272	68,421	113,896	5.2	3,930,592	8,142	514,008	14,501,376	85,600,895
Illinois	192	36,309	1,615,269	8,326,561	13,698,545	22,908	37,681	5.2	1,174,945	2,768	172,338	4,699,328	26,511,316
Nonmetropolitan	72	6,254	193,137	1,215,117	2,547,427	3,330	6,995	6.3	160,517	416	16,076	773,472	4,467,717
Metropolitan	120	30,055	1,422,132	7,111,444	11,151,118	19,578	30,686	5.0	1,014,428	2,352	156,262	3,925,856	22,043,599
Bloomington-Normal	2	395	16,362	68,600	115,097	188	316	4.2	13,494	33	2,322	57,892	248,075
Champaign-Urbana	2	620	23,938	159,321	212,772	437	583	6.7	17,113	50	3,168	77,323	170,979
Chicago	84	22,020	1,104,903	5,422,847	8,324,571	14,950	22,940	4.9	727,527	1,776	124,221	2,864,213	16,410,386
Davenport-Moline-Rock Island	4	631	28,107	134,485	253,507	369	694	4.8	21,278	83	2,421	87,192	486,869
Decatur	2	434	20,094	107,694	239,493	295	656	5.4	22,768	36	1,654	66,647	381,883
Kankakee	2	710	19,717	94,499	162,362	259	444	4.8	20,838	41	1,639	59,273	434,299
Peoria-Pekin	5	1,225	51,641	290,205	464,871	795	1,274	5.6	50,546	74	4,871	209,210	1,505,069
Rockford	5	961	44,151	216,150	341,359	592	935	4.9	30,793	61	5,096	135,818	495,868
Springfield	3	1,095	44,537	235,555	344,664	645	945	5.3	46,839	60	3,504	106,973	645,009
St. Louis	11	1,964	68,682	382,088	692,422	1,048	1,899	5.6	63,232	138	7,366	261,315	1,265,162
Indiana	112	18,961	715,936	4,077,032	7,257,112	11,169	19,885	5.7	615,920	1,592	78,921	2,437,268	14,087,435
Nonmetropolitan	45	3,687	130,157	628,215	1,502,386	1,721	4,120	4.8	130,173	421	14,146	632,275	3,718,001
Metropolitan	67	15,274	585,779	3,448,817	5,754,726	9,448	15,765	5.9	485,747	1,171	64,775	1,804,993	10,369,434
Bloomington	1	811	17,896	226,158	323,242	620	886	12.6	10,885	40	1,899	52,965	314,721
Cincinnati	1	87	4,213	18,097	45,451	50	125	4.3	6,691	10	505	17,906	114,448
Elkhart-Goshen	2	450	19,137	90,574	166,850	248	457	4.7	16,038	39	3,009	75,357	256,461
Evansville-Henderson	6	1,215	41,094	281,486	428,965	770	1,176	6.8	20,534	43	4,286	115,196	525,553
Fort Wayne	10	1,639	65,749	359,452	618,199	984	1,693	5.5	49,830	154	8,188	212,928	730,999
Gary	8	2,535	102,528	567,662	876,527	1,555	2,402	5.5	61,992	266	8,508	221,817	1,119,162
Indianapolis	19	5,246	200,890	1,199,706	2,021,141	3,287	5,538	6.0	181,344	355	22,302	655,966	4,962,740
Kokomo	4	442	14,285	96,507	213,875	264	586	6.8	17,440	42	1,659	47,634	440,582
Lafayette	2	504	19,779	100,359	172,531	275	472	5.1	14,691	34	3,213	79,539	281,911
Louisville	6	651	25,980	137,271	283,568	376	776	5.3	32,446	51	2,660	105,966	508,409
Muncie	1	393	18,659	100,353	173,109	275	474	5.4	19,450	20	1,591	47,796	336,438
South Bend	3	722	31,885	155,568	240,715	427	659	4.9	33,907	57	4,658	98,470	368,967
Terre Haute	4	579	23,684	115,624	190,553	317	521	4.9	20,499	60	2,297	73,453	409,043
Michigan	145	26,130	1,163,157	6,296,654	11,849,369	17,251	32,468	5.4	1,086,519	2,010	127,754	4,029,309	25,866,365
Nonmetropolitan	59	4,562	147,781	892,040	2,559,772	2,446	7,013	6.0	167,918	381	15,130	726,718	4,894,361
Metropolitan	86	21,568	1,015,376	5,404,614	9,289,597	14,805	25,455	5.3	918,601	1,629	112,624	3,302,591	20,972,004
Ann Arbor	8	1,731	89,362	451,125	796,205	1,237	2,181	5.0	95,617	110	9,647	267,856	2,532,133
Benton Harbor	2	414	17,646	75,160	139,269	206	382	4.3	14,386	51	2,110	72,432	372,141
Detroit	41	10,775	539,730	2,798,392	4,698,522	7,663	12,874	5.2	474,739	822	57,287	1,705,827	9,598,964
Flint	3	1,281	65,013	326,947	519,171	896	1,423	5.0	39,072	103	6,730	211,540	1,659,449
Grand Rapids-Muskegon-Holland	11	2,656	112,393	599,141	1,046,504	1,642	2,868	5.3	118,769	272	17,051	386,822	2,018,404
Jackson	2	442	18,081	83,608	182,387	229	499	4.6	13,114	24	1,859	62,151	363,898
Kalamazoo-Battle Creek	8	1,448	55,865	347,482	677,671	952	1,858	6.2	54,133	113	6,901	225,567	1,437,101
Lansing-East Lansing	5	1,133	48,783	313,391	627,421	858	1,720	6.4	43,874	56	6,026	185,644	1,646,983
Saginaw-Bay City-Midland	6	1,688	68,503	409,368	602,447	1,122	1,650	6.0	64,897	78	5,013	184,752	1,342,931

Table continues

TABLE 8

U.S. CENSUS DIVISION 4, EAST NORTH CENTRAL

U.S. Community Hospitals
(Nonfederal, short-term general and other special hospitals)

2002 Utilization, Personnel and Finances

FULL-TIME EQUIVALENT PERSONNEL					FULL-TIME EQUIV. TRAINEES			EXPENSES						
								LABOR				TOTAL		
Physicians and Dentists	Registered Nurses	Licensed Practical Nurses	Other Salaried Personnel	Total Personnel	Medical and Dental Residents	Other Trainees	Total Trainees	Payroll (in thousands)	Employee Benefits (in thousands)	Total (in thousands)	Percent of Total	Amount (in thousands)	Adjusted per Admission	Adjusted per Inpatient Day
72,823	988,139	125,865	2,882,668	4,069,495	78,715	5,463	84,178	$175,961,479	$40,049,573	$216,011,067	51.9	$416,591,059	$7,354.60	$1,289.87
8,448	145,133	36,374	479,821	669,776	1,763	161	1,924	24,016,766	5,768,570	29,785,337	53.7	55,454,326	5,047.87	767.32
64,375	843,006	89,491	2,402,847	3,399,719	76,952	5,302	82,254	151,944,713	34,281,003	186,225,730	51.6	361,136,733	7,909.61	1,440.51
14,586	166,178	16,038	503,811	700,613	15,976	960	16,936	30,280,325	6,874,047	37,154,368	52.2	71,241,902	7,266.93	1,344.50
1,607	22,885	4,214	78,974	107,680	190	61	251	4,091,204	1,052,390	5,143,589	54.5	9,442,223	5,190.33	823.82
12,979	143,293	11,824	424,837	592,933	15,786	899	16,685	26,189,121	5,821,657	32,010,779	51.8	61,799,678	7,740.08	1,488.21
4,396	45,656	3,286	138,465	191,803	4,770	303	5,073	8,376,296	1,836,687	10,212,983	52.1	19,597,944	7,434.48	1,430.66
289	5,169	1,080	16,585	23,123	43	2	45	829,164	217,260	1,046,424	53.8	1,946,202	4,857.39	763.99
4,107	40,487	2,206	121,880	168,680	4,727	301	5,028	7,547,132	1,619,427	9,166,559	51.9	17,651,742	7,896.39	1,582.96
53	461	42	1,755	2,311	4	0	4	80,407	20,355	100,762	48.5	207,670	7,578.91	1,804.30
0	645	30	2,207	2,882	17	0	17	97,839	21,758	119,597	47.1	253,713	7,802.94	1,192.42
3,605	31,663	1,275	92,403	128,946	4,303	256	4,559	6,007,778	1,244,517	7,252,294	52.1	13,929,490	8,185.43	1,673.30
31	666	46	2,227	2,970	0	0	0	115,355	22,880	138,235	51.8	267,106	5,250.96	1,053.64
31	413	154	2,493	3,091	15	0	15	93,295	25,727	119,022	50.4	236,020	5,200.51	985.50
32	479	65	1,555	2,131	1	2	3	83,197	21,890	105,087	51.5	204,027	5,992.86	1,256.62
161	1,741	106	5,076	7,084	169	24	193	307,630	67,785	375,416	51.3	731,890	8,811.16	1,574.39
151	1,560	124	4,321	6,156	0	19	19	257,959	62,154	320,114	53.6	597,114	8,591.19	1,749.22
4	1,047	185	3,949	5,185	209	0	209	227,801	60,789	288,590	50.4	572,540	8,784.93	1,661.15
39	1,812	179	5,894	7,924	9	0	9	275,870	71,572	347,442	53.3	652,174	5,187.35	941.87
1,444	22,952	3,110	68,675	96,181	972	193	1,165	3,955,455	927,380	4,882,833	52.7	9,272,855	7,101.10	1,277.76
306	3,892	817	14,646	19,661	15	33	48	689,620	174,960	864,578	55.1	1,568,422	5,124.04	1,043.95
1,138	19,060	2,293	54,029	76,520	957	160	1,117	3,265,836	752,419	4,018,255	52.2	7,704,433	7,706.41	1,338.80
73	610	44	1,877	2,604	117	5	122	89,027	19,665	108,692	51.7	210,113	8,214.58	650.02
0	108	30	416	554	0	0	0	21,448	5,530	26,978	56.5	47,717	4,509.71	1,049.86
26	673	49	1,852	2,600	0	1	1	98,974	32,844	131,818	53.7	245,554	6,903.40	1,471.70
104	1,100	102	4,171	5,477	38	21	59	209,209	44,222	253,431	52.6	481,492	7,550.33	1,122.45
13	2,310	248	5,110	7,681	0	6	6	332,335	82,759	415,095	51.0	814,610	7,126.13	1,317.71
201	2,935	279	8,084	11,499	149	51	200	498,609	113,650	612,261	53.3	1,148,320	7,176.87	1,310.08
558	7,414	908	21,390	30,270	478	70	548	1,373,649	300,653	1,674,300	52.2	3,207,779	9,294.92	1,587.11
11	475	59	1,652	2,197	0	0	0	83,043	19,633	102,676	53.8	190,854	5,968.30	892.36
8	643	75	1,370	2,096	0	0	0	92,242	25,711	117,953	54.6	216,120	6,236.50	1,252.64
16	685	126	2,335	3,162	0	4	4	121,645	24,265	145,910	55.2	264,482	4,643.38	932.69
13	471	107	1,304	1,895	88	0	88	82,299	19,697	101,996	49.2	207,504	6,446.82	1,198.69
87	929	106	2,649	3,771	69	2	71	162,833	37,327	200,161	47.4	422,509	8,568.95	1,755.23
28	707	160	1,819	2,714	18	0	18	100,522	26,462	126,984	51.3	247,379	6,226.36	1,298.22
3,591	34,616	3,167	107,819	149,193	4,161	230	4,391	6,573,511	1,480,607	8,054,121	52.6	15,321,065	7,172.14	1,292.99
482	4,593	989	17,312	23,376	59	16	75	880,942	225,616	1,106,558	56.1	1,971,064	5,553.14	770.02
3,109	30,023	2,178	90,507	125,817	4,102	214	4,316	5,692,569	1,254,991	6,947,563	52.0	13,350,001	7,494.75	1,437.09
116	3,394	219	9,680	13,409	1,063	9	1,072	642,605	169,932	812,537	55.2	1,576,595	9,823.81	1,980.14
5	586	75	1,821	2,487	0	0	0	86,213	24,333	110,546	55.2	200,353	6,129.99	1,438.60
2,138	15,469	643	44,597	62,847	2,220	166	2,386	2,898,308	594,174	3,492,483	51.5	6,780,285	7,402.22	1,443.07
138	1,768	190	4,734	6,830	327	3	330	346,101	79,135	425,237	55.6	764,730	7,397.27	1,472.98
328	3,230	483	11,195	15,236	133	27	160	625,825	133,059	758,886	52.1	1,457,271	6,877.97	1,392.51
13	386	61	1,676	2,136	0	0	0	92,457	19,670	112,128	47.6	235,515	5,956.84	1,291.30
97	1,796	130	5,761	7,784	0	0	0	335,712	81,174	416,886	51.4	810,505	7,723.29	1,196.02
147	1,650	98	4,824	6,719	204	2	206	325,105	68,352	393,457	56.0	703,190	6,790.30	1,120.76
127	1,744	279	6,219	8,369	155	7	162	340,242	85,161	425,403	51.8	821,558	7,550.87	1,363.70

Table continues

MSAs

TABLE **8**

U.S. CENSUS DIVISION 4, EAST NORTH CENTRAL CONTINUED

U.S. Community Hospitals
(Nonfederal, short-term general and other special hospitals)

2002 Utilization, Personnel and Finances

MSAs

CLASSIFICATION	Hospitals	Beds	Admissions	Inpatient Days	Adjusted Patient Days	Average Daily Census	Adjusted Average Daily Census	Average Stay (days)	Surgical Operations	NEWBORNS		OUTPATIENT VISITS	
										Bassinets	Births	Emergency	Total
Ohio	168	33,706	1,475,630	7,657,394	13,417,186	20,980	36,751	5.2	1,241,582	2,664	150,298	5,125,829	28,355,387
Nonmetropolitan	52	4,937	183,767	850,874	1,855,672	2,332	5,086	4.6	174,412	551	21,121	948,029	4,383,268
Metropolitan	116	28,769	1,291,863	6,806,520	11,561,514	18,648	31,665	5.3	1,067,170	2,113	129,177	4,177,800	23,972,119
Akron	7	1,810	89,478	483,141	804,753	1,323	2,204	5.4	75,874	125	8,416	312,154	1,595,210
Canton-Massillon	5	1,385	56,980	333,205	566,859	913	1,553	5.8	51,976	103	5,016	199,105	1,276,584
Cincinnati	14	3,347	171,438	832,210	1,386,772	2,280	3,799	4.9	132,798	241	19,206	509,176	2,308,625
Cleveland-Lorain-Elyria	34	8,222	333,574	1,997,322	3,424,591	5,471	9,378	6.0	326,765	515	30,440	979,277	8,124,510
Columbus	13	4,322	219,131	1,026,883	1,654,006	2,814	4,530	4.7	162,177	318	26,575	667,940	3,258,372
Dayton-Springfield	10	2,847	129,678	640,238	1,075,307	1,755	2,946	4.9	108,930	267	13,415	447,253	2,313,548
Hamilton-Middletown	4	620	33,031	132,602	253,984	364	695	4.0	19,661	72	4,298	152,613	456,492
Lima	3	645	28,886	134,355	255,650	368	700	4.7	18,099	66	2,729	113,845	681,710
Mansfield	3	522	19,212	108,318	213,912	297	586	5.6	13,665	51	1,811	95,396	315,345
Parkersburg-Marietta	2	222	8,393	35,900	83,035	98	227	4.3	7,202	21	624	40,483	176,210
Steubenville-Weirton	1	350	13,082	78,344	153,077	215	419	6.0	7,372	17	439	57,705	206,581
Toledo	10	2,517	104,443	567,288	930,829	1,555	2,549	5.4	82,732	163	9,452	329,799	1,807,733
Wheeling	3	278	8,487	69,102	139,199	189	381	8.1	6,804	10	436	28,576	256,884
Youngstown-Warren	7	1,682	76,050	367,612	619,540	1,006	1,698	4.8	53,115	144	6,320	244,478	1,194,315
Wisconsin	120	14,610	579,830	3,396,381	6,765,578	9,302	18,531	5.9	570,553	1,263	65,588	1,833,344	11,612,237
Nonmetropolitan	65	5,156	142,345	1,226,495	2,996,261	3,360	8,206	8.6	125,907	386	14,418	543,208	3,368,498
Metropolitan	55	9,454	437,485	2,169,886	3,769,317	5,942	10,325	5.0	444,646	877	51,170	1,290,136	8,243,739
Appleton-Oshkosh-Neenah	6	779	35,237	150,931	293,240	413	804	4.3	52,184	90	4,979	97,372	411,972
Duluth-Superior	1	31	942	2,961	9,327	8	26	3.1	1,120	0	0	15,831	63,371
Eau Claire	5	608	22,959	121,933	241,258	333	661	5.3	17,085	47	2,209	65,695	392,607
Green Bay	3	554	25,959	113,896	209,823	313	575	4.4	30,275	54	3,722	114,771	507,529
Janesville-Beloit	3	405	14,173	103,756	197,153	284	541	7.3	15,463	33	2,006	59,030	931,659
Kenosha	2	194	10,517	41,064	77,384	113	212	3.9	11,259	31	1,357	80,047	396,292
La Crosse	2	481	22,306	94,448	154,184	259	422	4.2	18,550	46	2,258	41,568	211,597
Madison	4	1,173	55,877	284,136	428,539	779	1,173	5.1	79,348	79	6,603	112,880	869,104
Milwaukee-Waukesha	18	4,058	198,963	985,299	1,654,661	2,697	4,532	5.0	169,332	370	22,071	542,621	3,592,693
Minneapolis-St. Paul	4	125	4,841	15,229	35,483	42	97	3.1	5,112	23	666	15,605	84,312
Racine	3	440	19,506	112,170	220,290	307	603	5.8	15,671	39	2,230	78,303	524,248
Sheboygan	3	391	11,893	83,799	158,051	229	433	7.0	16,719	37	1,669	41,236	170,811
Wausau	1	215	14,312	60,264	89,924	165	246	4.2	12,528	28	1,400	25,177	87,544

TABLE 8

U.S. CENSUS DIVISION 4, EAST NORTH CENTRAL CONTINUED

U.S. Community Hospitals
(Nonfederal, short-term general and other special hospitals)

2002 Utilization, Personnel and Finances

FULL-TIME EQUIVALENT PERSONNEL					FULL-TIME EQUIV. TRAINEES			EXPENSES						
								LABOR				TOTAL		
Physicians and Dentists	Registered Nurses	Licensed Practical Nurses	Other Salaried Personnel	Total Personnel	Medical and Dental Residents	Other Trainees	Total Trainees	Payroll (in thousands)	Employee Benefits (in thousands)	Total (in thousands)	Percent of Total	Amount (in thousands)	Adjusted per Admission	Adjusted per Inpatient Day
4,155	46,274	5,118	133,403	188,950	5,410	233	5,643	8,214,606	1,840,585	10,055,186	52.6	19,132,293	7,281.95	1,425.95
251	5,386	862	16,849	23,348	73	10	83	892,541	236,070	1,128,607	52.7	2,142,120	5,109.98	1,154.36
3,904	40,888	4,256	116,554	165,602	5,337	223	5,560	7,322,065	1,604,515	8,926,579	52.5	16,990,173	7,694.29	1,469.55
250	3,522	484	8,238	12,494	381	0	381	459,330	108,469	567,798	53.6	1,059,007	7,073.77	1,315.94
51	1,951	325	4,533	6,860	93	0	93	282,306	65,033	347,339	53.5	648,978	6,729.83	1,144.87
553	5,223	173	14,515	20,464	854	140	994	827,930	150,872	978,802	47.3	2,068,035	7,139.01	1,491.26
1,789	10,037	1,251	33,534	46,611	1,994	25	2,019	2,444,549	520,376	2,964,923	56.2	5,275,817	9,023.50	1,540.57
854	6,863	339	18,282	26,338	1,094	23	1,117	1,105,963	243,899	1,349,860	48.1	2,808,013	7,899.28	1,697.70
67	4,024	365	12,931	17,387	383	4	387	701,102	146,167	847,268	53.3	1,590,533	7,282.86	1,479.14
2	877	63	2,239	3,181	3	1	4	131,514	24,901	156,417	51.1	306,187	4,784.09	1,205.54
6	901	158	2,507	3,572	2	0	2	141,149	42,146	183,295	54.1	338,555	6,157.34	1,324.29
8	592	151	1,787	2,538	0	0	0	97,894	32,481	130,376	54.3	240,021	6,419.03	1,122.05
2	442	91	628	1,163	4	0	4	44,260	12,628	56,888	53.6	106,079	5,479.30	1,277.52
12	439	37	1,209	1,697	0	0	0	60,639	19,817	80,455	52.9	144,113	5,638.02	941.44
167	3,607	409	9,656	13,839	400	25	425	620,748	142,422	763,172	52.9	1,442,203	8,584.39	1,549.37
21	292	61	785	1,159	0	0	0	37,795	8,632	46,427	55.3	83,990	4,936.24	603.38
122	2,118	349	5,710	8,299	129	5	134	366,887	86,673	453,559	51.6	878,642	6,892.99	1,418.22
1,000	16,680	1,357	55,449	74,486	663	1	664	3,160,456	788,788	3,949,245	49.9	7,917,745	7,210.42	1,170.30
279	3,845	466	13,582	18,172	0	0	0	798,938	198,484	997,422	55.0	1,814,415	5,363.54	605.56
721	12,835	891	41,867	56,314	663	1	664	2,361,518	590,305	2,951,823	48.4	6,103,329	8,032.69	1,619.21
23	795	84	2,915	3,817	0	0	0	177,167	39,437	216,605	52.9	409,129	5,932.25	1,395.20
0	25	5	115	145	0	0	0	6,341	1,263	7,605	60.6	12,542	4,227.26	1,344.73
2	652	44	2,120	2,818	0	0	0	105,889	24,837	130,725	55.9	234,009	5,519.99	969.95
43	1,005	117	2,978	4,143	0	0	0	190,879	41,334	232,213	57.9	401,151	8,205.34	1,911.85
187	613	51	2,175	3,026	18	0	18	85,525	21,995	107,520	37.8	284,395	10,542.53	1,442.51
28	350	52	1,082	1,512	5	1	6	72,456	16,621	89,076	52.8	168,739	8,320.46	2,180.54
147	627	106	2,522	3,402	24	0	24	113,055	35,729	148,784	56.4	263,867	7,277.67	1,711.37
13	1,732	68	5,473	7,286	460	0	460	338,432	98,738	437,171	52.5	833,012	10,105.93	1,943.84
172	5,582	241	17,708	23,703	156	0	156	1,035,368	254,163	1,289,532	44.3	2,914,155	8,646.04	1,761.08
0	111	7	475	593	0	0	0	23,923	4,174	28,097	47.2	59,508	5,230.54	1,677.08
102	708	72	2,111	2,993	0	0	0	97,467	23,713	121,181	51.1	237,011	6,159.18	1,075.91
2	325	27	1,090	1,444	0	0	0	51,407	12,270	63,676	53.1	119,943	5,357.21	758.88
2	310	17	1,103	1,432	0	0	0	63,608	16,031	79,638	48.0	165,869	7,766.84	1,844.54

TABLE 8

U.S. CENSUS DIVISION 5, EAST SOUTH CENTRAL

U.S. Community Hospitals
(Nonfederal, short-term general and other special hospitals)

2002 Utilization, Personnel and Finances

CLASSIFICATION	Hospitals	Beds	Admissions	Inpatient Days	Adjusted Patient Days	Average Daily Census	Adjusted Average Daily Census	Average Stay (days)	Surgical Operations	NEWBORNS Bassinets	Births	OUTPATIENT VISITS Emergency	Total
UNITED STATES	4,927	820,653	34,478,280	196,690,099	322,970,965	539,685	885,994	5.7	27,576,675	59,974	3,870,191	109,951,738	556,404,212
Nonmetropolitan	2,178	171,591	5,382,463	35,210,002	72,269,855	96,579	198,275	6.5	4,598,958	13,757	531,940	23,038,926	114,101,059
Metropolitan	2,749	649,062	29,095,817	161,480,097	250,701,110	443,106	687,719	5.5	22,977,717	46,217	3,338,251	86,912,812	442,303,153
CENSUS DIVISION 5, EAST SOUTH CENTRAL	426	64,591	2,492,114	13,856,950	22,936,323	37,963	62,836	5.6	1,954,497	4,549	224,418	8,643,710	32,639,748
Nonmetropolitan	258	24,574	809,941	4,749,331	8,942,882	13,013	24,499	5.9	614,833	1,742	66,182	3,508,934	11,792,294
Metropolitan	168	40,017	1,682,173	9,107,619	13,993,441	24,950	38,337	5.4	1,339,664	2,807	158,236	5,134,776	20,847,454
Alabama	106	15,935	676,337	3,244,123	4,991,657	8,884	13,671	4.8	517,883	1,394	55,677	2,162,011	10,045,515
Nonmetropolitan	49	3,545	132,466	495,625	969,534	1,356	2,654	3.7	114,416	350	10,303	589,922	2,351,326
Metropolitan	57	12,390	543,871	2,748,498	4,022,123	7,528	11,017	5.1	403,467	1,044	45,374	1,572,089	7,694,189
Anniston	3	447	20,579	88,101	132,678	241	364	4.3	14,353	40	1,953	91,186	240,649
Auburn-Opelika	1	284	16,066	74,590	122,580	204	336	4.6	10,342	36	1,510	40,002	90,137
Birmingham	17	4,358	193,662	1,007,343	1,398,727	2,760	3,831	5.2	148,458	252	12,836	512,160	2,717,380
Decatur	4	558	17,552	73,324	115,681	201	317	4.2	14,014	42	1,971	67,248	283,807
Dothan	3	673	35,308	154,346	241,323	423	661	4.4	22,948	67	2,476	90,364	958,200
Florence	3	577	26,024	121,422	185,689	332	508	4.7	22,109	55	2,086	86,478	213,556
Gadsden	2	529	20,216	96,218	132,172	264	362	4.8	17,155	47	1,266	54,647	289,093
Huntsville	4	988	47,300	233,300	373,736	638	1,025	4.9	37,345	113	5,553	159,434	680,494
Mobile	10	2,353	83,558	472,604	698,860	1,295	1,913	5.7	61,476	248	7,653	227,567	1,316,506
Montgomery	8	1,040	47,208	237,049	368,789	649	1,010	5.0	34,823	100	5,241	131,054	492,794
Tuscaloosa	2	583	36,398	190,201	251,888	521	690	5.2	20,444	44	2,829	111,949	411,573
Kentucky	104	15,066	601,644	3,393,525	5,849,808	9,294	16,030	5.6	543,125	1,023	52,098	2,109,556	8,646,112
Nonmetropolitan	72	7,742	275,107	1,583,846	2,962,985	4,336	8,118	5.8	218,307	539	21,068	1,077,559	4,701,898
Metropolitan	32	7,324	326,537	1,809,679	2,886,823	4,958	7,912	5.5	324,818	484	31,030	1,031,997	3,944,214
Cincinnati	5	905	43,927	207,226	359,585	567	986	4.7	28,330	77	4,870	194,561	689,989
Clarksville-Hopkinsville	1	139	6,104	26,693	55,041	73	151	4.4	5,390	18	619	24,467	82,824
Evansville-Henderson	1	209	8,116	37,273	58,695	102	161	4.6	10,613	12	790	31,327	155,361
Huntington-Ashland	2	738	28,668	142,118	225,292	389	617	5.0	33,775	29	1,607	95,468	341,081
Lexington	12	1,987	82,496	471,805	764,802	1,293	2,097	5.7	82,086	129	8,418	238,911	1,103,679
Louisville	10	3,001	137,038	835,165	1,285,197	2,289	3,521	6.1	144,401	185	12,882	367,000	1,305,957
Owensboro	1	345	20,188	89,399	138,211	245	379	4.4	20,223	34	1,844	80,263	265,323
Mississippi	91	13,144	416,815	2,745,516	4,505,180	7,522	12,339	6.6	273,882	832	39,553	1,556,488	3,996,380
Nonmetropolitan	73	7,899	229,213	1,638,570	2,847,223	4,491	7,798	7.1	139,792	495	20,633	980,925	2,212,951
Metropolitan	18	5,245	187,602	1,106,946	1,657,957	3,031	4,541	5.9	134,090	337	18,920	575,563	1,783,429
Biloxi-Gulfport-Pascagoula	6	1,380	51,658	274,673	437,360	752	1,198	5.3	46,017	129	4,321	204,089	873,295
Hattiesburg	2	748	33,759	173,451	261,873	475	717	5.1	16,498	35	3,597	114,545	198,452
Jackson	9	2,798	92,065	567,773	830,473	1,555	2,275	6.2	66,546	140	9,450	241,842	637,020
Memphis	1	319	10,120	91,049	128,251	249	351	9.0	5,029	33	1,552	15,087	74,662
Tennessee	125	20,446	797,318	4,473,786	7,589,678	12,263	20,796	5.6	619,607	1,300	77,090	2,815,655	9,951,741
Nonmetropolitan	64	5,388	173,155	1,031,290	2,163,140	2,830	5,929	6.0	142,318	358	14,178	860,528	2,526,119
Metropolitan	61	15,058	624,163	3,442,496	5,426,538	9,433	14,867	5.5	477,289	942	62,912	1,955,127	7,425,622
Chattanooga	6	1,594	65,253	336,716	523,247	922	1,434	5.2	59,314	59	5,679	207,066	780,204
Clarksville-Hopkinsville	1	201	9,834	40,700	79,806	112	219	4.1	5,855	16	1,452	45,564	151,331
Jackson	2	747	28,452	168,648	273,622	462	750	5.9	19,467	42	3,362	78,242	184,845
Johnson City-Kingsport-Bristol	11	2,016	68,027	376,801	607,790	1,034	1,666	5.5	47,578	136	5,272	272,520	977,809
Knoxville	10	2,617	109,088	581,439	961,384	1,592	2,634	5.3	93,688	164	11,287	399,153	1,507,428
Memphis	13	3,573	151,925	967,580	1,397,428	2,653	3,828	6.4	93,291	231	17,089	436,554	1,360,644
Nashville	18	4,310	191,584	970,612	1,583,261	2,658	4,336	5.1	158,096	294	18,771	516,028	2,463,361

TABLE 8

U.S. CENSUS DIVISION 5, EAST SOUTH CENTRAL

U.S. Community Hospitals
(Nonfederal, short-term general and other special hospitals)

2002 Utilization, Personnel and Finances

FULL-TIME EQUIVALENT PERSONNEL					FULL-TIME EQUIV. TRAINEES			EXPENSES						
								LABOR				TOTAL		
Physicians and Dentists	Registered Nurses	Licensed Practical Nurses	Other Salaried Personnel	Total Personnel	Medical and Dental Residents	Other Trainees	Total Trainees	Payroll (in thousands)	Employee Benefits (in thousands)	Total (in thousands)	Percent of Total	Amount (in thousands)	Adjusted per Admission	Adjusted per inpatient Day
72,823	988,139	125,865	2,882,668	4,069,495	78,715	5,463	84,178	$175,961,479	$40,049,573	$216,011,067	51.9	$416,591,059	$7,354.60	$1,289.87
8,448	145,133	36,374	479,821	669,776	1,763	161	1,924	24,016,766	5,768,570	29,785,337	53.7	55,454,326	5,047.87	767.32
64,375	843,006	89,491	2,402,847	3,399,719	76,952	5,302	82,254	151,944,713	34,281,003	186,225,730	51.6	361,136,733	7,909.61	1,440.51
1,934	67,378	12,482	188,115	269,909	2,521	406	2,927	9,772,024	2,220,851	11,992,884	49.4	24,262,442	5,841.99	1,057.82
837	18,156	5,513	57,700	82,206	101	12	113	2,725,572	671,901	3,397,480	51.6	6,585,720	4,278.92	736.42
1,097	49,222	6,969	130,415	187,703	2,420	394	2,814	7,046,451	1,548,950	8,595,404	48.6	17,676,722	6,762.33	1,263.21
465	18,022	3,054	47,839	69,380	1,064	33	1,097	2,383,083	530,256	2,913,344	50.5	5,767,179	5,399.64	1,155.36
72	2,555	614	7,452	10,693	9	2	11	348,191	87,269	435,460	51.6	844,087	3,237.66	870.61
393	15,467	2,440	40,387	58,687	1,055	31	1,086	2,034,892	442,987	2,477,884	50.3	4,923,093	6,097.77	1,224.00
2	516	92	1,120	1,730	13	0	13	58,765	13,423	72,189	53.7	134,360	4,332.25	1,012.68
7	400	48	1,382	1,837	0	0	0	62,879	12,187	75,067	50.7	148,194	5,612.77	1,208.96
108	5,753	807	14,741	21,409	612	0	612	804,918	167,054	971,973	48.1	2,020,729	7,305.02	1,444.69
13	433	91	1,267	1,804	47	2	49	67,915	15,936	83,852	50.2	166,959	6,020.00	1,443.27
22	778	254	2,492	3,546	5	0	5	120,996	23,616	144,613	52.6	274,674	4,948.90	1,138.20
22	638	142	1,977	2,779	23	0	23	68,828	21,301	90,129	54.2	166,332	4,147.00	895.76
5	490	66	1,077	1,638	7	0	7	58,450	12,074	70,524	45.9	153,769	5,537.22	1,163.40
37	1,371	190	3,299	4,897	1	0	1	199,747	53,124	252,871	53.1	476,319	6,241.00	1,274.48
89	2,717	357	6,475	9,638	292	4	296	303,163	67,977	371,141	53.2	697,816	5,700.41	998.51
82	1,576	222	4,351	6,231	55	5	60	162,786	34,230	197,017	48.6	405,425	5,393.87	1,099.34
6	795	171	2,206	3,178	0	20	20	126,444	22,064	148,508	53.3	278,516	5,765.78	1,105.71
565	16,402	2,722	46,563	66,252	134	23	157	2,480,637	553,535	3,034,172	48.9	6,201,408	5,892.33	1,060.10
343	6,454	1,699	20,369	28,865	86	8	94	997,467	242,493	1,239,960	51.2	2,423,309	4,616.62	817.86
222	9,948	1,023	26,194	37,387	48	15	63	1,483,171	311,042	1,794,212	47.5	3,778,099	7,161.68	1,308.74
57	1,201	137	2,735	4,130	24	15	39	192,600	40,225	232,826	53.1	438,327	5,634.39	1,218.98
0	151	44	382	577	0	0	0	19,807	4,526	24,333	40.6	59,864	4,756.43	1,087.63
24	342	38	1,050	1,454	13	0	13	29,914	6,841	36,759	52.4	70,091	5,484.40	1,194.15
32	719	144	1,888	2,783	8	0	8	116,645	30,915	147,560	49.4	298,525	6,568.79	1,325.06
24	3,078	219	6,540	9,861	3	0	3	391,195	79,404	470,599	46.7	1,008,529	7,431.61	1,318.68
80	3,893	382	12,350	16,705	0	0	0	664,296	134,450	798,746	46.0	1,736,504	8,190.36	1,351.16
5	564	59	1,249	1,877	0	0	0	68,709	14,680	83,389	50.2	166,258	5,326.90	1,202.93
408	11,045	2,233	31,790	45,476	364	2	366	1,592,376	376,165	1,968,543	50.4	3,907,204	5,755.57	867.27
330	5,308	1,595	17,282	24,515	1	0	1	810,505	199,635	1,010,142	51.2	1,973,009	5,001.40	692.96
78	5,737	638	14,508	20,961	363	2	365	781,871	176,531	958,401	49.6	1,934,195	6,801.80	1,166.61
21	1,738	111	3,830	5,700	0	0	0	229,956	52,248	282,204	50.9	554,286	6,724.41	1,267.35
26	897	122	2,538	3,583	0	0	0	123,424	34,975	158,399	47.7	332,090	6,526.66	1,268.13
31	2,864	346	7,494	10,735	363	0	363	394,724	81,423	476,147	49.6	960,817	7,023.56	1,156.95
0	238	59	646	943	0	2	2	33,767	7,884	41,651	47.9	87,002	6,103.29	678.38
496	21,909	4,473	61,923	88,801	959	348	1,307	3,315,928	760,896	4,076,825	48.6	8,386,650	6,195.21	1,105.01
92	3,839	1,605	12,597	18,133	5	2	7	569,410	142,505	711,918	52.9	1,345,314	3,747.40	621.93
404	18,070	2,868	49,326	70,668	954	346	1,300	2,746,518	618,390	3,364,907	47.8	7,041,336	7,078.63	1,297.57
38	2,039	238	5,707	8,022	136	0	136	304,463	69,863	374,325	49.5	755,502	7,337.17	1,443.87
2	219	68	690	979	0	0	0	37,909	8,300	46,209	54.8	84,390	4,376.41	1,057.44
30	714	208	2,927	3,879	3	0	3	133,572	33,042	166,614	51.3	324,484	7,016.01	1,185.88
2	1,910	366	4,868	7,146	0	16	16	265,179	60,831	326,008	46.2	705,564	6,219.27	1,160.87
112	2,863	479	9,584	13,038	112	4	116	474,239	113,801	588,042	47.8	1,228,937	6,937.23	1,278.30
38	4,808	696	11,311	16,853	120	315	435	670,243	142,941	813,182	46.5	1,748,814	7,958.09	1,251.45
182	5,517	813	14,239	20,751	583	11	594	860,915	189,611	1,050,527	47.9	2,193,645	6,944.57	1,385.52

MSAs

2002 Utilization, Personnel and Finances

CLASSIFICATION	Hospitals	Beds	Admissions	Inpatient Days	Adjusted Patient Days	Average Daily Census	Adjusted Average Daily Census	Average Stay (days)	Surgical Operations	NEWBORNS Bassinets	NEWBORNS Births	OUTPATIENT VISITS Emergency	OUTPATIENT VISITS Total
UNITED STATES	4,927	820,653	34,478,280	196,690,099	322,970,965	539,685	885,994	5.7	27,576,675	59,974	3,870,191	109,951,738	556,404,212
Nonmetropolitan	2,178	171,591	5,382,463	35,210,002	72,269,855	96,579	198,275	6.5	4,598,958	13,757	531,940	23,038,926	114,101,059
Metropolitan	2,749	649,062	29,095,817	161,480,097	250,701,110	443,106	687,719	5.5	22,977,717	46,217	3,338,251	86,912,812	442,303,153
CENSUS DIVISION 6, WEST NORTH CENTRAL	679	74,277	2,509,141	16,581,836	30,354,532	45,577	83,423	6.6	2,190,501	5,246	261,872	7,108,385	45,699,586
Nonmetropolitan	499	32,865	733,849	6,845,933	14,607,048	18,843	40,209	9.3	648,721	2,562	73,533	2,631,463	18,436,881
Metropolitan	180	41,412	1,775,292	9,735,903	15,747,484	26,734	43,214	5.5	1,541,780	2,684	188,339	4,476,922	27,262,705
Iowa	116	11,267	370,968	2,447,672	4,997,646	6,716	13,704	6.6	409,982	793	37,342	1,072,319	9,330,676
Nonmetropolitan	95	5,834	144,482	1,234,870	2,936,294	3,389	8,045	8.5	150,455	428	12,665	500,279	4,212,384
Metropolitan	21	5,433	226,486	1,212,802	2,061,352	3,327	5,659	5.4	259,527	365	24,677	572,040	5,118,292
Cedar Rapids	2	729	27,308	155,363	291,712	426	799	5.7	37,562	55	3,401	87,995	588,091
Davenport-Moline-Rock Island	2	525	21,352	115,243	180,638	315	495	5.4	13,775	32	2,529	64,265	221,349
Des Moines	6	1,441	69,248	349,712	540,466	963	1,493	5.1	50,288	111	8,601	170,431	1,577,559
Dubuque	2	509	15,599	85,127	143,598	234	393	5.5	16,378	42	1,596	45,442	128,959
Iowa City	2	880	32,052	221,101	359,866	606	986	6.9	86,324	38	2,662	55,063	1,034,596
Omaha	2	319	12,299	58,497	101,940	160	279	4.8	13,874	22	1,100	40,994	154,211
Sioux City	2	469	23,549	114,086	176,813	312	485	4.8	17,712	30	2,508	49,110	445,390
Waterloo-Cedar Falls	3	561	25,079	113,673	266,319	311	729	4.5	23,614	35	2,280	58,740	968,137
Kansas	132	10,850	328,987	2,165,195	3,995,790	5,954	10,991	6.6	244,669	789	38,591	940,408	5,675,015
Nonmetropolitan	107	6,043	132,173	1,133,053	2,367,521	3,126	6,530	8.6	97,919	501	11,932	410,150	3,007,946
Metropolitan	25	4,807	196,814	1,032,142	1,628,269	2,828	4,461	5.2	146,750	288	26,659	530,258	2,667,069
Kansas City	12	2,031	84,288	423,484	694,982	1,160	1,902	5.0	74,710	161	12,790	228,848	1,313,585
Lawrence	1	102	7,112	29,990	75,546	82	207	4.2	4,718	13	1,076	28,204	148,275
Topeka	3	659	25,425	122,356	225,006	335	617	4.8	20,449	36	3,129	85,668	427,492
Wichita	9	2,015	79,989	456,312	632,735	1,251	1,735	5.7	46,873	78	9,664	187,538	777,717
Minnesota	133	16,659	598,852	4,162,994	7,622,091	11,397	20,884	7.0	458,224	1,334	68,220	1,605,237	8,901,898
Nonmetropolitan	87	6,957	126,920	1,660,408	3,515,289	4,544	9,633	13.1	117,588	491	16,855	508,266	2,965,501
Metropolitan	46	9,702	471,932	2,502,586	4,106,802	6,853	11,251	5.3	340,636	843	51,365	1,096,971	5,936,397
Duluth-Superior	8	1,229	43,056	312,608	530,396	856	1,452	7.3	40,119	89	3,387	100,719	465,479
Grand Forks	2	289	2,530	76,279	244,045	209	669	30.1	1,785	17	175	3,390	68,938
Minneapolis-St. Paul	28	6,023	330,233	1,485,480	2,338,021	4,068	6,406	4.5	246,190	633	42,976	829,524	4,479,327
Rochester	3	1,195	71,364	354,876	520,400	972	1,426	5.0	37,753	47	2,254	96,401	516,970
St. Cloud	5	966	24,749	273,343	473,940	748	1,298	11.0	14,789	57	2,573	66,937	405,683
Missouri	119	18,891	809,355	4,235,298	7,294,584	11,649	20,061	5.2	603,500	1,241	74,815	2,476,194	14,904,088
Nonmetropolitan	58	4,483	173,350	872,274	1,825,829	2,403	5,030	5.0	134,751	430	15,497	741,381	4,687,438
Metropolitan	61	14,408	636,005	3,363,024	5,468,755	9,246	15,031	5.3	468,749	811	59,318	1,734,813	10,216,650
Columbia	4	923	34,431	194,063	293,747	532	804	5.6	33,721	46	3,197	61,026	808,850
Joplin	4	764	36,887	175,298	307,735	479	844	4.8	23,395	52	3,637	138,838	779,509
Kansas City	21	3,611	154,118	874,082	1,461,956	2,397	4,006	5.7	112,212	212	15,852	517,706	2,385,778
Springfield	3	1,380	58,974	285,720	458,257	784	1,256	4.8	48,841	78	5,767	160,699	1,623,124
St. Joseph	1	460	17,300	70,058	110,231	192	302	4.0	7,034	20	1,491	43,794	486,296
St. Louis	28	7,270	334,295	1,763,803	2,836,829	4,862	7,819	5.3	243,546	403	29,374	812,750	4,133,093
Nebraska	86	8,106	206,208	1,723,683	3,098,166	4,730	8,519	8.4	203,137	617	24,030	511,085	3,467,037
Nonmetropolitan	72	4,130	82,272	783,757	1,679,569	2,156	4,633	9.5	88,749	395	9,191	226,369	1,846,521
Metropolitan	14	3,976	123,936	939,926	1,418,597	2,574	3,886	7.6	114,388	222	14,839	284,716	1,620,516
Lincoln	3	1,080	37,993	246,752	319,136	675	874	6.5	27,471	72	4,473	84,731	379,292
Omaha	11	2,896	85,943	693,174	1,099,461	1,899	3,012	8.1	86,917	150	10,366	199,985	1,241,224
North Dakota	42	3,880	94,630	845,194	1,640,386	2,331	4,519	8.9	75,863	229	9,337	295,074	1,916,774
Nonmetropolitan	35	2,329	32,381	496,367	1,030,570	1,375	2,849	15.3	27,883	124	3,281	130,974	808,758
Metropolitan	7	1,551	62,249	348,827	609,816	956	1,670	5.6	47,980	105	6,056	164,100	1,108,016
Bismarck	2	509	18,511	94,010	183,524	257	503	5.1	17,791	15	1,620	32,722	629,819
Fargo-Moorhead	3	692	31,898	168,590	245,098	462	671	5.3	20,821	66	3,100	95,846	394,281
Grand Forks	2	350	11,840	86,227	181,194	237	496	7.3	9,368	24	1,336	35,532	83,916
South Dakota	51	4,624	100,141	1,001,800	1,705,869	2,800	4,745	10.0	195,126	243	9,537	208,068	1,504,098
Nonmetropolitan	45	3,089	42,271	665,204	1,251,976	1,850	3,489	15.7	31,376	193	4,112	114,044	908,333
Metropolitan	6	1,535	57,870	336,596	453,893	950	1,256	5.8	163,750	50	5,425	94,024	595,765
Rapid City	1	372	16,866	87,715	126,558	240	347	5.2	8,130	12	1,919	43,237	153,564
Sioux Falls	5	1,163	41,004	248,881	327,335	710	909	6.1	155,620	38	3,506	50,787	442,201

MSAs

TABLE 8

U.S. CENSUS DIVISION 6, WEST NORTH CENTRAL

U.S. Community Hospitals
(Nonfederal, short-term general and other special hospitals)

2002 Utilization, Personnel and Finances

FULL-TIME EQUIVALENT PERSONNEL					FULL-TIME EQUIV. TRAINEES			EXPENSES						
								LABOR				TOTAL		
Physicians and Dentists	Registered Nurses	Licensed Practical Nurses	Other Salaried Personnel	Total Personnel	Medical and Dental Residents	Other Trainees	Total Trainees	Payroll (in thousands)	Employee Benefits (in thousands)	Total (in thousands)	Percent of Total	Amount (in thousands)	Adjusted per Admission	Adjusted per Inpatient Day
72,823	988,139	125,865	2,882,668	4,069,495	78,715	5,463	84,178	$175,961,479	$40,049,573	$216,011,067	51.9	$416,591,059	$7,354.60	$1,289.87
8,448	145,133	36,374	479,821	669,776	1,763	161	1,924	24,016,766	5,768,570	29,785,337	53.7	55,454,326	5,047.87	767.32
64,375	843,006	89,491	2,402,847	3,399,719	76,952	5,302	82,254	151,944,713	34,281,003	186,225,730	51.6	361,136,733	7,909.61	1,440.51
5,369	78,817	11,582	237,072	332,840	3,156	182	3,338	13,492,674	2,910,218	16,402,885	52.7	31,131,082	6,992.48	1,025.58
1,600	22,865	6,133	79,880	110,478	99	14	113	3,690,794	808,800	4,499,586	54.6	8,234,243	5,194.14	563.72
3,769	55,952	5,449	157,192	222,362	3,057	168	3,225	9,801,880	2,101,417	11,903,299	52.0	22,896,838	7,986.94	1,454.00
823	12,666	1,417	38,524	53,430	548	24	572	1,940,204	455,218	2,395,423	53.4	4,483,595	6,141.42	897.14
251	4,879	821	16,181	22,132	22	0	22	706,800	160,552	867,352	54.1	1,603,574	4,682.34	546.12
572	7,787	596	22,343	31,298	526	24	550	1,233,404	294,666	1,528,071	53.1	2,880,021	7,430.68	1,397.15
4	967	98	2,363	3,432	0	16	16	123,099	30,043	153,143	51.5	297,607	5,872.63	1,020.21
2	613	36	1,676	2,327	7	0	7	91,933	20,923	112,856	46.2	244,092	7,257.73	1,351.28
290	2,376	92	6,990	9,748	153	0	153	385,195	84,077	469,273	54.7	858,586	7,957.10	1,588.60
14	568	36	1,257	1,875	0	0	0	64,788	13,216	78,004	50.5	154,400	5,686.51	1,075.22
78	1,514	32	4,376	6,000	363	8	371	265,763	81,845	347,608	53.4	651,165	12,437.72	1,809.46
7	336	34	871	1,248	0	0	0	54,664	11,089	65,753	53.3	123,290	5,755.01	1,209.43
73	686	81	2,236	3,076	0	0	0	115,209	26,618	141,827	54.2	261,767	7,105.52	1,480.48
104	727	187	2,574	3,592	3	0	3	132,753	26,854	159,607	55.2	289,114	5,018.90	1,085.59
551	9,640	1,411	29,193	40,795	130	16	146	1,582,427	311,390	1,893,818	53.0	3,576,366	6,171.61	895.03
184	3,843	844	13,396	18,267	9	14	23	601,654	121,751	723,406	55.8	1,295,857	4,930.68	547.35
367	5,797	567	15,797	22,528	121	2	123	980,773	189,639	1,170,412	51.3	2,280,509	7,201.49	1,400.57
132	2,723	119	6,570	9,544	0	2	2	427,693	83,662	511,355	50.2	1,018,576	7,322.57	1,465.62
15	203	29	636	883	0	0	0	37,017	6,820	43,837	53.4	82,163	4,586.30	1,087.60
152	973	277	2,884	4,286	0	0	0	180,272	31,164	211,435	58.6	361,016	7,432.13	1,604.47
68	1,898	142	5,707	7,815	121	0	121	335,792	67,992	403,785	49.3	818,754	7,370.78	1,293.99
1,220	17,067	2,602	51,989	72,878	657	51	708	3,579,760	809,980	4,389,741	55.7	7,883,927	7,671.84	1,034.35
322	3,876	1,395	14,954	20,547	15	0	15	745,631	170,160	915,792	56.8	1,612,386	5,749.88	458.68
898	13,191	1,207	37,035	52,331	642	51	693	2,834,129	639,820	3,473,949	55.4	6,271,541	8,393.12	1,527.11
94	1,088	266	3,908	5,356	2	0	2	241,111	60,612	301,722	58.1	519,352	7,461.85	979.18
2	83	63	379	527	0	0	0	17,358	3,711	21,069	63.4	33,253	4,151.45	136.26
590	9,460	631	26,279	36,960	443	25	468	2,110,192	472,401	2,582,595	55.8	4,627,012	8,805.25	1,979.00
127	1,722	137	3,986	5,972	94	19	113	330,908	73,731	404,638	52.0	777,566	7,367.50	1,494.17
85	838	110	2,483	3,516	103	7	110	134,560	29,365	163,925	52.1	314,358	8,146.10	663.29
1,718	24,945	3,630	71,532	101,825	1,679	66	1,745	3,992,276	841,950	4,834,221	49.6	9,747,671	7,017.15	1,336.29
441	4,723	1,555	15,596	22,315	40	0	40	758,073	167,611	925,680	51.1	1,811,207	5,034.59	991.99
1,277	20,222	2,075	55,936	79,510	1,639	66	1,705	3,234,202	674,339	3,908,541	49.2	7,936,463	7,710.03	1,451.24
31	1,263	276	3,953	5,523	332	0	332	189,087	40,599	229,686	43.1	532,802	10,042.07	1,813.81
185	1,099	192	3,275	4,751	7	0	7	206,978	41,839	248,817	56.4	441,217	6,832.85	1,433.76
222	5,139	441	13,251	19,053	158	52	210	834,670	158,019	992,689	50.4	1,970,605	8,020.31	1,347.92
145	1,961	222	7,670	9,998	24	1	25	214,801	78,424	293,225	37.8	776,026	8,228.99	1,693.43
54	516	157	1,512	2,239	0	0	0	112,179	24,367	136,546	58.4	233,640	8,583.39	2,119.55
640	10,244	787	26,275	37,946	1,118	13	1,131	1,676,487	331,091	2,007,578	50.4	3,982,172	7,313.29	1,403.74
359	7,629	1,331	22,440	31,759	69	25	94	1,220,798	269,049	1,489,849	51.5	2,892,566	7,823.05	933.64
171	2,940	833	9,742	13,686	11	0	11	451,594	102,983	554,578	54.1	1,025,488	5,755.25	610.57
188	4,689	498	12,698	18,073	58	25	83	769,204	166,066	935,271	50.1	1,867,078	9,746.40	1,316.14
52	1,422	241	4,174	5,889	0	0	0	218,336	51,798	270,133	53.1	508,546	9,640.86	1,593.51
136	3,267	257	8,524	12,184	58	25	83	550,868	114,268	665,138	49.0	1,358,532	9,786.50	1,235.63
500	3,109	826	11,871	16,306	54	0	54	633,851	113,733	747,582	55.3	1,351,763	7,147.61	824.05
167	1,155	442	5,022	6,786	0	0	0	214,089	38,282	252,369	58.3	433,124	5,660.86	420.28
333	1,954	384	6,849	9,520	54	0	54	419,762	75,451	495,213	53.9	918,639	8,157.78	1,506.42
144	585	135	2,103	2,967	0	0	0	139,676	18,679	158,354	55.8	283,890	7,857.90	1,546.88
4	1,009	184	2,689	3,886	54	0	54	144,821	31,302	176,123	45.9	383,670	8,298.08	1,565.37
185	360	65	2,057	2,667	0	0	0	135,266	25,470	160,736	64.0	251,079	8,301.50	1,385.69
198	3,761	365	11,523	15,847	19	0	19	543,359	108,897	652,251	54.6	1,195,194	7,161.18	700.64
64	1,449	243	4,989	6,745	2	0	2	212,953	47,462	260,409	57.5	452,606	5,316.21	361.51
134	2,312	122	6,534	9,102	17	0	17	330,406	61,436	391,842	52.8	742,587	9,082.30	1,636.04
9	663	78	1,984	2,734	17	0	17	95,924	11,420	107,344	49.8	215,617	8,860.35	1,703.70
125	1,649	44	4,550	6,368	0	0	0	234,481	50,016	284,498	54.0	526,971	9,176.36	1,609.88

MSAs

TABLE 8

U.S. CENSUS DIVISION 7, WEST SOUTH CENTRAL

U.S. Community Hospitals
(Nonfederal, short-term general and other special hospitals)

2002 Utilization, Personnel and Finances

CLASSIFICATION	Hospitals	Beds	Admissions	Inpatient Days	Adjusted Patient Days	Average Daily Census	Adjusted Average Daily Census	Average Stay (days)	Surgical Operations	NEWBORNS Bassinets	Births	OUTPATIENT VISITS Emergency	Total
UNITED STATES	4,927	820,653	34,478,280	196,690,099	322,970,965	539,685	885,994	5.7	27,576,675	59,974	3,870,191	109,951,738	556,404,212
Nonmetropolitan	2,178	171,591	5,382,463	35,210,002	72,269,855	96,579	198,275	6.5	4,598,958	13,757	531,940	23,038,926	114,101,059
Metropolitan	2,749	649,062	29,095,817	161,480,097	250,701,110	443,106	687,719	5.5	22,977,717	46,217	3,338,251	86,912,812	442,303,153
CENSUS DIVISION 7, WEST SOUTH CENTRAL	736	95,764	4,055,293	21,541,966	33,588,503	59,164	92,220	5.3	2,875,702	7,737	510,996	13,229,179	53,875,529
Nonmetropolitan	335	19,141	671,156	3,286,305	6,176,892	9,014	16,949	4.9	415,212	1,571	59,560	2,709,859	11,563,553
Metropolitan	401	76,623	3,384,137	18,255,661	27,411,611	50,150	75,271	5.4	2,460,490	6,166	451,436	10,519,320	42,311,976
Arkansas	87	9,942	383,509	2,110,323	3,469,990	5,779	9,510	5.5	278,792	771	38,191	1,224,053	4,838,504
Nonmetropolitan	56	4,335	146,399	821,033	1,509,327	2,247	4,139	5.6	94,294	318	12,167	543,857	2,277,162
Metropolitan	31	5,607	237,110	1,289,290	1,960,663	3,532	5,371	5.4	184,498	453	26,024	680,196	2,561,342
Fayetteville-Springdale-Rogers	8	840	39,432	177,049	272,936	484	748	4.5	26,643	83	5,989	148,072	250,625
Fort Smith	4	870	36,689	204,534	284,188	561	778	5.6	43,905	67	3,581	121,725	273,585
Jonesboro	3	479	22,390	125,707	202,347	344	554	5.6	16,710	32	2,071	58,626	249,798
Little Rock-North Little Rock	14	2,922	121,040	689,167	1,060,295	1,889	2,905	5.7	84,947	235	12,361	294,315	1,584,864
Memphis	1	119	4,521	20,594	28,094	56	77	4.6	5,487	11	675	21,808	42,192
Pine Bluff	1	377	13,038	72,239	112,803	198	309	5.5	6,806	25	1,347	35,650	160,278
Louisiana	128	17,867	692,011	3,873,634	6,047,704	10,618	16,570	5.6	467,940	1,231	57,564	2,468,832	10,731,627
Nonmetropolitan	51	2,974	106,789	557,596	1,004,740	1,531	2,753	5.2	65,080	166	6,952	498,165	1,564,203
Metropolitan	77	14,893	585,222	3,316,038	5,042,964	9,087	13,817	5.7	402,860	1,065	50,612	1,970,667	9,167,424
Alexandria	5	705	34,483	177,574	281,543	486	772	5.1	21,612	65	3,199	131,521	389,070
Baton Rouge	9	1,918	81,460	465,540	713,805	1,276	1,955	5.7	60,511	119	9,703	262,772	846,952
Houma	5	699	30,492	136,690	245,326	375	673	4.5	24,939	69	3,392	127,732	422,379
Lafayette	13	1,562	58,275	315,766	503,180	867	1,379	5.4	51,319	142	4,852	225,372	728,645
Lake Charles	6	960	33,054	164,552	280,103	451	766	5.0	22,256	65	2,720	119,954	419,899
Monroe	5	981	42,864	243,143	338,135	667	926	5.7	22,082	101	3,467	119,586	419,288
New Orleans	24	5,729	215,186	1,294,635	1,933,154	3,546	5,296	6.0	142,981	354	18,712	785,622	4,821,194
Shreveport-Bossier City	10	2,339	89,408	518,138	747,718	1,419	2,050	5.8	57,160	150	4,567	198,108	1,119,997
Oklahoma	105	11,122	445,952	2,371,009	3,745,249	6,496	10,264	5.3	282,800	833	43,564	1,292,652	4,802,763
Nonmetropolitan	67	4,100	140,577	711,725	1,314,860	1,949	3,604	5.1	87,166	374	12,725	474,010	1,617,117
Metropolitan	38	7,022	305,375	1,659,284	2,430,389	4,547	6,660	5.4	195,634	459	30,839	818,642	3,185,646
Enid	2	332	12,673	81,294	125,087	223	343	6.4	6,092	16	928	26,181	107,733
Fort Smith	1	25	620	2,325	12,369	6	34	3.8	277	1	4	15,240	15,499
Lawton	2	440	14,513	84,031	149,035	230	409	5.8	10,256	37	1,462	50,125	166,292
Oklahoma City	18	3,598	160,316	860,707	1,231,785	2,360	3,375	5.4	98,592	256	15,653	454,503	1,644,776
Tulsa	15	2,627	117,253	630,927	912,113	1,728	2,499	5.4	80,417	149	12,792	272,593	1,251,346
Texas	416	56,833	2,533,821	13,187,000	20,325,560	36,271	55,876	5.2	1,846,170	4,902	371,677	8,243,642	33,502,635
Nonmetropolitan	161	7,732	277,391	1,195,951	2,347,965	3,287	6,453	4.3	168,672	713	27,716	1,193,827	6,105,071
Metropolitan	255	49,101	2,256,430	11,991,049	17,977,595	32,984	49,423	5.3	1,677,498	4,189	343,961	7,049,815	27,397,564
Abilene	2	533	22,713	120,156	189,082	329	519	5.3	14,108	46	2,696	67,907	321,394
Amarillo	4	856	42,067	222,947	318,064	610	871	5.3	29,625	54	4,467	102,514	343,395
Austin-San Marcos	15	2,402	107,078	585,323	951,820	1,603	2,607	5.5	91,204	242	23,074	465,618	1,261,837
Beaumont-Port Arthur	10	1,413	61,261	333,067	491,204	912	1,346	5.4	38,122	90	5,204	151,729	624,773
Brazoria	3	234	9,199	33,108	82,741	91	227	3.6	8,813	32	1,266	52,113	171,668
Brownsville-Harlingen-San Benito	5	895	49,917	228,780	313,513	626	858	4.6	25,457	89	9,404	98,846	300,569
Bryan-College Station	2	402	20,136	94,901	143,474	260	393	4.7	15,293	60	3,360	64,539	260,415
Corpus Christi	7	1,169	52,993	280,304	411,371	768	1,127	5.3	35,824	110	7,084	155,673	557,748
Dallas	46	8,094	386,923	1,993,204	2,976,877	5,462	8,152	5.2	287,332	749	66,514	1,331,030	4,752,347
El Paso	8	1,680	75,240	374,995	561,647	1,027	1,539	5.0	39,897	204	14,882	229,340	1,173,987
Fort Worth-Arlington	24	3,774	177,740	943,012	1,441,582	2,688	4,099	5.3	147,732	378	29,990	694,525	2,115,262
Galveston-Texas City	3	974	40,958	227,587	374,303	624	1,026	5.6	31,456	48	6,187	104,945	955,666
Houston	53	11,271	506,686	2,834,117	4,149,517	7,791	11,391	5.6	375,410	935	77,755	1,422,261	6,234,060
Killeen-Temple	4	890	35,095	183,721	429,107	504	1,176	5.2	28,219	40	3,786	115,897	1,788,688
Laredo	2	604	24,532	123,302	188,342	338	516	5.0	16,545	85	6,679	64,795	248,278
Longview-Marshall	4	686	31,282	140,102	228,448	385	627	4.5	18,496	68	3,593	131,853	341,041
Lubbock	6	1,710	75,021	427,121	613,732	1,170	1,681	5.7	49,336	65	6,581	217,885	1,122,559
McAllen-Edinburg-Mission	7	1,332	76,258	387,145	497,013	1,059	1,362	5.1	38,063	109	15,142	109,597	343,164
Odessa-Midland	4	806	32,549	173,034	255,306	475	700	5.3	31,824	80	5,364	116,276	362,551
San Angelo	2	375	18,555	84,982	141,742	233	388	4.6	18,051	39	2,013	61,580	184,658
San Antonio	23	4,973	241,801	1,243,410	1,788,719	3,407	4,900	5.1	212,361	415	33,019	681,788	1,942,075
Sherman-Denison	3	590	27,274	144,634	221,221	396	607	5.3	15,118	46	2,300	174,945	348,285
Texarkana	5	684	28,627	170,934	241,727	469	663	6.0	13,974	50	2,385	100,062	294,480
Tyler	5	923	45,996	247,691	359,814	679	985	5.4	29,626	49	3,384	126,835	636,607
Victoria	2	638	21,352	104,921	158,475	288	434	4.9	18,900	43	2,096	50,842	201,938
Waco	2	722	26,342	186,000	289,403	509	793	7.1	25,495	51	3,476	86,146	341,074
Wichita Falls	4	471	18,656	102,551	159,351	281	436	5.5	21,217	12	2,260	70,274	169,045

TABLE 8

U.S. CENSUS DIVISION 7, WEST SOUTH CENTRAL

U.S. Community Hospitals
(Nonfederal, short-term general and other special hospitals)

2002 Utilization, Personnel and Finances

FULL-TIME EQUIVALENT PERSONNEL					FULL-TIME EQUIV. TRAINEES			EXPENSES						
								LABOR				TOTAL		
Physicians and Dentists	Registered Nurses	Licensed Practical Nurses	Other Salaried Personnel	Total Personnel	Medical and Dental Residents	Other Trainees	Total Trainees	Payroll (in thousands)	Employee Benefits (in thousands)	Total (in thousands)	Percent of Total	Amount (in thousands)	Adjusted per Admission	Adjusted per Inpatient Day
72,823	988,139	125,865	2,882,668	4,069,495	78,715	5,463	84,178	$175,961,479	$40,049,573	$216,011,067	51.9	$416,591,059	$7,354.60	$1,289.87
8,448	145,133	36,374	479,821	669,776	1,763	161	1,924	24,016,766	5,768,570	29,785,337	53.7	55,454,326	5,047.87	767.32
64,375	843,006	89,491	2,402,847	3,399,719	76,952	5,302	82,254	151,944,713	34,281,003	186,225,730	51.6	361,136,733	7,909.61	1,440.51
3,177	106,664	23,322	303,168	436,331	5,408	1,297	6,705	17,351,001	3,771,190	21,122,201	49.3	42,808,056	6,621.16	1,274.49
453	14,009	7,178	49,158	70,798	38	0	38	2,225,998	499,705	2,725,699	52.2	5,225,006	4,049.23	845.90
2,724	92,655	16,144	254,010	365,533	5,370	1,297	6,667	15,125,003	3,271,486	18,396,502	48.9	37,583,050	7,262.47	1,371.06
301	10,290	3,205	29,076	42,872	13	2	15	1,477,611	318,583	1,796,197	49.7	3,612,280	5,666.97	1,041.01
161	3,417	1,645	10,420	15,643	3	0	3	488,956	108,189	597,147	52.3	1,142,723	4,200.48	757.11
140	6,873	1,560	18,656	27,229	10	2	12	988,654	210,394	1,199,050	48.6	2,469,557	6,758.85	1,259.55
61	1,048	288	3,044	4,441	0	0	0	133,994	26,674	160,668	51.9	309,849	5,052.98	1,135.24
1	1,007	242	2,854	4,104	0	0	0	132,224	30,799	163,023	51.9	314,133	6,030.82	1,105.37
1	577	244	1,516	2,338	0	0	0	65,941	14,612	80,553	41.1	196,081	5,306.22	969.03
74	3,852	655	9,835	14,416	10	2	12	587,421	122,620	710,042	47.8	1,484,274	7,874.38	1,399.87
2	97	42	339	480	0	0	0	20,281	2,522	22,804	54.8	41,612	6,747.58	1,481.18
1	292	89	1,068	1,450	0	0	0	48,792	13,168	61,960	50.1	123,607	6,071.39	1,095.78
1,069	18,308	3,642	55,426	78,445	910	44	954	2,763,791	608,933	3,372,727	50.0	6,751,804	6,145.66	1,116.42
130	2,328	872	8,343	11,673	5	0	5	358,661	76,532	435,193	53.6	811,374	4,078.26	807.55
939	15,980	2,770	47,083	66,772	905	44	949	2,405,130	532,400	2,937,534	49.4	5,940,430	6,602.83	1,177.96
36	881	173	2,158	3,248	15	9	24	121,501	28,102	149,602	48.2	310,322	5,841.57	1,102.22
86	2,016	276	6,346	8,724	27	0	27	337,267	69,073	406,340	50.2	808,962	6,456.35	1,133.31
30	738	144	2,270	3,182	1	0	1	101,806	24,280	126,087	42.6	295,673	5,407.83	1,205.23
39	1,505	474	4,900	6,918	12	0	12	223,569	50,186	273,755	48.2	568,007	6,077.41	1,128.83
66	859	140	2,600	3,665	26	2	28	116,910	25,690	142,601	52.4	271,934	4,829.15	970.84
61	1,075	242	3,074	4,452	36	0	36	146,801	35,578	182,378	44.9	406,372	6,708.13	1,201.80
227	6,665	992	19,074	26,958	261	28	289	1,026,315	232,553	1,258,871	49.6	2,538,917	7,843.33	1,313.35
394	2,241	329	6,661	9,625	527	5	532	330,961	66,938	397,900	53.8	740,243	5,585.56	990.00
440	10,475	2,651	34,178	47,744	246	35	281	1,617,667	335,619	1,953,284	49.0	3,986,181	5,596.86	1,064.33
132	2,882	1,244	10,421	14,679	27	0	27	441,272	99,556	540,825	53.0	1,019,936	3,881.94	775.70
308	7,593	1,407	23,757	33,065	219	35	254	1,176,395	236,063	1,412,459	47.6	2,966,245	6,599.31	1,220.48
12	279	60	932	1,283	4	0	4	46,146	7,819	53,965	47.0	114,878	5,941.47	918.39
0	12	8	167	187	0	0	0	3,285	815	4,100	56.7	7,233	2,193.09	584.75
61	266	222	1,525	2,074	0	0	0	69,307	13,890	83,197	44.2	188,420	7,257.25	1,264.27
210	4,111	657	12,008	16,986	99	3	102	622,887	130,346	753,235	47.4	1,588,333	6,879.77	1,289.46
25	2,925	460	9,125	12,535	116	32	148	434,770	83,194	517,962	48.5	1,067,380	6,278.26	1,170.23
1,367	67,591	13,824	184,488	267,270	4,239	1,216	5,455	11,491,932	2,508,055	13,999,993	49.2	28,457,792	7,084.22	1,400.10
30	5,382	3,417	19,974	28,803	3	0	3	937,108	215,427	1,152,534	51.2	2,250,972	4,043.90	958.69
1,337	62,209	10,407	164,514	238,467	4,236	1,216	5,452	10,554,823	2,292,628	12,847,459	49.0	26,206,819	7,573.28	1,457.75
2	682	218	1,904	2,806	0	49	49	93,782	18,086	111,869	45.6	224,767	6,309.60	1,188.73
10	1,294	225	2,792	4,321	0	0	0	157,820	35,210	193,030	45.6	422,989	6,876.98	1,329.89
50	2,823	345	6,886	10,104	99	0	99	494,673	81,381	576,053	49.3	1,169,537	6,626.76	1,228.74
0	1,550	393	3,581	5,524	2	1	3	212,734	47,761	260,500	50.4	517,255	5,563.43	1,053.03
0	190	50	595	835	0	0	0	32,625	8,417	41,042	49.6	82,806	3,574.32	1,000.79
18	785	331	2,661	3,795	23	2	25	173,469	45,546	219,015	49.6	441,873	6,406.75	1,409.43
0	496	179	1,449	2,124	0	0	0	70,920	17,203	88,123	47.4	185,835	6,109.57	1,295.25
6	1,303	285	3,731	5,325	109	4	113	200,931	47,594	248,525	48.3	514,583	6,636.62	1,250.90
224	11,846	1,064	28,505	41,639	1,049	34	1,083	1,966,711	386,257	2,352,968	46.5	5,058,098	8,418.87	1,699.13
1	1,794	190	5,131	7,116	0	0	0	278,494	61,372	339,867	40.9	830,978	7,321.72	1,479.54
19	5,789	935	13,289	20,032	253	0	253	847,314	190,084	1,037,401	49.7	2,087,092	7,451.34	1,447.78
0	1,405	153	4,049	5,607	549	0	549	203,327	53,512	256,839	43.0	596,656	8,930.24	1,594.05
804	14,638	1,952	43,997	61,391	1,078	834	1,912	2,965,343	658,119	3,623,463	55.0	6,588,871	8,573.04	1,587.86
0	905	253	2,578	3,736	300	265	565	346,215	97,689	443,904	61.9	717,261	9,104.95	1,671.52
0	398	77	1,619	2,094	0	0	0	79,351	15,533	94,884	47.8	198,381	5,300.77	1,053.30
0	819	120	2,089	3,028	0	7	7	111,409	30,690	142,099	49.5	287,100	5,502.54	1,256.74
55	2,244	391	5,641	8,331	69	3	72	365,091	80,555	445,646	48.2	925,357	8,471.40	1,507.75
0	1,639	378	3,606	5,623	0	0	0	217,883	35,130	253,014	46.1	549,254	5,506.14	1,105.11
1	853	219	2,427	3,500	0	1	1	130,306	45,670	175,976	45.8	384,050	8,001.70	1,504.27
0	371	101	1,322	1,794	0	0	0	65,175	16,120	81,294	48.1	169,167	5,458.92	1,193.48
35	5,943	1,133	13,107	20,218	685	0	685	889,363	167,589	1,056,950	41.6	2,542,366	7,214.82	1,421.33
16	665	174	1,962	2,817	1	0	1	104,515	27,146	131,662	49.5	265,776	6,356.31	1,201.41
0	819	251	1,754	2,824	0	16	16	104,152	22,392	126,545	47.1	268,498	6,313.59	1,110.75
77	1,323	355	5,307	7,062	19	0	19	213,229	56,426	269,656	44.8	601,946	8,959.53	1,672.94
0	524	154	1,151	1,829	0	0	0	64,643	13,659	78,301	48.6	161,260	4,997.97	1,017.57
19	681	208	1,934	2,842	0	0	0	93,910	17,470	111,379	46.6	238,863	5,823.93	825.36
0	430	273	1,447	2,150	0	0	0	71,435	16,017	87,454	49.6	176,201	5,786.74	1,105.74

MSAs

TABLE 8

U.S. CENSUS DIVISION 8, MOUNTAIN

U.S. Community Hospitals
(Nonfederal, short-term general and other special hospitals)

2002 Utilization, Personnel and Finances

CLASSIFICATION	Hospitals	Beds	Admissions	Inpatient Days	Adjusted Patient Days	Average Daily Census	Adjusted Average Daily Census	Average Stay (days)	Surgical Operations	NEWBORNS Bassinets	Births	OUTPATIENT VISITS Emergency	Total
UNITED STATES	4,927	820,653	34,478,280	196,690,099	322,970,965	539,685	885,994	5.7	27,576,675	59,974	3,870,191	109,951,738	556,404,212
Nonmetropolitan	2,178	171,591	5,382,463	35,210,002	72,269,855	96,579	198,275	6.5	4,598,958	13,757	531,940	23,038,926	114,101,059
Metropolitan	2,749	649,062	29,095,817	161,480,097	250,701,110	443,106	687,719	5.5	22,977,717	46,217	3,338,251	86,912,812	442,303,153
CENSUS DIVISION 8, MOUNTAIN . . .	349	42,499	1,894,701	9,643,564	15,902,359	26,427	43,589	5.1	1,442,820	3,901	292,890	6,124,812	29,549,308
Nonmetropolitan	206	12,130	342,807	2,396,981	4,877,109	6,575	13,390	7.0	295,325	1,149	52,288	1,547,242	8,036,845
Metropolitan	143	30,369	1,551,894	7,246,583	11,025,250	19,852	30,199	4.7	1,147,495	2,752	240,602	4,577,570	21,512,463
Arizona.	61	10,930	591,094	2,544,370	3,854,956	6,970	10,560	4.3	359,279	1,043	85,418	1,559,078	5,136,881
Nonmetropolitan	15	867	38,713	166,377	343,694	456	943	4.3	29,705	90	6,142	163,130	768,862
Metropolitan.	46	10,063	552,381	2,377,993	3,511,262	6,514	9,617	4.3	329,574	953	79,276	1,395,948	4,368,019
Flagstaff	2	317	11,938	57,848	91,036	159	249	4.8	7,588	34	1,398	35,418	91,230
Las Vegas	3	381	19,101	81,062	125,748	222	345	4.2	13,551	32	1,874	64,448	193,637
Phoenix-Mesa	31	6,992	387,344	1,683,193	2,460,794	4,611	6,740	4.3	225,686	698	58,610	942,822	2,857,817
Tucson	9	2,097	117,082	484,950	726,044	1,328	1,988	4.1	70,929	170	14,108	306,052	1,066,743
Yuma	1	276	16,916	70,940	107,640	194	295	4.2	11,820	19	3,286	47,208	158,592
Colorado.	68	9,575	426,560	2,172,074	3,635,014	5,949	9,959	5.1	314,731	835	65,284	1,501,013	7,012,498
Nonmetropolitan	36	1,841	46,481	353,103	806,072	966	2,210	7.6	47,788	163	7,160	229,956	1,360,717
Metropolitan.	32	7,734	380,079	1,818,971	2,828,942	4,983	7,749	4.8	266,943	672	58,124	1,271,057	5,651,781
Boulder-Longmont	3	412	23,804	93,892	171,489	257	470	3.9	19,097	63	5,477	100,116	644,751
Colorado Springs	2	775	48,212	189,756	301,226	519	825	3.9	33,393	120	7,404	187,006	545,860
Denver	18	4,624	230,267	1,128,735	1,713,074	3,093	4,692	4.9	159,133	349	35,347	704,946	2,709,707
Fort Collins-Loveland.	3	443	22,699	96,247	162,099	264	444	4.2	16,506	54	3,494	68,483	451,967
Grand Junction	3	661	18,138	140,196	222,806	384	611	7.7	14,746	18	1,882	94,158	639,309
Greeley	1	276	15,016	65,404	97,559	179	267	4.4	7,998	23	2,292	43,603	327,977
Pueblo.	2	543	21,943	104,741	160,689	287	440	4.8	16,070	45	2,228	72,745	332,210
Idaho	39	3,349	123,046	648,640	1,135,877	1,779	3,116	5.3	101,442	292	19,601	445,100	2,388,086
Nonmetropolitan	33	2,005	63,765	375,997	712,752	1,031	1,956	5.9	53,857	184	9,813	251,590	1,134,112
Metropolitan.	6	1,344	59,281	272,643	423,125	748	1,160	4.6	47,585	108	9,788	193,510	1,253,974
Boise City	5	1,109	52,954	219,166	338,204	601	927	4.1	43,838	92	8,495	163,961	1,087,351
Pocatello	1	235	6,327	53,477	84,921	147	233	8.5	3,747	16	1,293	29,549	166,623
Montana	53	4,263	106,758	1,071,834	1,971,371	2,932	5,401	10.0	71,135	275	9,963	276,829	2,658,735
Nonmetropolitan	48	2,909	49,193	708,410	1,358,706	1,937	3,723	14.4	29,418	174	4,752	168,671	1,220,058
Metropolitan.	5	1,354	57,565	363,424	612,665	995	1,678	6.3	41,717	101	5,211	108,158	1,438,677
Billings	2	624	26,940	169,743	333,185	465	913	6.3	21,056	36	2,191	43,602	1,074,853
Great Falls	1	393	13,563	115,139	157,753	315	432	8.5	8,406	44	1,466	29,815	117,106
Missoula	2	337	17,062	78,542	121,727	215	333	4.6	12,255	21	1,554	34,741	246,718
Nevada	26	4,495	211,657	1,110,583	1,590,812	3,053	4,378	5.2	162,563	241	29,709	626,330	2,462,224
Nonmetropolitan	9	470	13,687	81,848	192,957	238	549	6.0	13,018	34	1,949	91,373	407,098
Metropolitan.	17	4,025	197,970	1,028,735	1,397,855	2,815	3,829	5.2	149,545	207	27,760	534,957	2,055,126
Las Vegas	12	3,014	157,471	809,628	1,087,640	2,216	2,979	5.1	118,571	149	22,023	404,267	1,503,059
Reno.	5	1,011	40,499	219,107	310,215	599	850	5.4	30,974	58	5,737	130,690	552,067
New Mexico.	36	3,602	180,041	849,396	1,507,036	2,328	4,128	4.7	162,822	399	28,178	705,643	4,187,662
Nonmetropolitan	22	1,598	63,421	267,021	521,159	732	1,429	4.2	52,303	188	9,558	297,811	1,412,991
Metropolitan.	14	2,004	116,620	582,375	985,877	1,596	2,699	5.0	110,519	211	18,620	407,832	2,774,671
Albuquerque	11	1,553	90,861	471,971	803,143	1,293	2,199	5.2	87,033	143	13,775	307,059	2,282,012
Las Cruces	1	240	13,264	60,430	97,620	166	267	4.6	11,664	35	2,841	27,291	266,826
Santa Fe	2	211	12,495	49,974	85,114	137	233	4.0	11,822	33	2,004	73,482	225,833
Utah	42	4,403	206,344	876,524	1,483,497	2,401	4,062	4.2	229,258	633	48,792	797,951	4,814,311
Nonmetropolitan	21	958	37,424	157,005	338,818	428	926	4.2	40,721	173	8,966	194,535	1,050,554
Metropolitan.	21	3,445	168,920	719,519	1,144,679	1,973	3,136	4.3	188,537	460	39,826	603,416	3,763,757
Flagstaff.	1	38	321	560	1,389	2	4	1.7	1,316	5	47	2,606	13,255
Provo-Orem	5	656	35,784	121,506	189,483	333	518	3.4	27,776	111	10,785	108,938	598,333
Salt Lake City-Ogden	15	2,751	132,815	597,453	953,807	1,638	2,614	4.5	159,445	344	28,994	491,872	3,152,169
Wyoming	24	1,882	49,201	370,143	723,796	1,015	1,985	7.5	41,590	183	5,945	212,868	888,911
Nonmetropolitan	22	1,482	30,123	287,220	602,951	787	1,654	9.5	28,515	143	3,948	150,176	682,453
Metropolitan.	2	400	19,078	82,923	120,845	228	331	4.3	13,075	40	1,997	62,692	206,458
Casper	1	205	8,989	37,782	55,361	104	152	4.2	5,527	24	930	33,808	73,520
Cheyenne.	1	195	10,089	45,141	65,484	124	179	4.5	7,548	16	1,067	28,884	132,938

FULL-TIME EQUIVALENT PERSONNEL					FULL-TIME EQUIV. TRAINEES			EXPENSES — LABOR				EXPENSES — TOTAL		
Physicians and Dentists	Registered Nurses	Licensed Practical Nurses	Other Salaried Personnel	Total Personnel	Medical and Dental Residents	Other Trainees	Total Trainees	Payroll (in thousands)	Employee Benefits (in thousands)	Total (in thousands)	Percent of Total	Amount (in thousands)	Adjusted per Admission	Adjusted per Inpatient Day
72,823	988,139	125,865	2,882,668	4,069,495	78,715	5,463	84,178	$175,961,479	$40,049,573	$216,011,067	51.9	$416,591,059	$7,354.60	$1,289.87
8,448	145,133	36,374	479,821	669,776	1,763	161	1,924	24,016,766	5,768,570	29,785,337	53.7	55,454,326	5,047.87	767.32
64,375	843,006	89,491	2,402,847	3,399,719	76,952	5,302	82,254	151,944,713	34,281,003	186,225,730	51.6	361,136,733	7,909.61	1,440.51
2,650	53,063	6,022	148,999	210,734	1,738	133	1,871	9,009,120	1,945,538	10,954,661	51.1	21,439,443	6,917.98	1,348.19
615	10,125	1,826	33,680	46,246	32	20	52	1,655,746	394,380	2,050,127	53.1	3,861,342	5,319.28	791.73
2,035	42,938	4,196	115,319	164,488	1,706	113	1,819	7,353,374	1,551,158	8,904,534	50.7	17,578,101	7,406.99	1,594.35
678	13,767	1,315	36,521	52,281	780	46	826	2,261,007	486,112	2,747,122	48.6	5,647,682	6,258.24	1,465.04
41	1,044	126	3,460	4,671	0	5	5	167,174	37,564	204,738	52.1	393,167	5,145.42	1,143.94
637	12,723	1,189	33,061	47,610	780	41	821	2,093,833	448,549	2,542,384	48.4	5,254,515	6,361.18	1,496.47
2	463	8	935	1,408	0	0	0	65,517	16,098	81,616	49.3	165,701	8,704.63	1,820.17
10	465	82	1,365	1,922	1	0	1	65,103	15,172	80,276	49.8	161,194	5,440.79	1,281.88
532	8,491	846	21,810	31,679	699	37	736	1,461,483	316,243	1,777,727	48.0	3,704,792	6,441.27	1,505.53
93	2,882	226	7,751	10,952	80	4	84	439,279	85,171	524,450	48.4	1,083,586	6,138.15	1,492.45
0	422	27	1,200	1,649	0	0	0	62,451	15,864	78,315	56.2	139,242	5,424.95	1,293.59
465	13,143	1,109	36,542	51,259	326	47	373	2,357,238	494,251	2,851,489	52.1	5,472,452	7,736.22	1,505.48
81	1,418	250	5,282	7,031	5	3	8	273,054	67,555	340,608	52.9	643,471	5,798.50	798.28
384	11,725	859	31,260	44,228	321	44	365	2,084,184	426,696	2,510,881	52.0	4,828,981	8,096.76	1,706.99
32	801	48	2,276	3,157	0	0	0	140,627	26,926	167,554	57.4	291,925	6,675.01	1,702.30
18	1,351	39	3,931	5,339	0	11	11	225,688	51,601	277,289	52.4	529,182	6,913.98	1,756.76
194	7,050	505	17,012	24,761	218	28	246	1,241,704	239,457	1,481,160	50.9	2,907,488	8,214.17	1,697.23
40	600	72	2,078	2,790	18	0	18	121,904	30,521	152,426	51.8	294,203	8,111.48	1,814.96
65	961	79	2,725	3,830	50	5	55	180,366	43,340	223,706	52.7	424,640	14,231.52	1,905.87
13	315	21	1,284	1,633	23	0	23	77,528	15,950	93,478	51.5	181,499	8,103.35	1,860.40
22	647	95	1,954	2,718	12	0	12	96,367	18,901	115,268	57.6	200,044	5,941.13	1,244.91
235	4,062	687	12,047	17,031	148	7	155	630,127	145,935	776,063	52.2	1,488,004	6,752.45	1,310.00
75	1,826	407	5,585	7,893	14	0	14	286,687	70,233	356,921	52.5	680,404	5,320.31	954.62
160	2,236	280	6,462	9,138	134	7	141	343,440	75,702	419,142	51.9	807,600	8,732.98	1,908.66
160	2,051	202	5,932	8,345	134	7	141	313,607	68,679	382,286	52.0	734,632	8,912.19	2,172.16
0	185	78	530	793	0	0	0	29,833	7,022	36,856	50.5	72,968	7,262.65	859.24
439	3,151	654	11,036	15,280	0	1	1	603,226	134,391	737,617	55.5	1,328,470	6,744.50	673.88
126	1,576	322	5,697	7,721	0	1	1	255,712	59,885	315,598	55.6	567,122	5,596.40	417.40
313	1,575	332	5,339	7,559	0	0	0	347,514	74,505	422,019	55.4	761,348	7,961.06	1,242.68
235	685	198	2,787	3,905	0	0	0	185,353	38,789	224,142	56.0	400,411	7,933.18	1,201.77
5	377	60	1,176	1,618	0	0	0	65,285	15,855	81,140	54.7	148,274	7,979.04	939.92
73	513	74	1,376	2,036	0	0	0	96,876	19,861	116,737	54.9	212,662	8,001.43	1,747.04
88	5,307	464	12,177	18,036	191	12	203	985,599	194,588	1,180,186	52.3	2,257,001	7,522.78	1,418.77
36	404	79	1,463	1,982	2	0	2	84,984	19,233	104,217	51.9	200,760	6,100.82	1,040.44
52	4,903	385	10,714	16,054	189	12	201	900,614	175,355	1,075,969	52.3	2,056,241	7,697.96	1,471.00
49	3,690	308	7,526	11,573	189	12	201	658,105	138,422	796,526	55.3	1,441,198	6,850.26	1,325.07
3	1,213	77	3,188	4,481	0	0	0	242,510	36,933	279,443	45.4	615,043	10,841.77	1,982.63
454	5,485	753	16,961	23,653	40	1	41	908,181	187,199	1,095,380	51.4	2,129,702	6,568.96	1,413.17
163	1,762	285	5,454	7,664	11	0	11	265,059	60,497	325,557	52.2	623,763	4,827.48	1,196.88
291	3,723	468	11,507	15,989	29	1	30	643,122	126,701	769,823	51.1	1,505,939	7,722.92	1,527.51
250	3,119	412	9,524	13,305	10	0	10	529,009	96,200	625,209	51.9	1,203,889	7,910.80	1,498.97
13	325	7	984	1,329	12	0	12	54,270	10,003	64,273	41.8	153,814	7,178.50	1,575.64
28	279	49	999	1,355	7	1	8	59,843	20,498	80,341	54.2	148,236	6,931.47	1,741.62
225	6,514	831	18,513	26,083	253	8	261	1,004,859	238,010	1,242,869	49.6	2,505,242	7,088.49	1,688.74
31	970	213	3,109	4,323	0	0	0	150,962	36,097	187,059	52.0	360,053	4,460.85	1,062.67
194	5,544	618	15,404	21,760	253	8	261	853,896	201,914	1,055,810	49.2	2,145,189	7,866.19	1,874.05
1	22	8	83	114	0	0	0	170	40	210	3.8	5,564	6,989.64	4,005.58
17	1,003	85	2,439	3,544	19	0	19	138,810	32,627	171,437	53.1	322,603	5,580.22	1,702.55
176	4,519	525	12,882	18,102	234	8	242	714,916	169,247	884,163	48.7	1,817,022	8,486.71	1,905.02
66	1,634	209	5,202	7,111	0	11	11	258,884	65,051	323,935	53.0	610,889	6,479.45	844.01
62	1,125	144	3,630	4,961	0	11	11	172,114	43,315	215,429	54.9	392,601	5,906.08	651.13
4	509	65	1,572	2,150	0	0	0	86,771	21,735	108,506	49.7	218,288	7,850.11	1,806.35
2	252	2	810	1,066	0	0	0	43,096	13,133	56,229	47.7	117,842	8,947.06	2,128.61
2	257	63	762	1,084	0	0	0	43,674	8,603	52,277	52.0	100,446	6,862.95	1,533.90

MSAs

TABLE **8**

U.S. CENSUS DIVISION 9, PACIFIC

U.S. Community Hospitals
(Nonfederal, short-term general and other special hospitals)

2002 Utilization, Personnel and Finances

CLASSIFICATION	Hospitals	Beds	Admissions	Inpatient Days	Adjusted Patient Days	Average Daily Census	Adjusted Average Daily Census	Average Stay (days)	Surgical Operations	NEWBORNS Bassinets	Births	OUTPATIENT VISITS Emergency	Total
UNITED STATES	4,927	820,653	34,478,280	196,690,099	322,970,965	539,685	885,994	5.7	27,576,675	59,974	3,870,191	109,951,738	556,404,212
Nonmetropolitan	2,178	171,591	5,382,463	35,210,002	72,269,855	96,579	198,275	6.5	4,598,958	13,757	531,940	23,038,926	114,101,059
Metropolitan	2,749	649,062	29,095,817	161,480,097	250,701,110	443,106	687,719	5.5	22,977,717	46,217	3,338,251	86,912,812	442,303,153
CENSUS DIVISION 9, PACIFIC	573	97,048	4,453,054	23,756,101	35,844,850	65,469	98,710	5.3	3,211,897	7,201	616,819	13,731,605	74,559,958
Nonmetropolitan	140	8,627	294,470	1,825,237	3,707,860	4,998	10,167	6.2	289,623	778	39,233	1,423,966	7,475,705
Metropolitan	433	88,421	4,158,584	21,930,864	32,136,990	60,471	88,543	5.3	2,922,274	6,423	577,586	12,307,639	67,084,253
Alaska	19	1,378	47,560	300,060	526,278	821	1,440	6.3	57,495	138	7,596	254,592	1,337,616
Nonmetropolitan	16	699	20,105	153,935	301,397	421	824	7.7	20,765	81	3,065	107,855	617,175
Metropolitan	3	679	27,455	146,125	224,881	400	616	5.3	36,730	57	4,531	146,737	720,441
Anchorage	3	679	27,455	146,125	224,881	400	616	5.3	36,730	57	4,531	146,737	720,441
California	383	74,343	3,430,241	18,591,536	26,638,364	51,324	73,488	5.4	2,320,864	5,050	475,383	10,111,529	53,333,448
Nonmetropolitan	40	2,265	80,482	487,487	981,099	1,339	2,698	6.1	88,603	198	11,422	486,743	2,603,920
Metropolitan	343	72,078	3,349,759	18,104,049	25,657,265	49,985	70,790	5.4	2,232,261	4,852	463,961	9,624,786	50,729,528
Bakersfield	10	1,291	56,287	330,657	448,451	906	1,230	5.9	36,697	96	9,587	175,718	637,958
Chico-Paradise	4	467	28,589	130,837	206,215	359	565	4.6	18,323	32	2,767	97,144	696,619
Fresno	15	2,024	107,403	551,238	852,087	1,512	2,335	5.1	81,202	187	11,912	374,364	2,719,434
Los Angeles-Long Beach	102	23,622	1,036,559	5,871,482	7,999,772	16,446	22,363	5.7	630,791	1,556	140,753	2,825,627	11,945,885
Merced	2	289	10,661	48,561	80,119	133	220	4.6	8,307	40	2,687	45,675	305,945
Modesto	4	1,121	47,069	320,689	509,431	878	1,395	6.8	29,803	74	8,444	187,068	371,324
Oakland	19	5,326	256,075	1,525,047	2,111,524	4,180	5,786	6.0	151,556	361	36,620	732,917	4,146,202
Orange County	32	5,955	273,733	1,293,840	1,805,703	3,543	4,948	4.7	186,882	406	39,362	729,605	3,227,725
Redding	3	563	21,069	131,293	192,151	359	527	6.2	15,070	11	2,004	81,151	335,202
Riverside-San Bernardino	32	6,081	319,445	1,532,950	2,138,001	4,223	5,896	4.8	189,810	447	42,797	1,098,039	3,633,880
Sacramento	13	3,408	194,701	984,094	1,437,089	2,695	3,937	5.1	135,681	238	20,499	435,623	3,690,210
Salinas	4	596	36,155	166,083	264,909	454	726	4.6	24,779	80	6,239	98,466	734,039
San Diego	19	6,141	284,944	1,599,237	2,181,830	4,379	5,977	5.6	209,018	361	41,184	597,104	3,231,257
San Francisco	19	4,572	176,819	1,146,606	1,720,365	3,140	4,714	6.5	139,465	160	18,271	485,767	4,789,616
San Jose	12	3,374	167,709	742,919	1,094,853	2,036	3,000	4.4	125,302	279	31,057	473,156	3,641,329
San Luis Obispo-Atascadero-Paso Robles	5	373	19,990	87,839	136,797	241	374	4.4	24,885	36	1,835	101,297	519,378
Santa Barbara-Santa Maria-Lompoc	7	945	36,990	232,891	366,020	638	1,002	6.3	29,613	84	5,731	120,802	537,341
Santa Cruz-Watsonville	3	374	21,608	90,340	130,342	247	358	4.2	13,297	25	1,252	66,713	225,530
Santa Rosa	9	1,048	44,379	228,766	360,744	633	996	5.2	40,108	75	5,587	156,361	1,342,149
Stockton-Lodi	7	1,065	54,053	277,743	390,116	761	1,068	5.1	34,138	71	9,300	195,076	1,193,687
Vallejo-Fairfield-Napa	6	886	39,760	199,815	303,776	548	833	5.0	25,748	57	5,492	126,613	621,885
Ventura	8	1,496	61,865	342,988	504,276	940	1,382	5.5	42,282	113	10,314	204,756	1,069,546
Visalia-Tulare-Porterville	4	689	33,192	185,986	281,339	509	771	5.6	20,359	35	6,379	148,422	596,194
Yolo	2	159	7,023	22,730	51,608	62	141	3.2	11,739	14	1,869	41,732	454,519
Yuba City	2	213	13,681	59,418	89,747	163	246	4.3	7,406	14	2,019	25,590	62,674
Hawaii	25	3,191	111,498	866,160	1,362,769	2,374	3,734	7.8	84,557	219	15,845	311,713	1,964,332
Nonmetropolitan	12	1,032	29,976	272,744	437,302	748	1,198	9.1	23,483	62	4,546	74,034	252,809
Metropolitan	13	2,159	81,522	593,416	925,467	1,626	2,536	7.3	61,074	157	11,299	237,679	1,711,523
Honolulu	13	2,159	81,522	593,416	925,467	1,626	2,536	7.3	61,074	157	11,299	237,679	1,711,523
Oregon	60	6,798	345,193	1,511,420	2,686,024	4,141	7,359	4.4	305,386	719	45,409	1,117,313	8,176,178
Nonmetropolitan	31	2,005	85,968	400,822	860,606	1,096	2,357	4.7	75,712	210	10,042	378,211	2,000,771
Metropolitan	29	4,793	259,225	1,110,598	1,825,418	3,045	5,002	4.3	229,674	509	35,367	739,102	6,175,407
Corvalis	1	163	8,656	33,331	53,870	91	148	3.9	7,275	24	1,020	17,745	207,814
Eugene-Springfield	4	581	32,689	134,365	194,867	369	533	4.1	27,130	60	3,581	102,454	370,274
Medford-Ashland	3	429	22,813	94,835	147,921	260	405	4.2	15,730	34	2,113	63,662	829,946
Portland-Vancouver	17	3,124	171,945	745,710	1,259,979	2,044	3,452	4.3	163,657	333	23,765	465,757	4,342,850
Salem	4	496	23,122	102,357	168,781	281	464	4.4	15,882	58	4,888	89,484	424,523
Washington	86	11,338	518,562	2,486,925	4,631,415	6,809	12,689	4.8	443,595	1,075	72,586	1,936,458	9,748,384
Nonmetropolitan	41	2,626	77,939	510,249	1,127,456	1,394	3,090	6.5	81,060	227	10,158	377,123	2,001,030
Metropolitan	45	8,712	440,623	1,976,676	3,503,959	5,415	9,599	4.5	362,535	848	62,428	1,559,335	7,747,354
Bellingham	1	208	13,747	57,198	89,761	157	246	4.2	8,338	30	1,874	49,642	98,066
Bremerton	1	239	13,435	51,143	77,816	140	213	3.8	11,727	18	1,769	51,542	129,886
Olympia	2	412	21,477	86,389	141,248	237	387	4.0	19,950	27	2,663	72,879	327,585
Portland-Vancouver	1	334	21,478	81,960	154,086	225	422	3.8	13,800	50	4,690	90,775	246,735
Richland-Kennewick-Pasco	4	425	17,055	79,524	165,032	219	452	4.7	13,255	53	3,562	91,626	244,853
Seattle-Bellevue-Everett	21	4,346	226,885	1,030,003	1,877,580	2,822	5,143	4.5	188,230	469	30,338	749,620	4,894,617
Spokane	6	1,239	52,867	283,430	423,086	776	1,159	5.4	52,741	77	6,043	128,882	478,514
Tacoma	5	997	53,213	228,648	438,561	625	1,202	4.3	42,052	81	7,703	208,702	812,476
Yakima	4	512	20,466	78,381	136,789	214	375	3.8	12,442	43	3,786	115,667	514,622

TABLE 8 — U.S. CENSUS DIVISION 9, PACIFIC

TABLE 8

U.S. CENSUS DIVISION 9, PACIFIC

U.S. Community Hospitals
(Nonfederal, short-term general and other special hospitals)

2002 Utilization, Personnel and Finances

FULL-TIME EQUIVALENT PERSONNEL					FULL-TIME EQUIV. TRAINEES			EXPENSES						
								LABOR				TOTAL		
Physicians and Dentists	Registered Nurses	Licensed Practical Nurses	Other Salaried Personnel	Total Personnel	Medical and Dental Residents	Other Trainees	Total Trainees	Payroll (in thousands)	Employee Benefits (in thousands)	Total (in thousands)	Percent of Total	Amount (in thousands)	Adjusted per Admission	Adjusted per Inpatient Day
72,823	988,139	125,865	2,882,668	4,069,495	78,715	5,463	84,178	$175,961,479	$40,049,573	$216,011,067	51.9	$416,591,059	$7,354.60	$1,289.87
8,448	145,133	36,374	479,821	669,776	1,763	161	1,924	24,016,766	5,768,570	29,785,337	53.7	55,454,326	5,047.87	767.32
64,375	843,006	89,491	2,402,847	3,399,719	76,952	5,302	82,254	151,944,713	34,281,003	186,225,730	51.6	361,136,733	7,909.61	1,440.51
10,319	123,362	13,417	346,347	493,445	9,825	676	10,501	23,844,148	6,282,893	30,127,047	52.5	57,386,669	8,485.65	1,600.97
440	8,947	1,355	29,130	39,872	31	21	52	1,684,693	471,358	2,156,052	55.7	3,874,138	6,496.43	1,044.84
9,879	114,415	12,062	317,217	453,573	9,794	655	10,449	22,159,455	5,811,535	27,970,995	52.3	53,512,532	8,678.02	1,665.14
295	2,109	172	5,890	8,466	56	37	93	409,466	100,773	510,239	54.1	942,612	11,345.56	1,791.09
82	812	121	2,727	3,742	1	0	1	190,153	50,448	240,602	56.1	428,786	10,533.22	1,422.66
213	1,297	51	3,163	4,724	55	37	92	219,313	50,324	269,637	52.5	513,826	12,125.96	2,284.88
213	1,297	51	3,163	4,724	55	37	92	219,313	50,324	269,637	52.5	513,826	12,125.96	2,284.88
7,122	90,455	10,451	249,377	357,405	8,123	534	8,657	17,375,987	4,715,950	22,091,940	52.0	42,504,560	8,620.72	1,595.61
56	2,393	460	7,756	10,665	2	0	2	431,489	146,280	577,770	54.4	1,062,935	6,624.67	1,083.41
7,066	88,062	9,991	241,621	346,740	8,121	534	8,655	16,944,498	4,569,670	21,514,170	51.9	41,441,625	8,687.87	1,615.20
56	1,213	239	4,111	5,619	29	0	29	232,681	64,316	296,998	52.8	562,481	7,545.02	1,254.28
47	742	113	2,415	3,317	23	0	23	118,926	49,447	168,374	56.0	300,704	6,687.23	1,458.21
314	2,697	365	10,235	13,611	213	8	221	515,052	116,697	631,747	52.1	1,213,179	7,147.20	1,423.77
3,072	27,759	3,248	74,082	108,161	3,423	87	3,510	5,091,760	1,272,945	6,364,705	49.8	12,791,409	9,037.64	1,598.97
19	209	31	733	992	6	0	6	39,989	13,820	53,809	56.2	95,664	5,444.40	1,194.02
0	1,661	123	3,545	5,329	0	0	0	230,000	69,338	299,337	52.9	565,432	7,945.82	1,109.93
470	6,161	837	17,807	25,275	539	41	580	1,580,408	466,471	2,046,877	56.5	3,625,390	10,069.58	1,716.95
100	6,856	724	19,247	26,927	133	3	136	1,190,140	308,617	1,498,758	48.7	3,079,145	7,986.18	1,705.23
14	736	74	1,757	2,581	26	0	26	107,564	33,770	141,334	47.0	300,863	10,491.45	1,565.76
385	7,975	953	20,468	29,781	752	82	834	1,206,733	309,439	1,516,171	48.9	3,099,439	6,924.56	1,449.69
889	4,902	464	15,835	22,090	675	9	684	1,176,859	307,540	1,484,400	59.8	2,481,753	8,676.06	1,726.93
54	969	183	3,066	4,272	35	0	35	217,904	86,222	304,126	56.1	542,141	9,464.25	2,046.52
215	7,283	646	17,393	25,537	744	11	755	1,225,668	300,097	1,525,766	51.0	2,992,058	7,668.82	1,371.35
703	6,077	489	14,791	22,060	491	241	732	1,425,959	354,752	1,780,712	54.1	3,292,533	12,243.45	1,913.86
442	5,009	399	13,014	18,864	802	46	848	1,120,843	372,239	1,493,083	53.3	2,798,892	11,263.05	2,556.41
20	413	64	1,224	1,721	2	0	2	75,969	22,625	98,595	49.6	198,590	6,352.22	1,451.71
36	968	105	2,733	3,842	63	4	67	153,104	47,919	201,022	49.2	408,934	7,513.16	1,117.25
7	396	64	1,237	1,704	0	0	0	97,670	28,638	126,308	58.4	216,351	6,670.90	1,659.87
52	911	124	2,766	3,853	60	2	62	198,316	77,515	275,831	52.9	521,203	7,369.01	1,444.80
96	1,305	198	3,994	5,593	70	0	70	250,677	77,848	328,526	56.2	584,625	7,677.89	1,498.59
34	834	90	2,554	3,512	14	0	14	183,901	56,269	240,170	51.7	464,326	7,648.89	1,528.51
20	1,713	179	4,264	6,176	16	0	16	283,920	70,816	354,736	50.3	705,301	7,774.49	1,398.64
2	757	167	2,586	3,512	0	0	0	134,273	40,864	175,136	53.1	329,786	6,432.22	1,172.20
13	241	29	674	957	4	0	4	37,435	10,235	47,669	34.5	138,055	8,670.19	2,675.08
6	275	83	1,090	1,454	1	0	1	48,747	11,233	59,980	45.0	133,370	6,563.50	1,486.07
278	4,005	467	10,367	15,117	33	8	41	703,501	161,084	864,586	52.7	1,640,542	9,387.18	1,203.83
25	896	145	2,394	3,460	11	0	11	138,180	33,661	171,841	53.3	322,182	6,768.81	736.75
253	3,109	322	7,973	11,657	22	8	30	565,321	127,423	692,745	52.5	1,318,360	10,367.24	1,424.53
253	3,109	322	7,973	11,657	22	8	30	565,321	127,423	692,745	52.5	1,318,360	10,367.24	1,424.53
1,345	10,842	833	30,620	43,640	563	35	598	1,885,217	505,977	2,391,193	53.5	4,468,834	7,348.94	1,663.74
130	2,367	249	8,139	10,885	3	16	19	440,571	123,553	564,124	56.5	998,178	5,713.80	1,159.85
1,215	8,475	584	22,481	32,755	560	19	579	1,444,645	382,423	1,827,069	52.6	3,470,656	8,008.05	1,901.29
27	230	9	764	1,030	0	0	0	50,611	9,795	60,405	54.3	111,170	7,946.36	2,063.66
5	1,011	66	2,437	3,519	0	1	1	159,722	41,520	201,242	52.7	381,611	7,933.37	1,958.31
40	672	68	1,924	2,704	4	0	4	116,862	41,172	158,034	54.1	291,859	8,141.11	1,973.07
1,118	5,879	377	15,224	22,598	556	18	574	986,400	257,144	1,243,544	51.7	2,404,705	8,112.38	1,908.53
25	683	64	2,132	2,904	0	0	0	131,050	32,794	163,844	58.2	281,312	7,207.60	1,666.73
1,279	15,951	1,494	50,093	68,817	1,050	62	1,112	3,469,978	799,110	4,269,089	54.5	7,830,121	8,102.82	1,690.65
147	2,479	380	8,114	11,120	14	5	19	484,299	117,416	601,715	56.7	1,062,057	6,142.75	941.99
1,132	13,472	1,114	41,979	57,697	1,036	57	1,093	2,985,679	681,694	3,667,374	54.2	6,768,064	8,529.93	1,931.55
8	382	7	1,057	1,454	0	0	0	66,376	15,944	82,320	54.0	152,434	7,065.98	1,698.23
0	0	0	1,136	1,136	0	0	0	61,903	16,568	78,471	59.1	132,842	6,498.48	1,707.13
21	549	66	1,645	2,281	33	17	50	113,173	26,285	139,458	56.6	246,432	6,985.83	1,744.68
42	730	34	1,507	2,313	18	0	18	122,694	30,417	153,111	59.0	259,348	6,422.84	1,683.10
11	572	48	1,299	1,930	0	0	0	88,845	19,989	108,833	50.1	217,140	6,416.47	1,315.74
810	7,410	478	23,950	32,648	668	35	703	1,754,324	400,598	2,154,922	53.0	4,065,098	9,618.28	2,165.07
123	1,780	156	4,966	7,025	242	5	247	312,668	70,078	382,746	52.3	731,315	9,111.48	1,728.53
94	1,467	250	4,496	6,307	75	0	75	360,422	75,067	435,489	62.3	699,245	6,789.05	1,594.41
23	582	75	1,923	2,603	0	0	0	105,274	26,749	132,024	50.0	264,210	7,331.84	1,931.52

MSAs

Glossary

This glossary explains specific terms as they are used in the tables and text of Hospital Statistics

Adjusted average daily census: An estimate of the average number of patients (both inpatients and outpatients) receiving care each day during the reporting period, which is usually 12 months. The figure is derived by dividing the number of inpatient day equivalents (also called adjusted inpatient days) by the number of days in the reporting period.

Adjusted inpatient days: An aggregate figure reflecting the number of days of inpatient care, plus an estimate of the volume of outpatient services, expressed in units equivalent to an inpatient day in terms of level of effort. The figure is derived by first multiplying the number of outpatient visits by the ratio of outpatient revenue per outpatient visit to inpatient revenue per inpatient day. The product (which represents the number of patient days attributable to outpatient services) is then added to the number of *inpatient days*. Originally, the purpose of this calculation was to summarize overall productivity and calculate a unit cost that would include both inpatient and outpatient activities.

Formula 1:

$$\frac{\text{total expenses}}{\text{inpatient days} + \text{outpatient visits}\left(\dfrac{\dfrac{\text{outpatient revenue}}{\text{per outpatient visit}}}{\dfrac{\text{inpatient revenue}}{\text{per inpatient day}}}\right)}$$

However, the value of this calculation has changed over the years as the outpatient share of total revenue has grown and third-party payers have exerted a greater influence on pricing.

Admissions: The number of patients, excluding newborns, accepted for inpatient service during the reporting period; the number includes patients who visit the emergency room and are later admitted for inpatient service.

Adult day care program: Program providing supervision, medical and psychological care, and social activities for older adults who live at home or in another family setting, but cannot be alone or prefer to be with others during the day. May include intake assessment, health monitoring, occupational therapy, personal care, noon meal, and transportation services.

Acute long term care: Providers specialized acute hospital care to medically complex patients who are critically ill, have multisystem complications and/or failure, and require hospitalization averaging 25 days, in a facility offering specialized treatment programs and therapeutic intervention on a 24 hour/7day a week basis.

Alcoholism-drug abuse or dependency inpatient care: Provides diagnosis and therapeutic services to patients with alcoholism or other drug dependencies. Includes care for inpatient/residential treatment for patients whose course of treatment involves more intensive care than provided in an outpatient setting or where patient requires supervised withdrawal.

Alcoholism-drug abuse or dependency outpatient services: Organized hospital services that provide medical care and/or rehabilitative treatment services to outpatients for whom the primary diagnosis is alcoholism or other chemical dependency.

Ambulance services: Provision of ambulance services to the ill and injured who require medical attention on a scheduled or unscheduled basis.

Angioplasty: The reconstruction or restructuring of a blood vessel by operative means or by nonsurgical techniques such as balloon dilation or laser.

Arthritis treatment center: Specifically equipped and staffed center for the diagnosis and treatment of arthritis and other joint disorders.

Assisted living: A special combination of housing, supportive services, personalized assistance and health care designed to respond to the individual needs of those who need help in activities of daily living and instrumental activities of daily living. Supportive services are available, 24 hours a day, to meet scheduled and unscheduled needs, in a way that promotes maximum independence and dignity for each resident and encourages the involvement of a resident's family, neighbor and friends.

Auxiliary: A volunteer community organization formed to assist the hospital in carrying out its purpose and to serve as a link between the institution and the community.

Average daily census: The average number of people served on an inpatient basis on a single day during the reporting period; the figure is calculated by dividing the number of inpatient days by the number of days in the reporting period.

Beds: Number of beds regularly maintained (set up and staffed for use) for inpatients as of the close of the reporting period. Excludes newborn bassinets.

Bed-size category: Hospitals are categorized by the number of beds set up and staffed for use at the end of the reporting period. The eight categories in Hospital Statistics are: 6 to 24 beds; 25 to 49; 50 to 99; 100 to 199; 200 to 299; 300 to 399; 400 to 499; and 500 or more.

Birthing room-LDR room-LDRP room: A single-room type of maternity care with a more homelike setting for families than the traditional three-room unit(labor/delivery/recovery) with a separate postpartum area. A birthing room combines labor and delivery in one room. An LDR room accommodates three stages in the birthing process—labor, delivery, and recovery. An LDRP room accommodates all four stages of the birth process—labor, delivery, recovery, and postpartum.

Births: Total number of infants born in the hospital during the reporting period. Births do not include infants transferred from other institutions, and are excluded from admission and discharge figures.

Breast cancer screening/mammograms: Mammography screening - The use of breast x-ray to detect unsuspected breast cancer in asymptomatic women. Diagnostic mammography - The x-ray imaging of breast tissue in symptomatic women who are considered to have a substantial likelihood of having breast cancer already.

Burn care: Provides care to severely burned patients. Severely burned patients are those with any of the following: (1) second-degree burns of more than 25% total body surface area for adults or 20% total body surface area for children: (2) third-degree burns of more than 10% total body surface area; (3) any

severe burns of the hands, face, eyes, ears, or feet; or (4) all inhalation injuries, electrical burns, complicated burn injuries involving fractures and other major traumas, and all other poor risk factors.

Capitation: An at-risk payment arrangement in which a health care organization receives a fixed, prearranged payment and in turn guarantees to deliver or arrange all medically necessary care required by enrollees in the capitated plan. Specified by contractual agreements between the payer and the organization, the amount of the fixed payment reflects an actuarial assessment of the services required by enrollees and the costs of providing these services.

Cardiac catheterization laboratory: Facilities offering special diagnostic procedures for cardiac patients. Available procedures must include, but need not be limited to, introduction of a catheter into the interior of the heart by way of a vein or artery or by direct needle puncture. Procedures must be performed in a laboratory or a special procedure room.

Cardiac intensive care: Provides patient care of a more specialized nature than the usual medical and surgical care, on the basis of physicians' orders and approved nursing care plans. The unit is staffed with specially trained nursing personnel and contains monitoring and specialized support or treatment equipment for patients who, because of heart seizure, open-heart surgery, or other life-threatening conditions, require intensified, comprehensive observation and care. May include myocardial infarction, pulmonary care, and heart transplant units.

Case management: A system of assessment, treatment planning, referral and follow-up that ensures the provision of comprehensive and continuous services and the coordination of payment and reimbursement for care.

Children wellness program: A program that encourages improved health status and a healthful lifestyle of children through health education, exercise, nutrition and health promotion.

Chiropractic services: An organized clinical service including spinal manipulation or adjustment and related diagnostic and therapeutic services.

Closed physician-hospital organization (Closed PHO): A joint venture between the hospital and physicians who have been selected on the basis of cost-effectiveness and/or high quality. The PHO can act as a unified agent in managed care contracting, own a managed care plan, own and operate ambulatory care centers or ancillary services projects, or provide administrative services to physician members.

Community hospitals: All nonfederal, short-term general, and special hospitals whose facilities and services are available to the public. (Special hospitals include obstetrics and gynecology; eye, ear, nose, and throat; rehabilitation; orthopedic; and other individually described specialty services.) Short-term general and special childrens hospitals are also considered to be community hospitals.

A hospital may include a nursing-home-type unit and still be classified as short-term, provided that the majority of its patients are admitted to units where the average length of stay is less than 30 days. Therefore, statistics for community hospitals often include some data about such nursing-home-type units. An example is furnished by Montana, where in 1995 63.6 percent of all hospitals classified as community hospitals include nursing-home-type units. Expense, revenue, utilization, and personnel data for these hospitals include data about their nursing-home-type units. Thus, total admissions to Montana community hospitals in 1995 were 96,154; total inpatient days, 997,759; total expenses, $791,806,393; and total payroll expenses, $352,583,331. If nursing-home-type unit data were excluded, these same items would be 94,034; 457,340; 752,567,865; and $328,911841, respectively.

Note that before 1972, hospital units of institutions such as prison and college infirmaries were included in the category of community hospitals. Including these units made this category equivalent to the short-term general and other special hospitals category. Although these hospital units are few in number and small in size, this change in definition should be taken into consideration when comparing data.

Community outreach: A program that systematically interacts with the community to identify those in need of services, alerting persons and their families to the availability of services, locating needed services, and enabling persons to enter the service delivery system.

Complementary Medicine Services: Organized hospital services or formal arrangements to providers that provide care or treatment not based solely on traditional western allopathic medical teachings as instructed in most U.S. medical schools. Includes any of the following: acupuncture, chiropractic, homeopathy, osteopathy, diet and lifestyle changes, herbal medicine, message therapy, etc.

Control: The type of organization responsible for establishing policy concerning the overall operation of hospitals. The three major categories are government (including federal, state, and local); nongovernment (nonprofit); and investor-owned (for-profit).

Crisis prevention: Services provided in order to promote physical and mental well being and the early identification of disease and ill health prior to the onset and recognition of symptoms so as to permit early treatment.

CT scanner: Computed tomographic scanner for head or whole body scans.

Deduction from revenue: The difference between revenue at full established rates (gross) and the payment actually received from payers (net).

Dental Services: An organized dental service or dentists on staff, not necessarily involving special facilities, providing dental or oral services to inpatients or outpatients.

Diagnostic radioisotope facility: The use of radioactive isotopes (Radiopharmaceuticals) as tracers or indicators to detect an abnormal condition or disease.

Emergency department: Hospital facilities for the provision of unscheduled outpatient services to patients whose conditions require immediate care.

Emergency room visits: The number of visits to the emergency unit. When emergency outpatients are admitted to the inpatient areas of the hospital, they are counted as emergency room visits and subsequently, as inpatient admissions.

Enabling services: A program that is designed to help the patient access health care services by offering any of the following: linguistic services, transportation services, and/or referrals to local social services agencies.

Enrollment assistance services: A program that provides enrollment assistance for patients who are potentially eligible for public health insurance programs such as Medicaid, State Children's Health Insurance, or local/state indigent care programs. The specific services offered could include explanation of benefits, assist applicants in completing the application and locating all relevant documents, conduct eligibility interviews, and/or forward applications and documentation to state/local social service or health agency.

Equity model: An arrangement that allows established practitioners to become shareholders in a professional corporation in exchange for tangible and intangible assets of their existing practices.

Expenses: Includes all expenses for the reporting period including payroll, non-payroll, bad debt, and all nonoperating expenses. *Payroll expenses* include all salaries and wages. *Non-payroll expenses* are all professional fees and those salary expenditures excluded from payroll. *Labor related expenses* are defined as payroll expenses plus employee benefits. *Non-labor related expenses* are all other non-payroll expenses. *Bad debt* has been reclassified from a "reduction in revenue" to an expense in accordance with the revised AICPA Audit Guide. However, for purposes of historical consistency, the expense total that appears throughout *Hospital Statistics does not include "bad debt" as an expense item.* Note: Financial data may not add due to rounding.

Extracorporeal shock wave lithotripter (ESWL): A medical device used for treating stones in the kidney or ureter. The device disintegrates kidney stones noninvasively through the transmission of acoustic shock waves directed at the stones.

Fitness center: Provides exercise, testing, or evaluation programs and fitness activities to the community and hospital employees.

Foundation: A corporation, organized as a hospital affiliate or subsidiary, that purchases both tangible and intangible assets of one or more medical group practices. Physicians remain in a separate corporate entity but sign a professional services agreement with the foundation.

General medical-surgical care: Provides acute care to patients in medical and surgical units on the basis of physicians' orders and approved nursing care plans.

Geriatric services: The branch of medicine dealing with the physiology of aging and the diagnosis and treatment of disease affecting the aged. Services could include: Adult day care; Alzheimer's diagnostic-assessment services; Comprehensive geriatric assessment; Emergency response system; Geriatric acute care unit; and/or Geriatric clinics.

Government, nonfederal, state, local: Controlled by an agency of state, county, or city government.

Gross inpatient revenue: Revenue from services rendered to inpatients at full established rates (also known as "charges").

Gross outpatient revenue: Revenue from services rendered to outpatients at full established rates.

Group practice without walls: In this organization, the hospital sponsors the formation of a physician group or provides capital to physicians to establish one. The group shares administrative expenses, although the physicians remain independent practitioners.

Group Purchasing Organization: An organization whose primary function is to negotiate contracts for the purpose of purchasing for members of the group or has a central supply site for its members.

Health fair: Community health education events that focus on the prevention of disease and promotion of health through such activities as audiovisual exhibits and free diagnostic services.

Health information center: Education which is directed at increasing the information of individuals and populations. It is intended to increase the ability to make informed personal, family and community health decisions by providing consumers with informed choices about health matters with the objective of improving health status.

Health maintenance organization (HMO): A health care organization that acts as both insurer and provider of comprehensive but specified medical services in return for prospective per capita (capitation) payments.

Health screening: A preliminary procedure such as a test or examination to detect the most characteristic sign or signs of a disorder that may require further investigation.

Hemodialysis: Provision of equipment and personnel for the treatment of renal insufficiency on an inpatient or outpatient basis.

HIV-AIDS services: (could include). *HIV-AIDS unit* - Special unit or team designated and equipped specifically for diagnosis, treatment, continuing care planning, and counseling services for HIV-AIDS patients and their families. *General inpatient care for HIV-AIDS* - Inpatient diagnosis and treatment for human immunodeficiency virus and acquired immun-odeficiency syndrome patients, but dedicated unit is not available. *Specialized outpatient program for HIV-AIDS* - Special outpatient program providing diagnostic, treatment, continuing care planning, and counseling for HIV-AIDS patients and their families.

Home health services: Service providing nursing, therapy, and health-related homemaker or social services in the patient's home.

Hospice: A program providing palliative care, chiefly medical relief of pain and supportive services, addressing the emotional, social, financial, and legal needs of terminally ill patients and their families. Care can be provided in a variety of settings, both inpatient and at home.

Hospital district or authority: A political subdivision of a state, county, or city created solely for the purpose of establishing and maintaining medical care or health-related care institutions.

Hospitals in a network: Hospitals participating in a group that may include other hospitals, physicians, other providers, insurers, and/or community agencies that work together to coordinate and deliver a broad spectrum of services to the community.

Hospitals in a system: Hospitals belonging to a corporate body that owns and/or manages health provider facilities or health-related subsidiaries; the system may also own non-health-related facilities.

Hospital unit: The hospital operation, excluding activity pertaining to nursing-home-type unit (as described below), for the following items: Admissions, Beds, FTEs (full-time, part-time, and total), Inpatient Days, Length of Stay, Net Revenue, and Total Expense.

Hospital unit of institutions: A hospital unit that is not open to the public and is contained within a nonhospital unit. An example is an infirmary that is contained within a college.

Indemnity fee for service: The traditional type of health insurance, in which the insured is reimbursed for covered expenses without regard to choice of provider. Payment up to a stated limit may be made either to the individual incurring and claiming the expense, or directly to providers.

Independent practice association (IPA): An IPA is a legal entity that holds managed care contracts and contracts with physicians, usually in solo practice, to provide care either on a fee-for-services or capitated basis. The purpose of an IPA is to assist solo physicians in obtaining managed care contracts.

Inpatient days: The number of adult and pediatric days of care, excluding newborn days of care, rendered during the entire reporting period.

Inpatient surgeries: Surgical services provided to patients who remain in the hospital overnight.

Insurance product: In tables 3 through 6, insurance product refers to a hospital-owned insurance product.

Integrated salary model: In this arrangement, physicians are salaried by the hospital or other entity of a health system to provide medical services for primary care and specialty care.

Intermediate nursing care: Provides health-related services (skilled nursing care and social services) to residents with a variety of physical conditions or functional disabilities. These residents do not require the care provided by a hospital or skilled nursing facility, but do need supervision and support services.

Investor-owned, for-profit: Investor-owned, for-profit hospitals are those controlled on a for-profit basis by an individual, partnership, or profit-making corporation.

Labor-related expenses: Payroll expenses plus employee benefits. *Non-labor-related expenses refers* to all other nonpayroll expenses, such as interest depreciation, supplies, purchased services, professional fees, and others.

Length of stay (LOS): LOS refers to the average number of days a patient stays at the facility. Short-term hospitals are those where the average LOS is less than 30 days. Long-term hospitals are those where the average LOS is 30 days or more. The figure is derived by dividing the number of inpatient days by the number of admissions.

Note that this publication carries two LOS variables: *total facility length of stay and hospital unit length of stay. Total facility* includes admissions and inpatient days from nursing-home-type units under control of the hospital. In *hospital unit length of stay*, nursing home utilization is subtracted.

Licensed practical nurse (LPN): A nurse who has graduated from an approved school of practical (vocational) nursing and works under the supervision of registered nurses and/or physicians.

Long-term: Hospitals are classified either short-term or long-term according to the average length of stay (LOS). A long-term hospital is one in which the average LOS is 30 days or more.

Magnetic resonance imaging (MRI): The use of a uniform magnetic field and radio frequencies to study tissue and structure of the body. This procedure enables the visualization of biochemical activity of the cell in vivo without the use of ionizing radiation, radioisotopic substances, or high-frequency sound.

Managed care: A term covering a broad spectrum of arrangements for health care delivery and financing, including managed indemnity plans (MIP), health maintenance organizations (HMO), preferred provider organizations (PPO), point-of-service plans (POS), and direct contracting arrangements between employers and providers.

Managed care contract: A contract between the hospital and a managed care organization.

Management services organization (MSO): A corporation owned by the hospital or a physician/hospital joint venture that provides management services to one or more medical group practices. As part of a full-service management agreement, the MSO purchases the tangible assets of the practices and leases them back, employs all non-physician staff, and provides all supplies/administrative systems for a fee.

Meals on wheels: A hospital sponsored program which delivers meals to people, usually the elderly, who are unable to prepare their own meals. Low cost, nutritional meals are delivered to individuals' homes on a regular basis.

Medical surgical intensive care: Provides patient care of a more intensive nature than the usual medical and surgical care, on the basis of physicians' orders and approved nursing care plans. These units are staffed with specially trained nursing personnel and contain monitoring and specialized support equipment for patients who, because of shock, trauma, or other life-threatening conditions, require intensified, comprehensive observation and care. Includes mixed intensive care units.

Neonatal intensive care: A unit that must be separate from the newborn nursery providing intensive care to all sick infants including those with the very lowest birth weights (less than 1500 grams). NICU has potential for providing mechanical ventilation, neonatal surgery, and special care for the sickest infants born in the hospital or transferred from another institution. A full-time neonatologist serves as director of the NICU.

Neonatal intermediate care: A unit that must be separate from the normal newborn nursery and that provides intermediate and/or recovery care and some specialized services, including immediate resuscitation, intravenous therapy, and capacity for prolonged oxygen therapy and monitoring.

Net patient revenue: The estimated net realizable amounts from patients, third-party payers, and others for services rendered. The number includes estimated retroactive adjustments called for by agreements with third-party payers; retroactive adjustments are accrued on an estimated basis in the period the related services are rendered and then adjusted later as final settlements are determined.

Net total revenue: Net patient revenue plus all other revenue, including contributions, endowment revenue, governmental grants, and all other payments not made on behalf of individual patients.

Nongovernment, nonprofit: Hospitals that are nongovernment, nonprofit are controlled by not-for-profit organizations, including religious organizations (Catholic hospitals, for example), fraternal societies, and others.

Nursing-home-type unit/facility: A unit/facility that primarily offers the following type of services to a majority of all admissions:

- *Skilled nursing*: The provision of medical and nursing care services, health-related services, and social services under the supervision of a registered nurse on a 24-hour basis.

- *Intermediate care*: The provision, on a regular basis, of health-related care and services to individuals who do not require the degree of care or treatment that a skilled nursing unit is designed to provide.

- *Personal care*: The provision of general supervision and direct personal care services for residents who require assistance in activities of daily living but who do not need nursing services or inpatient care. Medical and nursing services are available as needed.

- *Sheltered/residential care*: The provision of general supervision and protective services for residents who do not need nursing services or continuous personal care services in the conduct of daily life. Medical and nursing services are available as needed.

Nutrition programs: Those services within a health care facility which are designed to provide inexpensive, nutritionally sound meals to patients.

Obstetrics: Levels should be designated: (1) unit provides services for uncomplicated maternity and newborn cases; (2) unit provides services for uncomplicated cases, the majority of complicated problems, and special neonatal services; and (3) unit provides services for all serious illnesses and abnormalities and is supervised by a full-time maternal/fetal specialist.

Occupational health services: Includes services designed to protect the safety of employees from hazards in the work environment.

Oncology services: An organized program for the treatment of cancer by the use of drugs or chemicals.

Open heart surgery: Heart surgery where the chest has been opened and the blood recirculated and oxygenated with the proper equipment and the necessary staff to perform the surgery.

Open physician hospital organization (Open PHO): A joint venture between the hospital and all members of the medical staff who wish to participate. The open PHO can act as a unified agent in managed care contracting, own a managed care plan, own and operate ambulatory care centers or ancillary services projects, or provide administrative services to physician members.

Osteopathic hospitals: Osteopathic medicine is a medical practice based on a theory that diseases are due chiefly to a loss of structural integrity, which can be restored by manipulation of the neuro-muscular and skeletal systems, supplemented by therapeutic measures (such as medicine or surgery).

Other Intensive Care: A distinct intensive care unit that is not one of the following types: medical/surgical, cardiac, pediatric and neonatal.

Other long term care: Provision of long term care other than skilled nursing care or intermediate care. This can include residential care-elderly housing services for those who do not require daily medical or nursing services, but may require some assistance in the activities of daily living, or sheltered care facilities for developmentally disabled.

Other special care: Provides care to patients requiring care more intensive than that provided in the acute area, yet not sufficiently intensive to require admission to an intensive care unit. Patients admitted to this area are usually transferred here from an intensive care unit once their condition has improved. These units are sometimes referred to as definitive observation, step-down, or progressive care units.

Outpatient care: Treatment provided to patients who do not remain in the hospital for overnight care. Hospitals may deliver outpatient care on site or through a facility owned and operated by the hospital, but physically separate from the hospital. In addition to treating minor illnesses or injuries, a free-standing center will stabilize seriously ill or injured patients before transporting them to a hospital. Laboratory and radiology services are usually available.

Outpatient care center (Freestanding): A facility owned and operated by the hospital, but physically separate from the hospital, that provides various medical treatments on an outpatient basis only. In addition to treating minor illnesses or injuries, the center will stabilize seriously ill or injured patients before transporting them to a hospital. Laboratory and radiology services are usually available.

Outpatient care center-services (Hospital-based): Organized hospital health care services offered by appointment on an ambulatory basis. Services may include outpatient surgery, examination, diagnosis, and treatment of a variety of medical conditions on a nonemergency basis, and laboratory and other diagnostic testing as ordered by staff or outside physician referral.

Outpatient surgeries: Scheduled surgical services provided to patients who do not remain in the hospital overnight. In the AHA Annual Survey, outpatient surgery may be performed in operating suites also used for inpatient surgery, specially designated surgical suites for outpatient surgery, or procedure rooms within an outpatient care facility.

Outpatient visit: A visit by a patient who is not lodged in the hospital while receiving medical, dental, or other services. Each visit an outpatient makes to a discrete unit constitutes one visit regardless of the number of diagnostic and/or therapeutic treatments that the patient receives. Total outpatient visits should include all clinic visits, referred visits, observation services, outpatient surgeries, and emergency room visits.

Pain management: A hospital wide formalized program that includes staff education for the management of chronic and acute pain based on guidelines and protocols like those developed by the Agency for Health Care Policy Research, etc.

Palliative care program: An organized program providing specialized medical care, drugs or therapies for the management of acute or chronic pain and/or the control of symptoms administered by specially trained physicians and other clinicians; and supportive care services, such as counseling on advanced directives, spiritual care, and social services, to patients with advanced disease and their families.

Patient education center: Written goals and objectives for the patient and/or family related to therapeutic regimens, medical procedures, and self care.

Patient representative services: Organized hospital services providing personnel through whom patients and staff can seek solutions to institutional problems affecting the delivery of high-quality care and services.

Payroll expenses: Includes all salaries and wages. All professional fees and salary expenditures excluded from payroll, such as employee benefits, are defined as nonpayroll expenses and are included in total expenses.

Pediatric intensive care: Provides care to pediatric patients that is of a more intensive nature than that usually provided to pediatric patients. The unit is staffed with specially trained personnel and contains monitoring and specialized support equipment for treatment of patients who, because of shock, trauma, or other life-threatening conditions, require intensified, comprehensive observation and care.

Pediatric medical-surgical care: Provides acute care to pediatric patients on the basis of physicians' orders and approved nursing care plans.

Personnel: Number of persons on the hospital payroll at the end of the reporting period. Personnel are recorded in *Hospital Statistics* as full-time equivalents (FTEs), which are cal-

culated by adding the number of full-time personnel to one-half the number of part-time personnel, excluding medical and dental residents, interns, and other trainees. *Per 100 adjusted census* indicates the ratio of personnel to adjusted average daily census, calculated on a per-100 basis.

Physical rehabilitation inpatient care: Provides care encompassing a comprehensive array of restoration services for the disabled and all support services necessary to help patients attain their maximum functional capacity.

Physical rehabilitation outpatient services: Outpatient program providing medical, health-related, therapy, social, and/or vocational services to help disabled persons attain or retain their maximum functional capacity.

Population: Population refers to the residential population of the United States. This includes both civilian and military personnel. Note that population is being used to calculate the values *for community health indicators per 1000 population.*

Positron emission tomography scanner (PET): A nuclear medicine imaging technology which uses radioactive (positron emitting) isotopes created in a cyclotron or generator and computers to produce composite pictures of the brain and heart at work. PET scanning produces sectional images depicting metabolic activity or blood flow rather than anatomy.

Preferred provider organization (PPO): A pre-set arrangement in which purchasers and providers agree to furnish specified health services to a group of employees/patients.

Primary care department: A unit or clinic within the hospital that provides primary care services (e.g. general pediatric care, general internal medicine, family practice, gynecology) through hospital-salaried medical and/or nursing staff, focusing on evaluating and diagnosing medical problems and providing medical treatment on an outpatient basis.

Psychiatric child-adolescent services: Provides care to emotionally disturbed children and adolescents, including those admitted for diagnosis and those admitted for treatment.

Psychiatric consultation-liaison services: Provides organized psychiatric consultation/liaison services to nonpsychiatric hospital staff and/or departments on psychological aspects of medical care that may be generic or specific to individual patients.

Psychiatric education services: Provides psychiatric educational services to community agencies and workers such as schools, police, courts, public health nurses, welfare agencies, clergy, and so forth. The purpose is to expand the mental health knowledge and competence of personnel not working in the mental health field and to promote good mental health through improved understanding, attitudes, and behavioral patterns.

Psychiatric emergency services: Services of facilities available on a 24-hour basis to provide immediate unscheduled outpatient care, diagnosis, evaluation, crisis intervention, and assistance to persons suffering acute emotional or mental distress.

Psychiatric geriatric services: Provides care to emotionally disturbed elderly patients, including those admitted for diagnosis and those admitted for treatment.

Psychiatric inpatient care: Provides acute or long-term care to emotionally disturbed patients, including patients admitted for diagnosis and those admitted for treatment of psychiatric problems, on the basis of physicians' orders and approved nursing care plans. Long-term care may include intensive supervision to the chronically mentally ill, mentally disordered, or other mentally incompetent persons.

Psychiatric outpatient services: Provides medical care, including diagnosis and treatment, of psychiatric outpatients.

Psychiatric partial hospitalization program: Organized hospital services of intensive day/evening outpatient services of three hours of more duration, distinguished from other outpatient visits of one hour.

Radiation therapy: The branch of medicine concerned with radioactive substances and using various techniques of visualization, with the diagnosis and treatment of disease using any of the various sources of radiant energy. Services could include: megavoltage radiation therapy; radioactive implants; stereotactic radiosurgery; therapeutic radioisotope facility; X-ray radiation therapy.

Registered nurse (RN): A nurse who has graduated from an approved school of nursing and who is currently registered by the state. RNs are responsible for the nature and quality of all nursing care that patients receive. In these tables, the number of RNs does not include those registered nurses more appropriately reported in other occupational categories, such as facility administrators, which are listed under *all other personnel* (Tables 1 and 2).

Rehabilitation services: A wide array of restoration services for disabled and recuperating patients, including all support services necessary to help them attain their maximum functional capacity.

Reproductive health (could include): *Fertility counseling* - A service that counsels and educates on infertility problems and includes laboratory and surgical workup and management for individuals having problems conceiving children. *In vitro fertilization* - Program providing for the induction of fertilization of a surgically removed ovum by donated sperm in a culture medium followed by a short incubation period. The embryo is then reimplanted in the womb.

Retirement housing: A facility which provides social activities to senior citizens, usually retired persons, who do not require health care but some short-term skilled nursing care may be provided. A retirement center may furnish housing and may also have acute hospital and long-term care facilities, or it may arrange for acute and long term care through affiliated institutions.

Rural: A rural hospital is located outside a metropolitan statistical area (MSA), as designated by the U.S. Office of Management and Budget, which is a geographically defined, integrated social and economic unit with a large population nucleus.

Single photon emission computerized tomography (SPECT): A nuclear medicine imaging technology that combines existing technology of gamma camera imaging with computed tomographic imaging technology to provide a more precise and clear image.

Skilled nursing care: Provides non-acute medical and skilled nursing care services, therapy, and social services under the supervision of a licensed registered nurse on a 24-hour basis.

Sleep Center: Specially equipped and staffed center for the diagnosis and treatment of sleep disorders.

Social work services (could include): Organized services that are properly directed and sufficiently staffed by qualified individuals who provide assistance and counseling to patients and their families in dealing with social, emotional, and environmental problems associated with illness or disability, often in the context of financial or discharge planning coordination.

Sports medicine: Provision of diagnostic screening and assessment and clinical and rehabilitation services for the prevention and treatment of sports-related injuries.

Support groups: A hospital sponsored program which allows a group of individuals with the same or similar problems who meet periodically to share experiences, problems, and solutions in order to support each other.

Surgical operations: Those surgical operations, whether major or minor, performed in the operating room(s). A surgical operation involving more than one surgical procedure is still considered only one surgical operation.

Tobacco treatment/cessation program: Organized hospital services with the purpose of ending tobacco-use habits of patients addicted to tobacco/nicotine.

Teen outreach services: A program focusing on the teenager which encourages an improved health status and a healthful lifestyle including physical, emotional, mental, social, spiritual and economic health through education, exercise, nutrition and health promotion.

Transplant services: The branch of medicine that transfers an organ or tissue from one person to another or from one body part to another to replace a diseased structure or to restore function or to change appearance. Services could include: Bone marrow transplant program; kidney transplant; organ transplant (other than kidney); tissue transplant.

Transportation to health facilities: A long-term care support service designed to assist the mobility of the elderly. Some programs offer improved financial access by offering reduced rates and barrier-free buses or vans with ramps and lifts to assist the elderly or handicapped; others offer subsidies for public transport systems or operate mini-bus services exclusively for use by senior citizens.

Trauma center (certified): A facility to provide emergency and specialized intensive care to critically ill and injured patients. **Level 1:** A regional resource trauma center, which is capable of providing total care for every aspect of injury and plays a leadership role in trauma research and education. **Level 2:** A community trauma center, which is capable of providing trauma care to all but the most severely injured patients who require highly specialized care. **Level 3:** A rural trauma hospital, which is capable of providing care to a large number of injury victims and can resuscitate and stabilize more severely injured patients so that they can be transported to Level 1 or 2 facilities.

Ultrasound: The use of acoustic waves above the range of 20,000 cycles per second to visualize internal body structures.

Urban: An urban hospital is located inside a Metropolitan Statistical Area (MSA), designated by the U.S. Office of Management and Budget, which is a geographically defined, integrated social and economic unit with a large population base.

Urgent care center: A facility that provides care and treatment for problems that are not life-threatening but require attention over the short term. These units function like emergency rooms but are separate from hospitals with which they may have backup affiliation arrangements.

Volunteer services department: An organized hospital department responsible for coordinating the services of volunteers working within the institution.

Women's health center/services: An area set aside for coordinated education and treatment services specifically for and promoted to women as provided by this special unit. Services may or may not include obstetrics but include a range of services other than OB.

2002 AHA Annual Survey
Health Forum, L.L.C.

A. REPORTING PERIOD (please refer to the instructions and definitions at the end of the questionnaire)

Report data for a full 12-month period, preferably your last completed fiscal year (365 days). (Be consistent in using the same reporting period for responses throughout various sections of this survey.)

1. Reporting Period used (beginning and ending date) ...... __ __ / __ __ / __ __ __ __   to __ __ / __ __ / __ __ __ __
   Month   Day   Year   Month   Day   Year

2. a. Were you in operation 12 full months

   at the end of your reporting period .... YES ☐   NO ☐

   b. Number of days open

   during reporting period .... _____

3. Indicate the beginning of your current fiscal year .... __ __ / __ __ / __ __ __ __
   Month   Day   Year

B. ORGANIZATIONAL STRUCTURE

1. CONTROL

Indicate the type of organization that is responsible for establishing policy for overall operation of your hospital. CHECK ONLY ONE:

Government, nonfederal
- ☐ 12 State
- ☐ 13 County
- ☐ 14 City
- ☐ 15 City-County
- ☐ 16 Hospital district or authority

Nongovernment, not-for profit (NFP)
- ☐ 21 Church-operated
- ☐ 23 Other not-for-profit (including NFP Corporation)

Investor-owned, for-profit
- ☐ 31 Individual
- ☐ 32 Partnership
- ☐ 33 Corporation

Government, federal
- ☐ 41 Air Force
- ☐ 42 Army
- ☐ 43 Navy
- ☐ 44 Public Health Service
- ☐ 45 Veterans' Affairs
- ☐ 46 Federal other than 41-45 or 47-48
- ☐ 47 PHS Indian Service
- ☐ 48 Department of Justice

2. SERVICE

Indicate the ONE category that BEST describes your hospital or the type of service it provides to the MAJORITY of admissions:
- ☐ 10 General medical and surgical
- ☐ 11 Hospital unit of an institution (prison hospital, college infirmary)
- ☐ 12 Hospital unit within an institution for the mentally retarded
- ☐ 22 Psychiatric
- ☐ 33 Tuberculosis and other respiratory diseases
- ☐ **41 Cancer**
- ☐ **42 Heart**
- ☐ 44 Obstetrics and gynecology
- ☐ 45 Eye, ear, nose, and throat
- ☐ 46 Rehabilitation
- ☐ 47 Orthopedic
- ☐ 48 Chronic disease
- ☐ 62 Institution for mentally retarded
- ☐ 82 Alcoholism and other chemical dependency
- ☐ **90 Acute Long-Term Care**

- ☐ 49 Other-specify treatment area: _____
  _____

3. OTHER

a. Does your hospital restrict admissions primarily to children? .... YES ☐   NO ☐

b. Is your hospital primarily osteopathic? .... YES ☐   NO ☐

B. ORGANIZATIONAL STRUCTURE (continued)

3. c. Is the hospital part of a health care system? YES ☐ No ☐

   d. Does the hospital itself operate subsidiary corporations? .... YES ☐ No ☐

   e. Is the hospital contract managed? If yes, please provide the name, city, and state of the organization ... YES ☐ No ☐
   Name: _____ City: _____ State: _____

   f. Is the hospital a participant in a network? If yes, please provide the name and telephone number........ YES ☐ No ☐
   of the network. If the hospital participates in more than one network, please provide the name, address, city, state and telephone number of the network(s) on page 8, under supplemental information.
   Name: _____ City: _____ State: _____ Telephone_____

   g. Does the hospital participate in a group purchasing arrangement? If yes, please provide the............. YES ☐ No ☐
   name, city, and state of the group purchasing organization:
   Name: _____ City: _____ State: _____

B. FACILITIES AND SERVICES

For each service or facility listed below, please check all the categories that describe how each item is provided as of the last day of the reporting period. Check all categories that apply for an item. Leave all categories blank for a facility or service that is not provided. Column 2 refers to the systems that were identified in section B, question 3c. Column 3 refers to the networks that were identified in section B, question 3f.

	(1) Owned or provided by my hospital or it's subsidiary	(2) Provided by my Health System (in my local community)	(3) Provided by my network (in my local community)	(4) Provided through a formal contractual arrangement or joint venture with another provider that is not in my system or network (in my local community)
1. General medical-surgical care	☐ (# Beds: _____)	☐	☐	☐
2. Pediatric medical-surgical care	☐ (# Beds: _____)	☐	☐	☐
3. Obstetrics [Level of unit (1-3): (_____)].........	☐ (# Beds: _____)	☐	☐	☐
4. Medical surgical intensive care	☐ (# Beds: _____)	☐	☐	☐
5. Cardiac intensive care	☐ (# Beds: _____)	☐	☐	☐
6. Neonatal intensive care	☐ (# Beds: _____)	☐	☐	☐
7. Neonatal intermediate care	☐ (# Beds: _____)	☐	☐	☐
8. Pediatric intensive care	☐ (# Beds: _____)	☐	☐	☐
9. Burn care	☐ (# Beds: _____)	☐	☐	☐
10. Other special care	☐ (# Beds: _____)	☐	☐	☐
11. Other intensive care (specify:_____)	☐ (# Beds: _____)	☐	☐	☐
12. Physical rehabilitation	☐ (# Beds: _____)	☐	☐	☐
13. Alcoholism-drug abuse or dependency care.	☐ (# Beds: _____)	☐	☐	☐
14. Psychiatric care	☐ (# Beds: _____)	☐	☐	☐
15. Skilled nursing care	☐ (# Beds: _____)	☐	☐	☐
16. Intermediate nursing care	☐ (# Beds: _____)	☐	☐	☐
17. Acute long term care	☐ (# Beds: _____)	☐	☐	☐
18. Other long term care	☐ (# Beds: _____)	☐	☐	☐
19. Other care (specify: _____)...	☐ (# Beds: _____)	☐	☐	☐

C. FACILITIES AND SERVICES (continued)

	(1) Owned or provided by my hospital or it's subsidiary	(2) Provided by my Health System (in my local community)	(3) Provided by my network (in my local community)	(4) Provided through a formal contractual arrangement or joint venture with another provider that is not in my system or network (in my local community)
20. Adult day care program	☐	☐	☐	☐
21. Airborne infection isolation room (# rooms_____)	☐	☐	☐	☐
22. Alcoholism-drug abuse or dependency outpatient services	☐	☐	☐	☐
23. Ambulance services	☐	☐	☐	☐
24. Angioplasty	☐	☐	☐	☐
25. Arthritis treatment center	☐	☐	☐	☐
26. Assisted living	☐	☐	☐	☐
27. Auxiliary	☐	☐	☐	☐
28. Bariatric/weight control services	☐	☐	☐	☐
29. Birthing room - LDR room -LDRP room	☐	☐	☐	☐
30. Breast cancer screening/mammograms	☐	☐	☐	☐
31. Cardiac catheterization laboratory	☐	☐	☐	☐
32. Case management	☐	☐	☐	☐
33. Chaplaincy/pastoral care services	☐	☐	☐	☐
34. Children wellness program	☐	☐	☐	☐
35. Chiropractic services	☐	☐	☐	☐
36. Community outreach	☐	☐	☐	☐
37. Complementary medicine services	☐	☐	☐	☐
38. Crisis prevention	☐	☐	☐	☐
39. Dental services	☐	☐	☐	☐
40. Emergency services				
a. Emergency department	☐	☐	☐	☐
b. Trauma center (certified) [Level of unit (1-3):] _____	☐	☐	☐	☐
41. Enabling services	☐	☐	☐	☐
42. End of life service				
a. Hospice program	☐	☐	☐	☐
b. Pain management program	☐	☐	☐	☐
c. Palliative care program	☐	☐	☐	☐
43. Enrollment assistance services	☐	☐	☐	☐
44. Extracorporeal shock wave lithotripter (ESWL)	☐	☐	☐	☐
45. Fitness center	☐	☐	☐	☐
46. Freestanding outpatient care center	☐	☐	☐	☐
47. Geriatric services	☐	☐	☐	☐
48. Health fair	☐	☐	☐	☐
49. Health information center	☐	☐	☐	☐
50. Health screenings	☐	☐	☐	☐
51. Hemodialysis	☐	☐	☐	☐
52. HIV-AIDS services	☐	☐	☐	☐
53. Home health services	☐	☐	☐	☐
54. Hospital-based outpatient care center-services	☐	☐	☐	☐
55. Linguistic/translation services	☐	☐	☐	☐
56. Meals on wheels	☐	☐	☐	☐

C. FACILITIES AND SERVICES (continued)

	(1) Owned or provided by my hospital or it's subsidiary	(2) Provided by my Health System (in my local community)	(3) Provided by my network (in my local community)	(4) Provided through a formal contractual arrangement or joint venture with another provider that is not in my system or network (in my local community)
57. Neurological services..	☐	☐	☐	☐
58. Nutrition programs	☐	☐	☐	☐
59. Occupational health services	☐	☐	☐	☐
60. Oncology services	☐	☐	☐	☐
61. Open heart surgery	☐	☐	☐	☐
62. Orthopedic services	☐	☐	☐	☐
63. Outpatient surgery	☐	☐	☐	☐
64. Patient education center	☐	☐	☐	☐
65. Patient representative services	☐	☐	☐	☐
66. Physical rehabilitation outpatient services	☐	☐	☐	☐
67. Primary care department	☐	☐	☐	☐
68. Psychiatric services				
a. Psychiatric child-adolescent services	☐	☐	☐	☐
b. Psychiatric consultation-liaison services	☐	☐	☐	☐
c. Psychiatric education services	☐	☐	☐	☐
d. Psychiatric emergency services	☐	☐	☐	☐
e. Psychiatric geriatric services	☐	☐	☐	☐
f. Psychiatric outpatient services	☐	☐	☐	☐
g. Psychiatric partial hospitalization program	☐	☐	☐	☐
69. Radiation therapy	☐	☐	☐	☐
70. Radiology, diagnostic				
a. CT scanner	☐	☐	☐	☐
b. Diagnostic radioisotope facility	☐	☐	☐	☐
c. Magnetic resonance imaging (MRI)	☐	☐	☐	☐
d. Positron emission tomography (PET)	☐	☐	☐	☐
e. Single photon emission computerized tomography (SPECT).	☐	☐	☐	☐
f. Ultrasound	☐	☐	☐	☐
71. Reproductive health	☐	☐	☐	☐
72. Retirement housing	☐	☐	☐	☐
73. Sleep Center	☐	☐	☐	☐
74. Social work services	☐	☐	☐	☐
75. Sports medicine	☐	☐	☐	☐
76. Support groups	☐	☐	☐	☐
77. Swing bed services	☐	☐	☐	☐
78. Teen outreach services	☐	☐	☐	☐
79. Tobacco Treatment/Cessation Program	☐	☐	☐	☐
80. Transplant services	☐	☐	☐	☐
81. Transportation to health facilities	☐	☐	☐	☐
82. Urgent care center	☐	☐	☐	☐
83. Volunteer services department	☐	☐	☐	☐
84. Women's health center/services	☐	☐	☐	☐
85. Wound Management Services	☐	☐	☐	☐

C. FACILITIES AND SERVICES (continued)

86. In which of the following physician arrangements does your hospital or system/network participate? Column 2 refers to the systems that were identified in section B, question 3c. Column 3 refers to the networks that were identified in section b, question 3f. For hospital level physician arrangements that are reported in column 1, please report the number of physicians involved.

	(1) My Hospital		(2) My Heatlh System	(3) My Health Network
a. Independent Practice Association	☐	(# of physicians _____)	☐	☐
b. Group practice without walls	☐	(# of physicians _____)	☐	☐
c. Open Physician-Hospital Organization (PHO)	☐	(# of physicians _____)	☐	☐
d. Closed Physician-Hospital Organization (PHO)	☐	(# of physicians _____)	☐	☐
e. Management Service Organization (MSO)	☐	(# of physicians _____)	☐	☐
f. Integrated Salary Model	☐	(# of physicians _____)	☐	☐
g. Equity Model	☐	(# of physicians _____)	☐	☐
h. Foundation	☐	(# of physicians _____)	☐	☐

Please provide a separate list of the name(s) and address(es) of the hospital's physician arrangements reported in column 1.

87. Does your hospital, health system or health network have an equity interest in any of the following insurance products? (Check all that apply) Contractual relationships with HMOs and PPOs should not be reported here but in Question 6. Column 2 refers to the systems that were identified in section B, question 3c. Column 3 refers to the networks that were identified in section B, question 3f.

	(1) My Hospital	(2) My Health System	(3) My Health Network	(4) Joint Venture With Insurer
a. Health Maintenance Organization	☐	☐	☐	☐
b. Preferred Provider Organization	☐	☐	☐	☐
c. Indemnity Fee For Service Plan	☐	☐	☐	☐

88. Does your hospital have a formal written contract that specifies the obligations of each party with:

a. Health maintenance organization (HMO) .... YES ☐   NO ☐   b. If YES, how many contracts? _____

c. Preferred provider organization (PPO) .... YES ☐   NO ☐   d. If YES, how many contracts? _____

89a. What percentage of the hospital's net patient revenue is paid on a capitated basis?
If the hospital does not participate in capitated arrangements, please enter "0")   _____ %

89b. What percentage of the hospital's net patient revenue is paid on a shared risk basis?   _____ %

90. Does your hospital contract directly with employers or a coalition of employers to provide care on a capitated, predetermined, or shared risk basis? ....YES ☐   NO ☐

91. If your hospital has arrangements to care for a specific group of enrollees in exchange for a capitated payment, how many lives are covered?   _____

D. COMMUNITY ORIENTATION

1. Does your hospital's mission statement include a focus on community benefit? .... YES ☐   NO ☐
2. Does your hospital have a long-term plan for improving the health of its community? .... YES ☐   NO ☐
3. Does your hospital have resources for its community benefit activities? .... YES ☐   NO ☐
4. Does your hospital work with other providers, public agencies, or community representatives to conduct a health status assessment of the community? .... YES ☐   NO ☐
5. Does your hospital use health status indicators (such as rates of health problems or surveys of self-reported health) for defined populations to design new services or modify existing services? .... YES ☐   NO ☐
6a. Does your hospital work with other local providers, public agencies, or community representatives to develop a written assessment of the appropriate capacity for health services in the community? .... YES ☐   NO ☐
6b. If yes, have you used the assessment to identify unmet health needs, excess capacity, or duplicative services in the community? .... YES ☐   NO ☐
7. Does your hospital work with other providers to collect, track, and communicate clinical and health information across cooperating organizations? .... YES ☐   NO ☐
8. Does your hospital either by itself or in conjunction with others disseminate reports to the community on the quality and costs of health care services? .... YES ☐   NO ☐
9. Does your hospital self-assess against Baldrige like criteria for sustained continuous improvement? .... YES ☐   NO ☐
10. Does your hospital gather information on a patient's race/ethnicity at any point during their stay?................ YES ☐   NO ☐
11. Does your hospital gather information on a patient's primary language at any point during their stay?.............YES ☐   NO ☐

E. TOTAL FACILITY BEDS, UTILIZATION, FINANCES, AND STAFFING

Please report beds, utilization, financial, and staffing data for a 12 month period that is consistent with the period reported on page 1. Report financial data for reporting period only. Include within your operations all activities that are wholly owned by the hospital, including subsidiary corporations regardless of where the activity is physically located. Please do not include within your operations distinct and separate divisions that may be owned by your hospital's parent corporation. If final figures are not available, please estimate. Round to the nearest dollar. Report all personnel who were on the payroll and whose payroll expenses are reported in E3f. (Please refer to specific definitions on pages 15-16.)

Fill out column (2) if hospital owns and operates a nursing home type unit/facility. Column (1) should be the combined total of hospital plus Nursing Home Unit/Facility.	(1) Total Facility	(2) Nursing Home Unit/Facility

1. BEDS AND UTILIZATION

a. Beds set up and staffed for use at the end of the reporting period .... _____ _____

b. Bassinets set up and staffed for use at the end of the reporting period .... _____ _____

c. Births (exclude fetal deaths) .... _____ _____

d. Admissions (exclude newborns, include neonatal & swing admissions) .... _____ _____

e. Inpatient days (exclude newborns, include neonatal & swing days) .... _____ _____

f. Emergency room visits .... _____ _____

g. Total outpatient visits (include emergency room visits & outpatient surgeries) .... _____ _____

h. Inpatient surgical operations .... _____ _____

   Number of operating rooms .... _____ _____

i. Outpatient surgical operations .... _____ _____

2. MEDICARE/MEDICAID UTILIZATION
(exclude newborns, include neonatal & swing days and deaths)

a1. Total Medicare (Title XVIII) inpatient discharges (including Medicare Managed Care) .... _____ _____

a2. How many Medicare inpatient discharges were Medicare Managed Care .... _____ _____

b1. Total Medicare (Title XVIII) inpatient days (including Medicare Managed Care) .... _____ _____

b2. How many Medicare inpatient days were Medicare Managed Care .... _____ _____

c1. Total Medicaid (Title XIX) inpatient discharges (including Medicaid Managed Care) .... _____ _____

c2. How many Medicaid inpatient discharges were Medicaid Managed Care .... _____ _____

d1. Total Medicaid (Title XIX) inpatient days (including Medicaid Managed Care) .... _____ _____

d2. How many Medicaid inpatient days were Medicaid Managed Care .... _____ _____

3. FINANCIAL

* a. Net patient revenue .... _____.00 _____.00

* b. Tax appropriations .... _____.00

* c. Other operating revenue .... _____.00

* d. Nonoperating revenue .... _____.00

* e. TOTAL REVENUE (add 3a thru 3d) .... _____.00 _____.00

f. PAYROLL EXPENSES (only) .... _____.00 _____.00

g. Employee benefits .... _____.00 _____.00

h. Depreciated expense (for reporting period only) .... _____.00

i. Interest expense .... _____.00

j. TOTAL EXPENSES (Payroll plus all non-payroll expenses, including bad debt) _____.00 _____.00

*4. REVENUE BY TYPE

a. Total gross inpatient revenue .... _____.00

b. Total gross outpatient revenue .... _____.00

c. Total gross patient revenue .... _____.00

*5. UNCOMPENSATED CARE

a. Bad debt expense .... _____.00

b. Charity (Revenue forgone at full established rates. Include in gross revenue) .... _____.00

*These data will be treated as confidential and not released without written permission. AHA will, however, share these data with your respective state hospital association and, if requested, with your appropriate metropolitan/regional association. For members of the Catholic Health Association of the United States (CHA), AHA will also share these data with CHA unless there are objections. The state/metropolitan/regional association may not release these data without written permission from the hospital.

E. TOTAL FACILITY BEDS, UTILIZATION, FINANCES, AND STAFFING (continued)

*6. REVENUE BY PAYOR (report total facility gross and net figures)
(E.6a(2a) should include Medicaid disproportionate payments in the net column (2)

			(1) Gross	(2) Net
*a. GOVERNMENT	(1) Medicare:			
		a) Routine patient revenue	.00	.00
		b) Managed care revenue	.00	.00
		c) **Total (a + b)**	**.00**	**.00**
	(2) Medicaid:			
		a) Routine patient revenue	.00	.00
		b) Managed care revenue	.00	.00
		c) **Total (a + b)**	**.00**	**.00**
	(3) Other government:		.00	.00
*b. NONGOVERNMENT	(1) Self-pay		.00	.00
	(2) Third-party payors:			
		a) Managed care (includes HMO and PPO)	.00	.00
		b) Other third-party payors	.00	.00
		c) **Total third-party payors (a + b)**	**.00**	**.00**
	(3) All Other nongovernment:		.00	.00
*c. TOTAL			.00	.00

(Total gross should equal 4c on page 6, total net should equal 3a on page 6.)

Are the financial data on pages 5 and 6 from your audited financial statement?	YES ☐	No ☐

7. FIXED ASSETS

a. Property, plant and equipment at cost	.00
b. Accumulated depreciation	.00
c. Net property, plant and equipment (a-b)	.00
d. Total gross square feet of your physical plant used for or in support of your healthcare activities	.00

8. **STAFFING**

Report full-time (35 hours or more) and part-time (less than 35 hours) personnel who were on the hospital/facility **payroll at the end of your reporting period.** Include members of religious orders for whom dollar equivalents were reported. Exclude private-duty nurses, volunteers, and all personnel whose salary is financed entirely by outside research grants. Exclude physicians and dentists who are paid on a fee basis. FTE is the total number of hours worked by all employees over the full (12 month) reporting period divided by the normal number of hours worked by a full-time employee for that same time period. For example, if your hospital considers a normal work week for a full-time employee to be 40 hours, a total of 2,080 would be worked over a full year (52 weeks). If the total number of hours worked by all employees on the payroll is 208,000, then the number of Full-Time Equivalents (FTE) is 100 (employees). The FTE calculation for a specific occupational category such as Registered nurses is exactly the same. The calculation for each occupational occupational category should be based on the number of hours worked by staff employed in that specific category.

	(1) Full-Time (35 hr/wk or more) On Payroll	(2) Part-Time (less than 35 hr/wk) On Payroll	(3) FTE
a. Physicians and dentists	_____	_____	_____
b. Medical and dental residents/interns	_____	_____	_____
c. Other trainees	_____	_____	_____
d. Registered nurses	_____	_____	_____
e. Licensed practical (vocational) nurses	_____	_____	_____
f. **Nursing assistive personnel**	_____	_____	_____
g. All other personnel	_____	_____	_____
h. Total facility personnel (add 8a through 8g) (Should include hospital plus nursing home type unit/facility personnel)	_____	_____	_____
i. Nursing home type unit/facility personnel (if applicable - please break out these personnel from the total facility number.)	_____	_____	_____

SUPPLEMENTAL INFORMATION

1. Does your hospital participate in any joint venture arrangements? .... YES ☐   NO ☐
   If yes, please provide a separate list of the name(s) and address(es) of the arrangements.

2. Does your hospital provide services through a satellite facility(s)? .... YES ☐   NO ☐
   If yes, please provide a separate list of the name(s) and address(es) of the satellite.

3. For the titles listed below, please indicate the name and the exact title of the person who holds the position in the hospital.

	Name	Title
a. Chief Financial Officer	_____	_____
b. Chief Information Officer	_____	_____
c. Vice President, Strategic Planning	_____	_____
d. Chief of the Medical Staff	_____	_____

Use this space or an additional sheet if more space is required for comments or to elaborate on any of the information supplied on this survey. Refer to the response by page, section, and item name. Also, use this space to describe your community benefit activities.

_____
_____
_____
_____
_____
_____
_____
_____
_____
_____
_____
_____
_____
_____
_____
_____
_____

As declared previously, hospital specific revenue data are treated as confidential. AHA's policy is not to release these data without written permission from your institution. The AHA will however, share these data with your respective state hospital association and if requested with your appropriate metropolitan/regional association.

On occasion, the AHA is asked to provide these data to external organizations, both public and private, for their use in analyzing crucial health care policy or research issues. The AHA is requesting your permission to allow us to release your confidential data to those requests that we consider legitimate and worthwhile. In every instance of disclosure, the receiving organization will be prohibited from releasing hospital specific information.

Please indicate below whether or not you agree to these types of disclosure:

[   ] I hereby grant AHA permission to release my hospital's revenue data to external users that the AHA determines have a legitimate and worthwhile need to gain access to these data subject to the user's agreement with the AHA not to release hospital specific information.

_____
Chief Executive Officer   Date

[   ] I do not grant AHA permission to release my confidential data.

_____
Chief Executive Officer   Date

I am a member of the Catholic Health Association of the United States and I do not want my confidential data shared with them.

[   ] I do not grant AHA permission to release my confidential data to CHA.

Does your hospital or health system have an Internet or Homepage address? Yes ☐ No ☐	
If yes, please provide the address: http:// _____	

Thank you for your cooperation in completing this survey. If there are any questions about your responses to this survey, who should be contacted?

_____   _____   _____
Name (please print)   Title   (Area Code) Telephone Number

____/____/____   _____   (   )
Date of Completion   Chief Executive Officer   Hospital's Main Fax Number

NOTE: PLEASE PHOTOCOPY THE INFORMATION FOR YOUR HOSPITAL FILE BEFORE RETURNING THE ORIGINAL FORM TO THE AMERICAN HOSPITAL ASSOCIATION. ALSO, PLEASE FORWARD A PHOTOCOPY OF THE COMPLETED QUESTIONNAIRE TO YOUR STATE HOSPITAL ASSOCIATION.

THANK YOU

SECTION A
REPORTING PERIOD
Instructions

INSTRUCTIONS AND DEFINITIONS FOR THE 2002 ANNUAL SURVEY

HOSPITAL. For purposes of this survey, a hospital is defined as the organization or corporate entity licensed or registered as a hospital by a state to provide diagnostic and therapeutic patient services for a variety of medical conditions, both surgical and nonsurgical.

1. **Reporting period used (beginning and ending date):** Record the beginning and ending dates of the reporting period in an eight-digit number: for example, January 1, 2002 should be shown as 01/01/2002. Number of days should equal the time span between the two dates that the hospital was open. If you are reporting for less than 365 days, utilization and finances should be presented for days reported only.
2. **Were you in operation 12 full months at the end of your reporting period?** If you are reporting for less than 365 days, utilization and finances should be presented for days reported only.
3. **Number of days open during reporting period:** Number of days should equal the time span between the two dates that the hospital was open.

SECTION B
ORGANIZATIONAL STRUCTURE
Instructions and Definitions

1. CONTROL
   Check the box to the left of the type of organization that is responsible for establishing policy for overall operation of the hospital.
   Government, nonfederal.
   State. Controlled by an agency of state government.
   County. Controlled by an agency of county government.
   City. Controlled by an agency of municipal government.
   City-County. Controlled jointly by agencies of municipal and county governments.
   Hospital district or authority. Controlled by a political subdivision of a state, county, or city created solely for the purpose of establishing and maintaining medical care or health-related care institutions.
   Nongovernment, not for profit. Hospitals controlled by not-for-profit organizations, including religious organizations (Catholic hospitals, for example), community hospitals, cooperative hospitals, hospitals operated by fraternal societies, and so forth.
   Investor owned, for profit. Hospitals controlled on a for profit basis by an individual, partnership, or a profit making corporation.
   Government, federal. Hospitals controlled by an agency or department of the federal government.
2. SERVICE
   Indicate the ONE category that best describes the type of service that your hospital provides to the majority of admissions.
   General medical and surgical. Provides diagnostic and therapeutic services to patients for a variety of medical conditions, both surgical and nonsurgical.
   Hospital unit of an institution. Provides diagnostic and therapeutic services to patients in an institution.
   Hospital unit within an institution for the mentally retarded. Provides diagnostic and therapeutic services to patients in an institution for the mentally retarded.
   Psychiatric. Provides diagnostic and therapeutic services to patients with mental or emotional disorders.
   Tuberculosis and other respiratory diseases. Provides medical care and rehabilitative services to patients for whom the primary diagnosis is tuberculosis or other respiratory diseases.
   Cancer. Provides medical care to patients for whom the primary diagnosis is cancer.
   Heart. Provides diagnosis and treatment of heart disease.
   Obstetrics and gynecology. Provides medical and surgical treatment to pregnant women and to mothers following delivery. Also provides diagnostic and therapeutic services to women with diseases or disorders of the reproductive organs.
   Eye, ear, nose, and throat. Provides diagnosis and treatment of diseases and injuries of the eyes, ears, nose, and throat.
   Rehabilitation. Provides a comprehensive array of restoration services for the disabled and all support services necessary to help them attain their maximum functional capacity.
   Orthopedic. Provides corrective treatment of deformities, diseases, and ailments of the locomotive apparatus, especially affecting the limbs, bones, muscles, and joints.
   Chronic disease. Provides medical and skilled nursing services to patients with long-term illnesses who are not in an acute phase, but who require an intensity of services not available in nursing homes.
   Institution for the mentally retarded. Provides health-related care on a regular basis to patients with psychiatric or developmental impairment who cannot be treated in a skilled nursing unit.
   Alcoholism and other chemical dependency. Provides diagnostic and therapeutic services to patients with alcoholism or other drug dependencies.
   Acute Long Term Care. Provides high acuity interdisciplinary services to medically complex patients that require more intensive recuperation and care than can be provided in a typical nursing facility.
3. OTHER
   a **Children admissions. A hospital whose primary focus is the health and treatment of children and adolescents.**
   b. **Osteopathic.** Osteopathic medicine is a medical practice based on a theory that diseases are due chiefly to a loss of structural integrity which can be restored by manipulation of the neuro-muscular and skeletal system, supplemented by therapeutic measures (as use of medicine or surgery).
   c. **Health care system.** A corporate body that owns, leases, religiously sponsors, and/or manages health provider facilities.
   d. **Subsidiary.** A company that is wholly controlled by another or one that is more than 50% owned by another organization.
   e. **Contract managed.** General day-to-day management of an entire organization by another organization under a formal contract. Managing organization reports directly to the board of trustees or owners of the managed organization; managed organization retains total legal responsibility and ownership of the facility's assets and liabilities.
   f. **Network.** A group of hospitals, physicians, other providers, insurers and/or community agencies that voluntarily work together to coordinate and deliver health services
   g. **Group Purchasing Organization.** An organization whose primary function is to negotiate contracts for the purpose of purchasing for members of the group or has a central supply site for its members.

SECTION C
FACILITIES AND SERVICES
Definitions

1. **General medical-surgical care.** Provides acute care to patients in medical and surgical units on the basis of physicians' orders and approved nursing care plans.
2. **Pediatric medical-surgical care.** Provides acute care to pediatric patients on the basis of physicians' orders and approved nursing care plans.
3. **Obstetrics.** Levels should be designated: (1) unit provides services for uncomplicated maternity and newborn cases; (2) unit provides services for uncomplicated cases, the majority of complicated problems, and special neonatal services; and (3) unit provides services for all serious illnesses and abnormalities and is supervised by a full-time maternal/fetal specialist.
4. **Medical surgical intensive care.** Provides patient care of a more intensive nature than the usual medical and surgical care, on the basis of physicians' orders and approved nursing care plans. These units are staffed with specially trained nursing personnel and contain monitoring and specialized support equipment for patients.
6. **Neonatal intensive care.** A unit that must be separate from the newborn nursery providing intensive care to all sick infants including those with the very lowest birth weights (less than 1500 grams). NICU has potential for providing mechanical ventilation, neonatal surgery, and special care for the sickest infants born in the hospital or transferred from another institution. A full-time neonatologist serves as director of the NICU.
7. **Neonatal intermediate care.** A unit that must be separate from the normal newborn nursery and that provides intermediate and/or recovercare and some specialized services, including immediate resuscitation, intravenous therapy, and capacity for prolonged oxygen therapy and monitoring.
8. **Pediatric intensive care.** Provides care to pediatric patients that is of a more intensive nature than that usually provided to pediatric patients. The unit is staffed with specially trained personnel and contains monitoring and specialized support equipment for treatment of patients who, because of shock, trauma, or other life-threatening conditions, require intensified, comprehensive observation and care.
9. **Burn care.** Provides care to severely burned patients. Severely burned patients are those with any of the following: (1) second-degree burns of more than 25% total body surface area for adults or 20% total body surface area for children: (2) third-degree burns of more than who, because of shock, trauma, or other life-threatening conditions, require intensified, comprehensive observation and care. Includes mixed intensive care units.
5. **Cardiac intensive care.** Provides patient care of a more specialized nature than the usual medical and surgical care, on the basis of physicians' orders and approved nursing care plans. The unit is staffed with specially trained nursing personnel and contains monitoring and specialized support or treatment equipment for patients who, because of heart seizure, open-heart surgery, or other life-threatening conditions, require intensified, comprehensive observation and care. May include myocardial infarction, pulmonary care, and heart transplant units. 10% total body surface area; (3) any severe burns of the hands, face, eyes, ears, or feet; or (4) all inhalation injuries, electrical burns, complicated burn injuries involving fractures and other major traumas, and all other poor risk factors.
10. **Other special care.** Provides care to patients requiring care more intensive than that provided in the acute area, yet not sufficiently intensive to require admission to an intensive care unit. Patients admitted to this area are usually transferred here from an intensive care unit once their condition has improved. These units are sometimes referred to as definitive observation, step-down, or progressive care units.
12. **Physical rehabilitation.** Provides care encompassing a comprehensive array of restoration services for the disabled and all support services necessary to help patients attain their maximum functional capacity.
13. **Alcoholism-drug abuse or dependency care.** Provides diagnosis and therapeutic services to patients with alcoholism or other drug dependencies. Includes care for inpatient/residential treatment for patients whose course of treatment involves more intensive care than provided in an outpatient setting or where patient requires supervised withdrawal.
14. **Psychiatric care.** Provides acute or long-term care to emotionally disturbed patients, including patients admitted for diagnosis and those admitted for treatment of psychiatric problems, on the basis of physicians' orders and approved nursing care plans. Long-term care may include intensive supervision to the chronically mentally ill, mentally disordered, or other mentally incompetent persons.
15. **Skilled nursing care.** Provides non-acute medical and skilled nursing care services, therapy, and social services under the supervision of a licensed registered nurse on a 24-hour basis.
16. **Intermediate nursing care.** Provides health-related services (skilled nursing care and social services) to residents with a variety of physical conditions or functional disabilities. These residents do not require the care provided by a hospital or skilled nursing facility, but do need supervision and support services.
17. **Acute long term care.** Provides specialized acute hospital care to medically complex patients who are critically ill, have multisystem complications and/or failure, and require hospitalization averaging 25 days, in a facility offering specialized treatment programs and therapeutic intervention on a 24 hour/7 day a week basis.
18. **Other long term care.** Provision of long term care other than skilled nursing care or intermediate care. This can include residential care-elderly housing services for those who do not require daily medical or nursing services, but may require some assistance in the activities of daily living, or sheltered care facilities for developmentally disabled.
19. **Other care.** (specify) Any type of care other than those listed above.
    Total beds. <u>The sum of the beds reported in this section should equal what you have reported in Section E for beds set up and staffed.</u>
20. **Adult day care program.** Program providing supervision, medical and psychological care, and social activities for older adults who live at home or in another family setting, but cannot be alone or prefer to be with others during the day. May include intake assessment, health monitoring, occupational therapy, personal care, noon meal, and transportation services.
21. **Alcoholism-drug abuse or dependency outpatient services.** Organized hospital services that provide medical care and/or rehabilitative treatment services to outpatients for whom the primary diagnosis is alcoholism or other chemical dependency.
22. **Airborne infection isolation room .** A single-occupancy room for patient care where environmental factors are controlled in an effort to minimize the transmission of those infectious agents, usually spread person to person by droplet nuclei associated with coughing and inhalation. Such rooms typically have specific ventilation requirements for controlled ventilation, air pressure and filtration.
23 **Ambulance services.** Provision of ambulance service to the ill and injured who require medical attention on a scheduled and unscheduled basis.
24. **Angioplasty.** The reconstruction or restructuring of a blood vessel by operative means or by nonsurgical techniques such as balloon dilation or laser.
25. **Arthritis treatment center.** Specifically equipped and staffed center for the diagnosis and treatment of arthritis and other joint disorders.
26. **Assisted living.** A special combination of housing, supportive services, personalized assistance and health care designed to respond to the individual needs of those who need help in activities of daily living and instrumental activities of daily living. Supportive services are available, 24 hours a day, to meet scheduled and unscheduled needs, in a way that promotes maximum independence an dignity for each resident and encourages the involvement of a resident's family, neighbor and friends.
27. **Auxiliary.** A volunteer community organization formed to assist the hospital in carrying out its purpose and to serve as a link between the institution and the community.

28. **Bariactric/weight control services.** Bariatrics is the medical practice of weight reduction.

29. **Birthing room/LDR room/LDRP room.** A single-room type of maternity care with a more homelike setting for families than the traditional three-room unit (labor/delivery/recovery) with a separate postpartum area. A birthing room combines labor and delivery in one room. An LDR room accommodates three stages in the birthing process – labor, delivery, and recovery. An LDRP room accommodates all four stages of the birth process – labor, delivery, recovery, and postpartum.

30. **Breast cancer screening/mammograms.** Mammography screening - The use of breast x-ray to detect unsuspected breast cancer in asymptomatic women. Diagnostic mammography - The x-ray imaging of breast tissue in symptomatic women who are considered to have a substantial likelihood of having breast cancer already.

31. **Cardiac catheterization laboratory.** Facilities offering special diagnostic procedures for cardiac patients. Available procedures must include, but need not be limited to, introduction of a catheter into the interior of the heart by way of a vein or artery or by direct needle puncture. Procedures must be performed in a laboratory or a special procedure room.

32. **Case management.** A system of assessment, treatment planning, referral and follow-up that ensures the provision of comprehensive and continuous services and the coordination of payment and reimbursement for care.

33. **Chaplaincy/pastoral care services.** A service ministering religious activities and providing pastoral counseling to patients, their families, and staff of a health care organization.

34. **Children wellness program.** A program that encourages improved health status and a healthful lifestyle of children through health education, exercise, nutrition and health promotion.

35. **Chiropractic services.** An organized clinical service including spinal manipulation or adjustment and related diagnostic and therapeutic services.

36. **Community outreach.** A program that systematically interacts with the community to identify those in need of services, alerting persons and their families to the availability of services, locating needed services, and enabling persons to enter the service delivery system.

37. **Complementary medicine services.** Organized hospital services or formal arrangements to providers that provide care or treatment not based solely on traditional western allopathic medical teachings as instructed in most U.S. medical schools. Includes any of the following: acupuncture, chiropractic, homeopathy, osteopathy, diet and lifestyle changes, herbal medicine, massage therapy, etc.

38. **Crisis prevention.** Services provided in order to promote physical and mental well being and the early identification of disease and ill health prior to the onset and recognition of symptoms so as to permit early treatment.

39. **Dental Services.** An organized dental service or dentists on staff, not necessarily involving special facilities, providing dental or oral services to inpatients or outpatients.

40. **Emergency services.** Health services that are provided after the onset of a medical condition that manifests itself by symptoms of sufficient severity, including severe pain, that the absence of immediate medical attention could reasonably be expected by a prudent layperson, who possesses an average knowledge of health and medicine, to result in placing the patient's health in serious jeopardy.

40a. **Emergency department.** Hospital facilities for the provision of unscheduled outpatient services to patients whose conditions require immediate care.

40b. **Trauma center (certified).** A facility to provide emergency and specialized intensive care to critically ill and injured patients. Level 1: A regional resource trauma center, which is capable of providing total care for every aspect of injury and plays a leadership role in trauma research and education. Level 2: A community trauma center, which is capable of providing trauma care to all but the most severely injured patients who require highly specialized care. Level 3: A rural trauma hospital, which is capable of providing care to a large number of injury victims and can resuscitate and stabilize more severely injured patients so that they can be transported to level 1 or 2 facilities. Please provide explanation on page 15 if necessary.

41. **Enabling services.** A program that is designed to help the patient access health care services by offering any of the following: transportation services, and/or referrals to local social services agencies.

42. **End of life services.**

42a. **Hospice Program.** A recognized clinical program with specific eligibility criteria that provides palliative medical care focused on relief of pain and symptom control and other services that address the emotional, social, financial and spiritual needs of terminally ill patients and their families. Hospice care can be provided either at home, in a hospital setting, or a free-standing facility.

42b. **Pain management program.** A recognized clinical service or program providing specialized medical care, drugs or therapies for the management of acute or chronic pain and other distressing symptoms, administered by specially trained physicians and other clinicians, to patients suffering from an acute illness of diverse causes.

42c. **Palliative care program.** An organized program providing specialized medical care, drugs or therapies for the management of acute or chronic pain and/or the control of symptoms administered by specially trained physicians and other clinicians; and supportive care services, such as counseling on advanced directives, spiritual care, and social services, to patients with advanced disease and their families.

43. **Enrollment assistance services.** A program that provides enrollment assistance for patients who are potentially eligible for public health insurance programs such as Medicaid, State Children's Health Insurance, or local/state indigent care programs. The specific services offered could include explanation of benefits, assist applicants in completing the application and locating all relevant documents, conduct eligibility interviews, and/or forward applications and documentation to state/local social service or health agency.

44. **Extracorporeal shock wave lithotripter (ESWL).** A medical device used for treating stones in the kidney or urether. The device disintegrates kidney stones noninvasively through the transmission of acoustic shock waves directed at the stones.

45. **Fitness center.** Provides exercise, testing, or evaluation programs and fitness activities to the community and hospital employees.

46. **Freestanding outpatient care center.** A facility owned and operated by the hospital, but physically separate from the hospital, that provides various medical treatments on an outpatient basis only. In addition to treating minor illnesses or injuries, the center will stabilize seriously ill or injured patients before transporting them to a hospital. Laboratory and radiology services are usually available.

47. **Geriatric services.** The branch of medicine dealing with the physiology of aging and the diagnosis and treatment of disease affecting the aged. Services could include: Adult day care; Alzheimer's diagnostic-assessment services; Comprehensive geriatric assessment; Emergency response system; Geriatric acute care unit; and/or Geriatric clinics.

48. **Health fair.** Community health education events that focus on the prevention of disease and promotion of health through such activities as audiovisual exhibits and free diagnostic services.

49. **Health information center.** Education which is directed at increasing the information of individuals and populations. It is intended to increase the ability to make informed personal, family and community health decisions by providing consumers with informed choices about health matters with the objective of improving health status.

50. **Health screening.** A preliminary procedure such as a test or examination to detect the most characteristic sign or signs of a disorder that may require further investigation.

51. **Hemodialysis:** Provision of equipment and personnel for the treatment of renal insufficiency on an inpatient or outpatient basis.

52. **HIV-AIDS services** (could include). HIV -AIDS unit-Special unit or team designated and equipped specifically for diagnosis, treatment, continuing care planning, and counseling services for HIV -AIDS patients and their families. General inpatient care for HIV -AIDS-Inpatient diagnosis and treatment for human immunodeficiency virus and acquired immunodeficiency syndrome patients, but dedicated unit is not available. Specialized outpatient program for HIV -AIDS-Special outpatient program providing diagnostic, treatment, continuing care planning, and counseling for HIV -AIDS patients and their families.

53. **Home health services.** Service providing nursing, therapy, and health-related homemaker or social services in the patient's home.

54. **Hospital-based outpatient care center-services.** Organized hospital health care services offered by appointment on an ambulatory basis. Services may include outpatient surgery, examination, diagnosis, and treatment of a variety of medical conditions on a nonemergency basis, and laboratory and other diagnostic testing as ordered by staff or outside physician referral.

55. **Linguistic/translation services.** Services provided by the hospital designed to make health care more accessible to non- English speaking patients and their physicans.

56. **Meals on wheels.** A hospital sponsored program which delivers meals to people, usually the elderly, who are unable to prepare their own meals. Low cost, nutritional meals are delivered to individuals' homes on a regular basis.

57. **Neurological services.** Services provided by the hospital dealing with the operative and nonoperative management of disorders of the central, peripheral, and autonomic nervous system.

58. **Nutrition programs**. Those services within a health care facility which are designed to provide inexpensive, nutritionally sound meals to patients.

59. **Occupational health services.** Includes services designed to protect the safety of employees from hazards in the work environment.

60. **Oncology services.** An organized program for the treatment of cancer by the use of drugs or chemicals.

61. **Open heart surgery.** Heart surgery where the chest has been opened and the blood recirculated and oxygenated with the proper equipment and the necessary staff to perform the surgery.

62. **Orthopedic services.** Services provided for the prevention or correction of injuries or disorders of the skeletal system and associated muscles, joints and ligaments.

63. **Outpatient surgery.** Scheduled surgical services provided to patientswho do not remain in the hospital overnight. The surgery may be performed in operating suites also used for inpatient surgery, specially designated surgical suites for outpatient surgery, or procedure rooms within an outpatient care facility.

64. **Patient education center.** Written goals and objectives for the patient and/or family related to therapeutic regimens, medical procedures, and self care.

65. **Patient representative services.** Organized hospital services providing personnel through whom patients and staff can seek solutions to institutional problems affecting the delivery of high-quality care and services.

66. **Physical rehabilitation outpatient services.** Outpatient program providing medical, health-related, therapy, social, and/or vocational services to help disabled persons attain or retain their maximum functional capacity.

67. **Primary care department.** A unit or clinic within the hospital that provides primary care services (e.g. general pediatric care, general internal medicine, family practice, gynecology) through hospital-salaried medical and/or nursing staff, focusing on evaluating and diagnosing medical problems and providing medical treatment on an outpatient basis.

68. **Psychiatric services:** Services provided by the hospital that offer immediate initial evaluation and treatment to patients with mental or emotional disorders.
    a. **Psychiatric child-adolescent services.** Provides care to emotionally disturbed children and adolescents, including those admitted for diagnosis and those admitted for treatment.
    b. **Psychiatric consultation-liaison services.** Provides organized psychiatric consultation/liaison services to nonpsychiatric hospital staff and/or departments on psychological aspects of medical care that may be generic or specific to individual patients.
    c. **Psychiatric education services.** Provides psychiatric educational services to community agencies and workers such as schools, police, courts, public health nurses, welfare agencies, clergy, and so forth. The purpose is to expand the mental health knowledge and competence of personnel not working in the mental health field and to promote good mental health through improved understanding, attitudes, and behavioral patterns.
    d. **Psychiatric emergency services.** Services of facilities available on a 24-hour basis to provide immediate unscheduled out-patient care, diagnosis, evaluation, crisis intervention, and assistance to persons suffering acute emotional or mental distress.
    e. **Psychiatric geriatric services.** Provides care to emotionally disturbed elderly patients, including those admitted for diagnosis and those admitted for treatment.
    f. **Psychiatric outpatient services.** Provides medical care, including diagnosis and treatment, of psychiatric outpatients.
    g. **Psychiatric partial hospitalization program.** Organized hospital services of intensive day/evening outpatient services of three hours of more duration, distinguished from other outpatient visits of one hour.

69. **Radiation therapy.** The branch of medicine concerned with radioactive substances and using various techniques of visualization, with the diagnosis and treatment of disease using any of the various sources of radiant energy. Services could include: megavoltage radiation therapy; radioactive implants; stereotactic radiosurgery; therapeutic radioisotope facility; X-ray radiation therapy.

70. **Radiology, diagnostic. The branch of radiology that deals with the utilization of all modalities of radiant energy in medical Diagnoses and therapeutic procedures using radiologic guidance. This includes, but is not restricted to, imaging techniques and methodologies utilizing radiation emitted by x-ray tubes, radionnuclides, and ultrasonographic devices and the radiofrequency electromagnetic radiation emitted by atoms.**
    a. **CT scanner.** Computed tomographic scanner for head or whole body scans.
    b. **Diagnostic radioisotope facility.** The use of radioactive isotopes (Radiopharmaceuticals) as tracers or indicators to detect an abnormal condition or disease.
    c. **Magnetic resonance imaging (MRI).** The use of a uniform magnetic field and radio frequencies to study tissue and structure of the body. This procedure enables the visualization of biochemical activity of the cell in vivo without the use of ionizing radiation, radioisotopic substances, or high-frequency sound.
    d. **PET.** Positron emission tomography scanner is a nuclear medicine imaging technology which uses radioactive (positron emitting) isotopes
    e. created in a cyclotron or generator and computers to produce composite pictures of the brain and heart at work. PET scanning produces sectional images depicting metabolic activity or blood flow rather than anatomy.
    f. **SPECT.** Single photon emission computerized tomography is a nuclear medicine imaging technology that combines existing technology of gamma camera imaging with computed tomographic imaging technology to provide a more precise and clear image.
    g. **Ultrasound.** The use of acoustic waves above the range of 20,000 cycles per second to visualize internal body structures.

71. **Reproductive health** (could include). Fertility counseling - A service that counsels and educates on infertility problems and includesl laboratory and surgical workup and management for individuals having problems conceiving children. In vitro fertilization - Program providing for the induction of fertilization of a surgically removed ovum by donated sperm in a culture medium followed by a short incubation period. The embryo is then reimplanted in the womb.

72. **Retirement housing.** A facility that provides social activities to senior citizens, usually retired persons, who do not require health care but some short-term skilled nursing care may be provided. A retirement center may furnish housing and may also have acute hospital and long-term care facilities, or it may arrange for acute and long-term care through affiliated institutions.

73. Respiratory Isolation Room.

74. **Sleep Center.** Specially equipped and staffed center for the diagnosis and treatment of sleep disorders.

75. **Social work services** (could include). Organized services that are properly directed and sufficiently staffed by qualified individuals who provide assistance and counseling to patients and their families in dealing with social, emotional, and environmental problems associated with illness or disability, often in the context of financial or discharge planning coordination.

76. **Sports medicine.** Provision of diagnostic screening and assessment and clinical and rehabilitation services for the prevention and treatment of sports-related injuries.

77. **Support groups.** A hospital sponsored program that allows a group of individuals with the same or similar problems who meet periodically to share experiences, problems, and solutions in order to support each other.

78. **Swing bed services. A hospital bed that can be used to provide either acute or long-term care depending on community or patient needs. To be eligible a hospital must have a Medicare provider agreement in place, have fewer than 100 beds, be located in a rural area, do not have a 24 hour nursing service waiver in effect, have not been terminated from the program in the prior two years, and meet various service conditions.**

79. **Teen outreach services.** A program focusing on the teenager which encourages an improved health status and a healthful lifestyle including physical, emotional, mental, social, spiritual and economic health through education, exercise, nutrition and health promotion.

80. **Tobacco Treatment/Cessation Program.** Organized hospital services with the purpose of ending tobacco-use habits of patients addicted to tobacco/nicotine.

81 **Transplant services.** The branch of medicine that transfers an organ or tissue from one person to another or from one body part to another to replace a diseased structure or to restore function or to change appearance. Services could include: Bone marrow transplant program; kidney transplant; organ transplant (other than kidney); tissue transplant.

82 **Transportation to health facilities.** A long-term care support service designed to assist the mobility of the elderly. Some programs offer improved financial access by offering reduced rates and barrier-free buses or vans with ramps and lifts to assist the elderly or handicapped; others offer subsidies for public transport systems or operate mini-bus services exclusively for use by senior citizens.

83. **Urgent care center.** A facility that provides care and treatment for problems that are not life-threatening but require attention over the short term. These units function like emergency rooms but are separate from hospitals with which they may have backup affiliation arrangements.

84. **Volunteer services department.** An organized hospital department responsible for coordinating the services of volunteers working within the institution.

84. **Women's health center/services. An area set aside for coordinated education and treatment services specifically for and promoted to women** as provided by this special unit. Services may or may not include obstetrics but include a range of services other than OB.

85. **Wound Management Services. Services for patients with chronic wounds and nonhealing wounds often resulting from diabetes, poor circulation, improper seating and immunocompromising conditions. The goals are to progress chronic wounds through stages of healing, reduce and eliminate infections, increase physical function to minimize complications from current wounds and prevent future chronic wounds. Wound management services are provided on an inpatient or outpatient basis, depending on the intensity of service needed.**

86a. **Independent practice association (IPA).** AN IPA is a legal entity that holds managed care contracts. The IPA then contracts with physicians, usually in solo practice, to provide care either on a fee-for-services or capitated basis. The purpose of an IPA is to assist solo physicians in obtaining managed care contracts.

86b. **Group practice without walls**. Hospital sponsors the formation of, or provides capital to physicians to establish, a "quasi" group to share administrative expenses while remaining independent practitioners.

86c. **Open physician-hospital organization (PHO).** A joint venture between the hospital and all members of the medical staff who wish to participate. The PHO can act as a unified agent in managed care contracting, own a managed care plan, own and operate ambulatory care centers or ancillary services projects, or provide administrative services to physician members.

86d. **Closed physician-hospital organization (PHO).** A PHO that restricts physician membership to those practitioners who meet criteria for cost effectiveness and/or high quality.

86e. **Management services organization (MSO).** A corporation, owned by the hospital or a physician/hospital joint venture, that provides management services to one or more medical group practices. The MSO purchases the tangible assets of the practices and leases them back as part of a full-service management agreement, under which the MSO employs all non-physician staff and provides all supplies/administrative systems for a fee.

86f. **Integrated salary model.** Physicians are salaried by the hospital or another entity of a health system to provide medical services for primary care and specialty care.

86g. **Equity model.** Allows established practitioners to become shareholders in a professional corporation in exchange for tangible and intangible assets of their existing practices.

86h. **Foundation.** A corporation, organized either as a hospital affiliate or subsidiary, which purchases both the tangible and intangible assets of one or more medical group practices. Physicians remain in a separate corporate entity but sign a professional services agreement with the foundation.

89a. **Capitation.** An at-risk payment arrangement in which an organization receives a fixed prearranged payment and in turn guarantees to deliver or arrange all medically necessary care required by enrollers in the capitated plan. The fixed amount is specified within contractual agreements between the payor and the involved organization. The fixed payment amount is based on an actuarial assessment of the services required by enrollees and the costs of providing these services, recognizing enrollees adjustment factors such as age, sex, and family size.

89b. **Shared risk payments.** A payment arrangement in which a hospital and a managed care organization share the risk of adverse claims experience. Methods for sharing risk could include: capitation with partial refunds or supplements if billed hospital charges or costs differ from capitated payments, and service or discharge-based payments with withholds and bonus payouts that depend on expenditure targets.

D. COMMUNITY ORIENTATION

1. **Mission statement. A general statement that describes a company's reason for existence, its vision and direction, its areas of expertise and its goals.**

5. **Health Status indicators. A tool used to quantify various aspects of a populations health status.**

9. **Self assessment** is an evaluation of an organization's management system through achievements in areas such as: leadership, strategic planning, human resource management, information management, process management, customer focus and satisfaction, and business results.

SECTION E
TOTAL FACILITY BEDS, UTILIZATION, FINANCES, AND STAFFING
Instructions and Definitions

1. For the purposes of this survey, nursing home type unit/facility provides care for the elderly and chronic care in a non-acute setting in any of the following categories: *Skilled nursing care *Intermediate care *Residential care/elderly housing (*see page 4 definitions)
The nursing home type units/facilities are to be owned an operated by the hospital. Only one legal entity may be vested with title to the physical property or operate under the authority of a duly executed lease of the physical property.

1a. Report the number of beds regularly available (those set up and staffed for use) at the end of the reporting period. Report only operating beds, not constructed bed capacity. Include all bed facilities that are set up and staffed for use by inpatients who have no other bed facilities, such as pediatric bassinets, isolation units, quiet rooms, and reception and observation units assigned to or reserved for them. Exclude newborn bassinets and bed facilities for patients receiving special procedures for a portion of their stay and who have other bed facilities assigned to or reserved for them. Exclude, for example, labor room, postanesthesia, or postoperative recovery room beds, psychiatric holding beds, and beds that are used only as holding facilities for patients prior to their transfer to another hospital.

b. Report the number of normal newborn **bassinets**. Do not include neonatal intensive care or intermediate care bassinets. These should be reported on page 3, C6 and C7.

c. Total **births** should exclude fetal deaths.

d. Include the number of adult and pediatric **admissions** only (exclude births). This figure should include all patients admitted during the reporting period, including neonatal and swing admissions.

e. Report the number of adult and pediatric days of care rendered during the entire reporting period. Do not include days of care rendered for normal infants born in the hospital, but do include those for their mothers. Include days of care for infants born in the hospital and transferred into a neonatal care unit. Also include swing bed inpatient days. **Inpatient day** of care (also commonly referred to as a **patient day** or a **census day**, or by some federal hospitals as an **occupied bed day**) is a period of service between the census-taking hours on two successive calendar days, the day of discharge being counted only when the patient was admitted the same day.

f. **Emergency room visits** should reflect the number of visits to the emergency unit. Emergency outpatients can be admitted to the inpatient areas of the hospital, but they are still counted as emergency visits and subsequently as inpatient admissions.

g. An **Outpatient visit** is a visit by a patient who is not lodged in the hospital while receiving medical, dental, or other services. Each appearance of an outpatient in each unit constitutes one visit regardless of the number of diagnostic and/or therapeutic treatments that the patient receives. Total outpatient visits should include all clinic visits, referred visits, observation services, outpatient surgeries, home health service visits, and emergency room visits.
Clinic visits should reflect total number of visits to each specialized medical unit that is responsible for the diagnosis and treatment of patients on an outpatient, nonemergency basis (i.e., alcoholism, dental, gynecology, etc.). Visits to the satellite clinics and primary group practices should be included if revenue is received by the hospital.
Referred visits should reflect total number of outpatient ancillary visits to each specialty unit of the hospital established for providing technical aid used in the diagnosis and treatment of patients. Examples of such units are diagnosticradiology, EKG, pharmacy, etc.
Observation services are those services furnished on a hospital's premises, including use of a bed and periodic monitoring by a hospital's nursing or other staff, which are reasonable and necessary to evaluate an outpatient's condition or determine the need for a possible admission to the hospital as an inpatient. Observation services usually do not exceed 24 hours. However, there is no hourly limit on the extent to which they may be used.
Home health service visits are visits by home health personnel to a patient's residence.
Also include the number of outpatient surgeries reported on line E1i. and the emergency room visits reported on line E1f.

h-I. Count each patient undergoing surgery as one surgical operation regardles s of the number of surgical procedures that were performed while the patient was in the operating or procedure room.

h-2. **Operating room. A unit/room of a hospital or other health care facility in which surgical procedures requiring anesthesia are performed.**
For outpatient surgical operations, please record operations performed on patients who do not remain in the hospital overnight. Include all operations whether performed in the inpatient operating rooms or in procedure rooms located in an outpatient facility. Include an endoscopy only when used as an operative tool and not when used for diagnosis alone.

2a2 **Managed Care Medicare Discharges.** A discharge day where a Medicare Managed Care Plan is the source of payment.
2b2 **Managed Care Medicare Inpatient Days.** An inpatient day where a Medicare Managed Care Plan is the source of payment.
2c2 **Managed Care Medicaid Discharges.** A discharge day where a Medicaid Managed Care Plan is the source of payment.
2d2 **Managed Care Medicaid Inpatient Days.** An inpatient day where a Medicaid Managed Care Plan is the source of payment.

3a. **Net patient revenue.** Reported at the estimated net realizable amounts from patients, third-party payors, and others for services rendered, including estimated retroactive adjustments under reimbursement agreements with third-party payors. Retroactive adjustments are accrued on an estimated basis in the period the related services are rendered and adjusted in future periods, as final settlements are determined.

3b. **Tax appropriations a predetermined amount set aside by the government from its taxing authority to support the operation of the hospital.**

c. **Other operating revenue.** Revenue from services other than health care provided to patients, as well as sales and services to nonpatients. Revenue that arises from the normal day-to-day operations from services other than health care provided to patients. Includes sales and services to nonpatients, and revenue from miscellaneous sources (rental of hospital space, sale of cafeteria meals, gift shop sales). Also include operating gains in this category.

d. **Nonoperating revenue.** Includes investment income, extraordinary gains and other nonoperating gains.

e. **Total revenue Add net patient revenue, tax appropriations, other operating revenue and nonoperating revenue.**

f. **Payroll expenses.** Include payroll for all personnel including medical and dental residents/interns and trainees.

g. **Employee benefits.** Includes social security, group insurance, retirement benefits, workman's compensation, unemployment insurance, etc.

h. **Depreciated expense (for reporting period only)** report only the depreciation expense applicable to the reporting period. The amount also Should be included in accumulated depreciation(E 7-b).

i. **Interest expense.** Report interest expense for the reporting period only.

j. Total expenses. Includes all payroll and non-payroll expenses (including bad debt) as well as any nonoperating losses (including extraordinary losses).

4a. **Total gross inpatient revenue. The hospitals full established rates(charges) for all services rendered to inpatients.**

4b. **Total gross outpatient revenue. The hospitals full established rates(charges) for all services rendered to outpatients.**

4c. **Total gross patient revenue.** Total gross patient revenue (add total gross inpatient revenue and total gross outpatient revenue).

5. Uncompensated care. Care for which no payment is expected or no charge is made. It is the sum of bad debt and charity care absorbed by a hospital or other health care organization in providing medical care for patients who are uninsured or are unable to pay.

5a. **Bad debt expense.** The provision for actual or expected uncollectibles resulting from the extension of credit. Because bad debts are reported as an expense and not a deduction from revenue, the gross charges that result in bad debts will remain in net revenue (E3a).

b. **Charity care.** Health services that were never expected to result in cash inflows. Charity care results from a provider's policy to provide health care services free of charge to individuals who meet certain financial criteria. **For purposes of this survey, charity care is measured on the basis of revenue forgone, at full established rates.**

E. TOTAL FACILITY BEDS, UTILIZATION, FINANCES, AND STAFFING (continued)

6a1 **Medicare.** Should agree with the Medicare utilization reported in questions E2a and b.

6a1a **Routine patient revenue.** Include traditional Medicare fee-for-service.

6a1c. **Total.** Medicare revenue (add Medicare routine patient revenue and Medicare managed care revenue).

6a2. **Medicaid.** Should agree with Medicaid utilization reported in questions E2c and d.

6a2a. **Routine patient revenue.** Include Medicaid disproportionate payments under Medicaid routine patient care (2a), in the net column (2).

6a2c. **Total** Medicaid revenue (add Medicaid routine Patient revenue and Medicaid managed care revenue).

6c. **Total** Total revenue (gross should equat E4c and net should equal E3a).

7. **Fixed Assets.** Represent land and physical properties that are consumed or used in the creation of economic activity by the health care entity. The historical or acquisition costs are used in recording fixed assets. Net plant, property, and equipment represent the original costs of these items less accumulated depreciation and amortization.

7d. **Gross Square Footage:** Include all inpatient, outpatient, office, and support space used for or in support of your health care activities. Exclude exterior, roof, and garage space in the figure.

Full-Time Equivalent (FTE) is the total number of hours worked by all employees over the full (12 month) reporting period divided by the normal number of hours worked by a full-time employee for that same time period. For example, if your hospital considers a normal work week for a full-time employee to be 40 hours, a total of 2,080 would be worked over a full year (52 weeks). If the total number of hours worked by all employees on the payroll is 208,000, then the number of Full-Time Equivalents (FTE) is 100 (employees). The FTE calculation for a specific occupational category such as Registered nurses is exactly the same. The calculation for each occupational category should be based on the number of hours worked by staff employed in that specific category.

8a. **Physicians and dentists.** Include only those physicians and dentists engaged in clinical practice and on the payroll. Those who hold administrative positions should be reported in "All other personnel."

c. **Other trainees.** A trainee is a person who has not completed the necessary requirements for certification or met the qualifications required for full salary under a related occupational category. Exclude medical and dental residents/interns who should be reported on line 7b.

d. **Registered nurses.** Nurses who have graduated from approved schools of nursing and who are currently registered by the state. They are responsible for the nature and quality of all nursing care that patients receive. Do not include any registered nurses more appropriately reported in other occupational categories, such as facility administrators, and therefore listed under "All other personnel."

e. **Licensed practical (vocational) nurses.** Nurses who have graduated from an approved school of practical (vocational) nursing who work under the supervision of registered nurses and physicians.

f. **Nursing assistive personnel.** Certified nursing assistant or equivalent unlicensed staff assigned to patient care units and reporting to nursing.

g. **All other personnel.** This should include all other personnel not already accounted for in other catergories.

h. **Total facility personnel.** This line is to include the total facility personnel - hospital plus nursing home type unit/facility personnel (for those hospitals that own and operate a nursing home type unit/facility).

i. **Nursing home type unit/facility personnel.** This line should be filled out only by hospitals that own and operate a nursing home type unit/ facility, where only one legal entity is vested with title to the physical property or operates under the authority of a duly executed lease of the physical property. If nursing home type unit/facility personnel are reported on the total facility personnel line, but cannot be broken out, please write "cannot break out" on this line.

SUPPLEMENTAL INFORMATION

1. Does your hospital participate in any joint venture arrangements? Joint Venture is a contractual arrangement between two or more parties forming an unincorporated business. The participants in the arrangement remain independent and separate outside of the ventures purpose.

2. Does your hospital provide services through a satellite facility(s)? Satellite Services are available at a facility geographically remote from the hospital campus.